Manual of Embryo Selection in Human Assisted Reproduction

Manual of Embryo Selection in Human Assisted Reproduction

Edited by

Catherine Racowsky
Hospital Foch

Jacques Cohen
VF 2.0, Guadalajara, Mexico and Althea Science, Hudson, New York, USA

Nick Macklon
London Women's Clinic

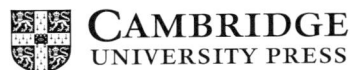
CAMBRIDGE
UNIVERSITY PRESS

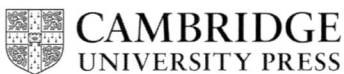

Shaftesbury Road, Cambridge CB2 8EA, United Kingdom

One Liberty Plaza, 20th Floor, New York, NY 10006, USA

477 Williamstown Road, Port Melbourne, VIC 3207, Australia

314–321, 3rd Floor, Plot 3, Splendor Forum, Jasola District Centre, New Delhi – 110025, India

103 Penang Road, #05–06/07, Visioncrest Commercial, Singapore 238467

Cambridge University Press is part of Cambridge University Press & Assessment, a department of the University of Cambridge.

We share the University's mission to contribute to society through the pursuit of education, learning and research at the highest international levels of excellence.

www.cambridge.org
Information on this title: www.cambridge.org/9781009016377

DOI: 10.1017/9781009025218

First published 2023

Printed in the United Kingdom by TJ Books Limited, Padstow Cornwall

A catalogue record for this publication is available from the British Library.

Library of Congress Cataloging-in-Publication Data
Names: Racowsky, Catherine, editor. | Cohen, Jacques, editor. |
   Macklon, Nick S., editor.
Title: Manual of embryo selection in human assisted reproduction / edited
   by Catherine Racowsky, Jacques Cohen, Nicholas Macklon.
Description: Cambridge, United Kingdom ; New York, NY : Cambridge
   University Press, 2022. | Includes bibliographical references and index.
Identifiers: LCCN 2022037927 (print) | LCCN 2022037928 (ebook) |
   ISBN 9781009016377 (paperback) | ISBN 9781009025218 (epub)
Subjects: MESH: Single Embryo Transfer–methods | Embryo Disposition |
   Embryo Implantation | Sperm-Ovum Interactions–physiology | Embryonic
   Development–physiology
Classification: LCC RG135 (print) | LCC RG135 (ebook) | NLM WQ 208 |
   DDC 618.1/780599–dc23/eng/20220912
LC record available at https://lccn.loc.gov/2022037927
LC ebook record available at https://lccn.loc.gov/2022037928

ISBN 978-1-009-01637-7 Paperback

Contents

Color plates can be found between pages 134 and 135.

Online resources

All videos mentioned in the book are available to view under the resources tab via:
www.cambridge.org/embryoselection
Password: EmbryoSelection23

Contributors

David F. Albertini, Bedford Research Foundation, Bedford, MA, USA

Silvia Azzena, SISMeR Reproductive Medicine Institute, Bologna, Italy

Nicoletta Barnocchi, G.EN.E.R.A. Umbria, G.EN.E.R.A. Centers for Reproductive Medicine, Umbertide, Italy

Virginia N. Bolton, King's College, London, UK

Andrea Borini, 9.baby, GeneraLife IVF, Bologna, Italy

Elena Borini, 9.baby, GeneraLife IVF, Bologna, Italy

Alison Campbell, CARE Fertility Group, Nottingham, UK

Danilo Cimadomo, G.EN.E.R.A. Umbria, G.EN.E.R.A. Centers for Reproductive Medicine, Umbertide, Italy, and Clinica Valle Giulia, G.EN.E.R.A. Centers for Reproductive Medicine, Rome, Italy

Jacques Cohen, IVF 2.0, Guadalajara, Mexico and Althea Science, Hudson, New York, USA

Giovanni Coticchio, 9.baby, GeneraLife IVF, Bologna, Italy

Thomas Ebner, Kepler University Hospital, MedCampus IV, Linz, Austria

Tracey A. Edgell, Hudson Institute of Medical Research and Monash University Department of Molecular and Translational Science, Clayton, Victoria, Australia

Jemma Evans, Hudson Institute of Medical Research and Monash University Department of Molecular and Translational Science, Clayton, Victoria, Australia

Laura Ferrick, School of BioSciences, University of Melbourne, Australia

Elpida Fragouli, Juno Genetics, Oxford, UK and Department of Life and Environmental Sciences, Bournemouth University, Bournemouth, UK

David K. Gardner, School of BioSciences, University of Melbourne, Australia and Melbourne IVF, Melbourne, Australia

Luca Gianaroli, SISMeR Reproductive Medicine Institute, Bologna, Italy

Russell P. Hayden, Department of Urology, Weill Cornell Medicine, New York, NY, USA

Federica Innocenti, G.EN.E.R.A. Umbria, G.EN.E.R.A. Centers for Reproductive Medicine, Umbertide, Italy, and Clinica Valle Giulia, G.EN.E.R.A. Centers for Reproductive Medicine, Rome, Italy

Rebecca L. Kelley, Melbourne IVF, Melbourne, Australia

Yee Shan Lisa Lee, Melbourne IVF, Melbourne, Australia

Kersti Lundin, Reproductive Medicine, Sahlgrenska University Hospital, Göteborg, Sweden

Nick Macklon, London Women's Clinic, London, UK

M. Cristina Magli, SISMeR Reproductive Medicine Institute, Bologna, Italy

Dean Morbeck, Department of Obstetrics and Gynecology, Monash University, Melbourne, AU

Sharon T. Mortimer, Oozoa Biomedical, Vancouver, Canada, and Division of Reproductive Endocrinology and Infertility, Department of Obstetrics and Gynaecology, Faculty of Medicine, University of British Columbia, Vancouver, Canada

Guiying Nie, Hudson Institute of Medical Research and Monash University Department of Molecular and Translational Science, Clayton, Victoria, Australia

Letizia Papini, G.EN.E.R.A. Umbria, G.EN.E.R.A. Centers for Reproductive Medicine, Umbertide, Italy

Nahid Punjani, Department of Urology, Weill Cornell Medicine, New York, NY, USA

Catherine Racowsky, Department of Obstetrics, Gynecology, and Reproductive Medicine, Hospital Foch, Suresnes, France

Laura Rienzi, G.EN.E.R.A. Umbria, G.EN.E.R.A. Centers for Reproductive Medicine, Umbertide, Italy and Clinica Valle Giulia, G.EN.E.R.A. Centers for Reproductive Medicine, Rome, Italy

Paolo Rinaudo, Department of Obstetrics, Gynecology, and Reproductive Sciences, University of California, San Francisco, CA, USA

Eleni Jaswa, Department of Obstetrics, Gynecology, and Reproductive Sciences, University of California San Francisco, CA, USA

Lois A. Salamonsen, Hudson Institute of Medical Research and Monash University Department of Molecular and Translational Science, Clayton, Victoria, Australia

Catello Scarica, Casa di Cura Villa Salaria – Institut Marques Reproductive Medicine, Rome, Italy

Peter N. Schlegel, Department of Urology, Weill Cornell Medicine, New York, NY, USA

Arne Sunde, Department of Clinical and Molecular Medicine, Norwegian University of Science and Technology, Trondheim, Norway

Filippo Maria Ubaldi, G.EN.E.R.A. Umbria, G.EN.E.R.A. Centers for Reproductive Medicine, Umbertide, Italy and Clinica Valle Giulia, G.EN.E.R.A. Centers for Reproductive Medicine, Rome, Italy

Jonathan Van Blerkom, Department of Molecular, Cellular and Developmental Biology, University of Colorado, Boulder, CO, USA

Dagan Wells, Juno Genetics, Oxford, UK and Nuffield Department of Women's and Reproductive Health, University of Oxford, John Radcliffe Hospital, Oxford, UK

Preface

Most of us remember the first time we witnessed an embryo being selected for transfer, whether this was as a trainee embryologist or as a clinician visiting the mysterious IVF laboratory. Watching the careful selection of an embryo over others for a chance of life can border on the astounding.

Yet, just as doctors are expected to bring a professional objective detachment to the care of their patients, so are embryologists to the care of the gametes and embryos in their charge. And they do this many times, every day, all around the world.

However, to succeed as an embryologist requires more than an ability to bring a forensic approach to decision-making. It requires exquisite hand–eye coordination and, among other attributes, a "feel" for what indicates is a viable embryo. That is why, even when specific criteria can be applied to assess quality, embryologists often have difficulty in describing how they use these. Identifying the best embryo has been described as recognizing a handwritten signature. You know whose it is, but you can't explain why.

Embryology and embryo selection have both evolved over the years. Although training as a clinical embryologist typically takes years of acquired knowledge, even then embryologists may not "know what they really know." While numerous studies have demonstrated reassuring correlations between the main scoring systems they employ and treatment outcomes, a number of developments in our field have put this approach under increasing pressure.

The most significant of these pressures has been the drive to reduce multiple pregnancies arising from IVF treatment. Agreement that the aim of treatment should no longer be a positive pregnancy test but a healthy singleton baby was an important milestone indicating the maturity of the discipline of IVF. However, this imposed a heavy and complex burden on embryologists. Reducing this most important risk of treatment while at the same time continuing the expected increase in success rates has without doubt brought to the forefront the continued central importance of embryo selection.

Embryology has responded to these challenges in a myriad of ways. Over the past 10 years, the speed and breadth of innovation in the field of embryo selection has been at times breathtaking. As with all rapid journeys, there have been notable bumps on the road and indeed the occasional wrong turn. As IVF waves to its second generation of children, the technologies that will lead us into the third generation are beginning to appear as valid and safe.

We hope that this manual will provide both embryologists and clinicians a clear and informative overview of the tools now available to assist in embryo selection, as well as evidence for their efficacy and safety and the broader considerations that must underlie these important clinical decisions.

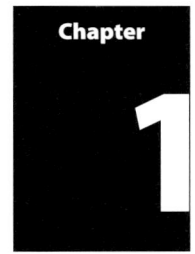

Chapter 1

Introduction
Why Do We Bother with Embryo Selection?

Arne Sunde and Kersti Lundin

1.1 The Early Days

When fertilization in vitro was developed by the pioneers – Dr. Robert G. (Bob) Edwards, Miss Jean Purdy, and Dr. Patrick Steptoe – their primary focus was to obtain oocytes that could be successfully fertilized in laboratory conditions. Embryo culture and embryo selection were just secondary aims at that time. In the early 1970s, the first attempts to obtain a pregnancy after IVF were in cycles in which ovarian stimulation was performed by administration of human menopausal gonadotropins (hMG) [1]. This resulted in multiple follicular growth and thus more than one oocyte available for fertilization. However, the first clinical pregnancy obtained was tubal. Suspecting that an hMG-stimulated cycle increased the likelihood of an ectopic pregnancy, the next attempts were made in natural cycles. Carrying out IVF in natural cycles presented several challenges including the requirement for careful monitoring of follicular growth by repeated measurements of pituitary and steroid hormones. A single follicle, or at most two, was then aspirated laparoscopically just prior to spontaneous ovulation. However, as remains the case today, not all follicular punctures resulted in an oocyte, not all oocytes were fertilized, and not all fertilized oocytes developed into an embryo capable of implantation [1]. With only one or two oocytes available, the success rate per attempt was therefore exceedingly low and only after more than 200 unsuccessful attempts [2], Louise Brown, the first child conceived in vitro, was born [3]. Because of the complexity and the low success rate performing IVF in a natural cycle, hMG-stimulated cycles were again introduced [4]. A timeline of important events in the development of IVF with associated technologies is shown in Figure 1.1.

1.2 Gametogenesis, Fertilization, and Embryo Quality

Follicular growth is a process that takes months; a recruited primordial follicle may take more than 180 days to develop into a preovulatory follicle [5]. The great majority of growing follicles arrest at various stages during development. From the approximately 300 000 follicles present in the ovary of a newborn girl, only around 450 will ultimately ovulate. Just prior to ovulation the cohort of mature follicles are still dependent on continuous follicle-stimulating hormone (FSH) stimulation. One of the follicles in the maturing cohort then starts to express factors that will inhibit the development of the other follicles in the cohort. This follicle now becomes dominant in the sense that it suppresses the maturation of the other follicles. Usually only this follicle is then able to respond to the luteinizing hormone (LH) surge and ovulate [6]. The rationale behind hormonal stimulation of the ovary is that continuous administration of FSH in the preovulatory period will rescue some of the follicles in the maturing cohort that otherwise would have undergone atresia, thereby resulting in multiple follicles from which to retrieve oocytes (Figure 1.2).

In fetal life, the oocytes, enclosed in primordial follicles, enter meiosis but shortly thereafter become arrested at the diplotene phase of prophase I. For some oocytes, this arrest will last for many years. The last oocytes that are ovulated just prior to menopause may have been in meiotic arrest for five decades. Resumption of meiosis is triggered by the LH surge and progression to metaphase II (MII) occurs over the ensuing 36 hours or so, in preparation for ovulation or, in an IVF cycle, for retrieval. Resumption of meiosis from MII to telophase II (TII) is triggered by the sperm and is finalized when the oocyte is fertilized.

Oogenesis in humans is far from a perfect process. It is complex and many oocytes that are ovulated do not have the correct number of chromosomes. The genetic quality of human oocytes in relation to the age of the woman has a u-shaped curve, lower in young and older women. The rate of aneuploid oocytes is lowest around the age of 30, at around 20%. In

Timeline of the Most Notable Advances in Clinical IVF

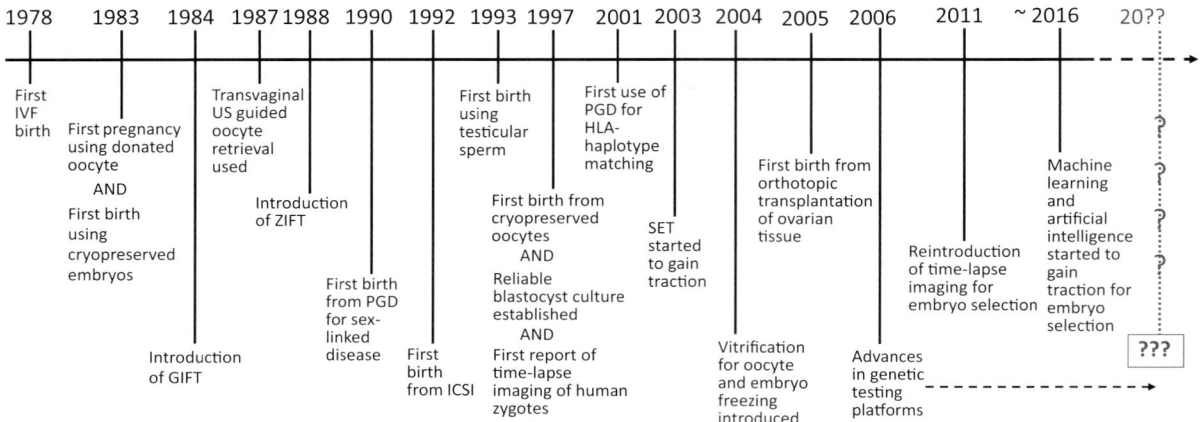

Figure 1.1 Timeline of the most notable advances in clinical IVF (Courtesy of Dr. Catherine Racowsky)

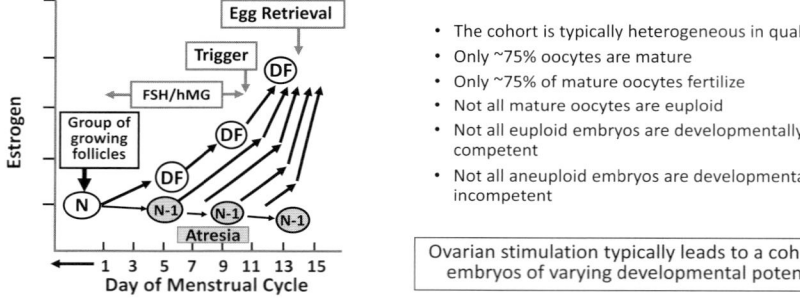

- The cohort is typically heterogeneous in quality
- Only ~75% oocytes are mature
- Only ~75% of mature oocytes fertilize
- Not all mature oocytes are euploid
- Not all euploid embryos are developmentally competent
- Not all aneuploid embryos are developmentally incompetent

Ovarian stimulation typically leads to a cohort of embryos of varying developmental potential

hCG = human chorionic gonadotropin; DF = dominant follicle; N = number of follicles in the cohort
FSH = follicle-stimulating hormone; hMG = human menopausal gonadotropin

Figure 1.2 Follicular maturation
Growth and maturation of human follicles is a complex process that takes over 180 days. The majority of the growing follicles will arrest and become atretic. Only 1 in 1 000 follicles in an ovary of a newborn will ever reach ovulation. Despite this seemingly strong selection of growing follicles, the frequency of aneuploid human oocytes is from 25% to 80% depending on the age of the woman. (Adapted from [7], with permission).

contrast, the rate of aneuploid MII oocytes in women who are very young is above 55% [8] and this reaches upward of 80% in women greater than 42 years of age [9]. In addition to the correct number of chromosomes, a competent MII oocyte must have undergone cytoplasmic maturation so that after fertilization it can support early embryogenesis.

Spermatogenesis takes on average 60 days from the germinal stem cell stage to ejaculated spermatozoa [10]. This is a complex process that involves several rounds of mitosis, followed by meiosis, and chromatin remodelling, and synthesis of m-RNA and proteins, all

packed into a highly specialized cell, the spermatozoa. As with oogenesis, nondisjunction may occur during spermatogenesis, resulting in an aneuploid sperm cell, although the frequency of aneuploid sperm is generally lower than for oocytes. It has been shown that in men with reduced semen quality the frequency of aneuploid spermatozoa is higher than in men with normal semen quality [11]. In addition, a range of other factors such as DNA fragmentation, chromatin structure, histones, protamines, epigenetic profiles, and Y-chromosome microdeletions may influence fertilization, embryo development, and/or embryo quality [11].

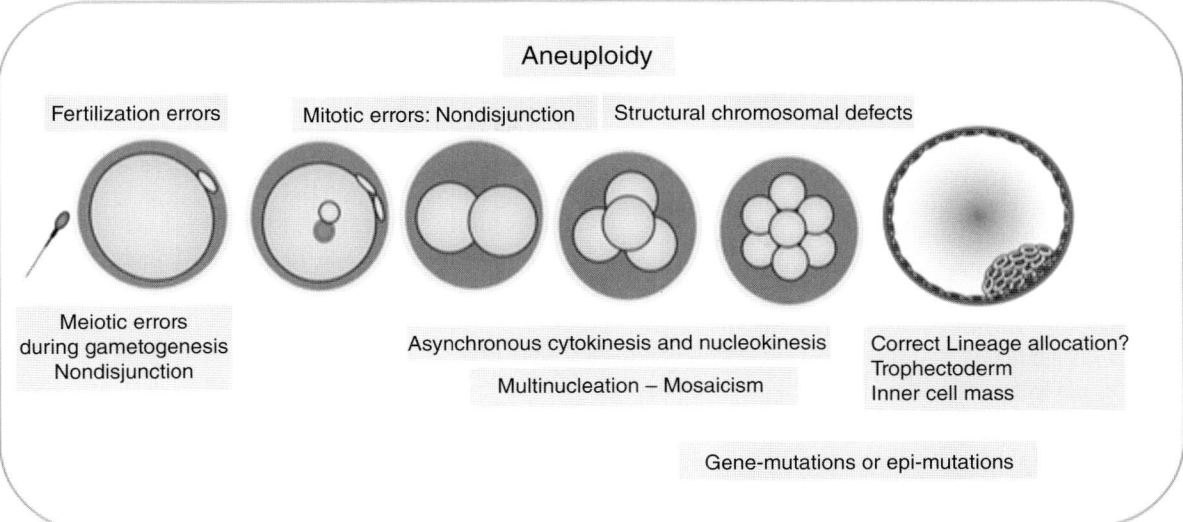

Figure 1.3 Errors in embryo development
Human gametogenesis is far from perfect and mature gametes may contain the wrong number of chromosomes (aneuploid). Fertilization and early cleavage may introduce new errors during mitosis (nondisjunction), frequently leading to embryos where at least one blastomere is aneuploid. Culture conditions may also have an influence on embryo viability. The embryologist working in clinical IVF is therefore faced with a situation where the embryos obtained may vary greatly with respect to implantation potential. The challenge therefore is to rank embryos so the best ones may be selected for fresh transfer and for cryopreservation.

Fertilization and early embryo development are complex processes where errors may occur that can compromise the developmental potential of the embryo (Figure 1.3). When this process takes place in vitro, iatrogenic factors can add to this. The proportion of embryos that are aneuploid or mosaic euploid/aneuploid at the cleavage stage and/or at the blastocyst stage varies according to the age of the woman and has been reported to be higher in cleavage stage embryos than in blastocysts [12]. Aneuploid embryos have been shown to have a lower implantation rate than euploid embryos [13].

Fecundity in the human is around 20% per cycle. This means that a couple with normal reproductive potential and regular intercourse have approximately a 20% chance per ovulation of obtaining a delivery. This is lower than most animal species, even when compared to the nonhuman primates such as the chimpanzee [14]. The low fecundity rate in humans may perhaps not come as a surprise when one considers that we have far from perfect gametes. There are reasons to believe that this has been the case for millennia and is part of being human and not due to a recent decline in the genetic quality of our gametes [14].

Even today, more than 40 years after the birth of Louise Brown, there are apparently still large differences in success rates between assisted reproduction technology (ART) laboratories and clinics as well as between countries. Laboratory variables such as the oxygen level, pH, osmolality, temperature control, air quality, and the culture media all have an influence on embryo development in vitro [15, 16, 17]. Suboptimal culture conditions will affect many steps of the process, and thereby reduce the likelihood of obtaining a delivery after IVF. As an example, a comparison of aneuploidy rates in embryos obtained after fertilization of oocytes from young oocyte donors show large differences between ART laboratories [18]. The cause of this is largely unknown but it cannot be ruled out that it is partly due to iatrogenic factors. However, prospective randomized studies have also shown that the composition of the culture media may influence the developmental speed and the epigenetic profile of embryos in vitro as well as have an influence on the phenotype of the children born [19, 20, 21].

3

1.3 Number of Transferred Embryos, Multiple Birth Rates, and Health of the Children

An attempt to obtain a delivery of a child using fertilization in vitro requires highly skilled professionals, expensive drugs, and a sophisticated laboratory. The financial burden and the emotional stress associated with assisted reproduction may be substantial. Couples that seek to be treated by assisted reproduction therefore obviously want to be offered a treatment with a high probability of success. Due to the poor results in the early days of IVF, several embryos were often transferred, to provide a reasonable chance of obtaining a pregnancy.

Reassuringly, now with more than 40 years of development of in vitro fertilization, implantation and live birth rates have been steadily improving. Data from the European Society of Human Reproduction and Embryology (ESHRE) European IVF-Monitoring Consortium (EIM) registry show an increase from a clinical pregnancy rate of 26% in 1997 (data from 18 countries; www.eshre.eu/Data-collection-and-research/Consortia/EIM/Publications) to 33% in 2018 (39 countries; [22]). This might seem like a rather modest increase for a 20-year period, but it is important to note that, during the same time, the single embryo transfer rate increased from 11% to 51%. Results from the United States reported a delivery rate of 23% for 1995 (www.cdc.gov/art/artdata/index.html) compared to 37% reported for 2019 [23].

Calculations from the ESHRE EIM datasets show that the implantation rate doubled during these years, from 12% in 1997 (mean numbers of embryos for transfer, 2.6) to 25% in 2014 (mean number of embryos transferred, 1.8). This considerable improvement can be attributed to several factors: improved stimulation strategies resulting in better oocyte quality and improved endometrial receptivity, improved handling and culture conditions for gametes and embryos, and optimization of assessment and selection of embryos. There are however considerable variations regarding results among countries, showing that there is still much room for improvement.

Unfortunately, the downside of the increased implantation rates was the dramatic increase of multiple births. The profession did not adjust the numbers of transferred embryos to the level of implantation quickly enough, and many clinics continued to transfer 3–4 or even more embryos, despite the improved implantation results. In the USA, data published by the Centers for Disease Control and Prevention (CDC) show that, in 2011, 46% of infants born from treatment with IVF were either twins or higher-order multiples (www.cdc.gov/art/artdata/index.html). The ESHRE EIM data show in the latest report (data from 2018) that although the mean multiple delivery rate has decreased from 29.6% to 12.5% for 2018, the variation is large, ranging from 1.9% to 27.4% [22]. It can be seen from these data that the multiple birth rate has a clear correlation with the number of embryos transferred, but interestingly not with improved delivery rates. The same trend has occurred in the USA where the CDC data show that the multiple delivery rate decreased to 22% in 2014, with a further decrease to 13% in 2018 without an obvious impact on live birth rates [23].

The increasing multiple delivery rates and the concurrent issues with health of the offspring have been established in many follow-up studies (e.g. [24–29]), highlighting the significant maternal, fetal, and neonatal risks associated with these pregnancies. The accumulated data finally led to regulation in many countries. In Europe, this development was led by Finland and Sweden. In 2003, the National Health Authorities in Sweden stated that transfer of a single embryo was strongly recommended, and that more than two embryos should not be transferred. This led to a dramatic decrease in national multiple rates, dropping from 25% to 5% in only four years [30]. Despite this, there has been a concurrent steady increase in live birth rates. In the USA, the Society for Assisted Reproductive Technology and the American Society for Reproductive Medicine have issued recommendations to lower the number of embryos for transfer. This has resulted in a single embryo transfer rate of 77% for 2019 in parallel with increasing live birth rates, but again with a large variation between states (www.cdc.gov/art/artdata/index.html; [23]).

The declining multiple birth rates have resulted in a positive impact for the health of the children. Follow-up studies of offspring have shown that perinatal risks for ART offspring have decreased and overall health has improved. An analysis of more than 92 000 children born from ART in Denmark, Finland, Norway, and Sweden from 1988 to 2007 found a decline in numbers of preterm birth, low or very low birthweight, stillbirths, and perinatal death [31].

1.4 Embryo Selection and Cumulative Results

When extended culture to the blastocyst stage began to be implemented, the slow freezing technique used at that time unfortunately resulted in limited survival of blastocysts after thawing. With the introduction into clinical IVF of the vitrification technique (which had been used in veterinary medicine for quite some time), blastocyst cryosurvival rates of over 90% were reported, with much increased implantation rates. This positive development in turn led to a further increased use of blastocyst culture in many clinics and countries, and in addition to an increased possibility and willingness from both patients and clinics to aim for single embryo transfer. In a high-quality ART program, culture of all excess embryos to day 5 or 6 for blastocyst cryopreservation results in >60% likelihood of at least one cryopreserved extra blastocyst (Ahlström and Lundin, personal observation). Thus, adopting this approach provides a good chance of a subsequent frozen thaw cycle adding to the likelihood of achieving at least one pregnancy from a single cohort of embryos.

Several studies have shown that for women considered to have a good prognosis, the cumulative live birth rate after single embryo transfer, followed by the transfer of a cryopreserved embryo in a subsequent cycle, is comparable to that after double embryo transfer, but with a significantly lower risk of multiple pregnancy (e.g. [32, 33, 34]). Thus, with the current excellent survival rates and improved implantation rates for cryopreserved blastocysts, we now have the possibility of transferring the embryos from one oocyte retrieval sequentially, one by one, without risk of them failing to survive during the freeze–thaw procedures. Somewhere along the way an embryo with good potential for implantation will presumably be transferred, and the cumulative pregnancy and delivery rate will be similar irrespective of embryo selection. However, for patients having a large number of good-quality embryos, transfer of them one by one without selection might in the end lead to a high number of transfers, possibly including a series of failed implantations and/or miscarriages, causing stress, as well as being expensive and time-consuming. There is currently a lack of good-quality studies investigating the relationship between embryo selection algorithms and early miscarriage and cumulative delivery rates. However, assessment, ranking, and selection of embryos will in most cases shorten the time to live birth as well as reduce stress and save resources for both the patient and the care provider.

An additional positive aspect from the extended culture of all extra embryos is that fewer embryos are discarded at an early stage. It has been shown that around 25–35% of so-called poor-quality embryos on day 2/3 can give rise to good-quality blastocysts [35–38], with potential for implantation and live birth equal to those of blastocysts from high-quality embryos. Thereby, today embryo/blastocyst assessment is more a method of ranking potential biological quality, instead of selecting at an early stage and discarding the rest. The ranked embryos/blastocysts can then be transferred one by one, starting with the one considered to be of highest viability.

1.5 Future Challenges

There has been a shift in how we assess, select, and utilize embryos. In the early days of IVF, due to suboptimal culture conditions, the most common practice was to transfer and to cryopreserve any extra-good-quality embryos, on day 2 or 3 postfertilization. Poorer-quality embryos were discarded. Gradually, as stated above, with improved culture media and culture conditions, it has become more common to extend culture until the blastocyst stage, so as to "select" the more viable embryos. However, it might be argued that our culture conditions in vitro are perhaps still not good enough to support development of all embryos and/or there might be differences between patients. It is possible that some embryos are more sensitive to the in vitro conditions and would still have been capable of developing and implanting if transferred at an earlier stage.

Thus, the challenge of embryo selection is how far to go, and how many "add-ons" we really need – and whether they are evidence based – to find the best embryo. Assessment of embryos is still mainly performed by embryologists scoring according to developmental and morphology criteria, either all the way from the gamete stage to the transfer/cryo stage, or only at certain predetermined times. Time-lapse (TL) methodology, which allows images to be taken and stored throughout the whole culture period, has enabled

1978	Defining the developmental timeline
1980s	Conventional morphology selection – cleavage stage
1990s	Conventional morphology selection – blastocyst stage
1990	PGT-M with FISH for X-linked disorder
1997	Time-lapse imaging of human zygotes
2001	PGT with blastomere biopsy
2005	PGT with trophectoderm biopsy and advanced sequencing platforms
2007	Metabolomics
2011	Time-lapse imaging reintroduced
2016	Machine learning and artificial intelligence started to gain traction
2016	PGT-A with cell-free DNA analyses
20??	………? ? ?

Courtesy of Dr Catherine Racowsky

Figure 1.4 Where are we with embryo selection going forward? (Courtesy of Dr. Catherine Racowsky)

the scoring of embryos at any time point. Although the TL technology thereby facilitates the work and the logistics of the IVF lab, it has so far not been conclusively demonstrated to improve embryo selection and downstream implantation or live birth rates [39, 40]. Still, TL imaging can reveal other developmental events that may reflect compromised implantation potential such as irregular cleavage patterns [41, 42]. In addition, the technology is useful for training staff and for validating introduction of a new constituent in the IVF laboratory, such as a culture medium.

Another highly debated method of selection is PGT-A screening. This technique to select euploid embryos has evolved much during the last few years. Despite the logical reasoning behind the method, its usefulness and value in specific patient groups is still under discussion and concerns regarding interference of mosaicism in interpretation of results prevail. Furthermore, the technique is quite invasive, with cells being removed from the embryo. Noninvasive methods, involving analysis of cell-free DNA in the spent culture medium [43, 44, 45) or blastocoelic fluid [46] are underway. However, currently no such methods are routinely applied for clinical use.

There is much interest in many areas of our society in machine learning, or so-called artificial intelligence. Indeed, this has evoked great interest in ART, and research is currently ongoing using datasets from time-lapse documentation to "feed" and train computers and to try to find patterns that correlate with embryo development and live birth [47, 48, 49]. If proven to have utility and application across clinics, this would effectively remove the bias of the current subjective assessment by the embryologist. If a highly predictive model could be generated, additional "add-ons" for selection might not even be needed in the future (Figure 1.4).

1.6 Summary

Gametogenesis, fertilization, and embryo development are all complex processes, which give rise to a heterogeneous cohort of embryos, with varying potential for implantation and live birth. The use of blastocyst vitrification has dramatically increased cryo-survival rates, whereby all embryos can be transferred sequentially, and the cumulative success rates will be similar irrespective of embryo selection. However, efficient embryo selection will shorten the time to pregnancy and live birth since the embryos with the highest potential will be transferred first. Embryo culture and selection algorithms may also have an influence on the utilization rate (embryos transferred fresh and cryopreserved counted per all embryos) and thereby on the resources utilized. An efficient embryo selection and ranking system will hopefully aid in continuing to lower the multiple birth rate from IVF and improve the health of the offspring.

Key Messages

- Gamete quality and culture conditions of gametes and embryos will influence the clinical success rate.
- A proportion of embryos resulting from an IVF procedure will not have the capacity to implant or sustain a pregnancy.
- Selection of embryos will shorten the time to live birth but not increase the cumulative success rate.
- Increasing success rates and cryosurvival rates will stimulate increased use of single-embryo transfer.
- Single-embryo transfers have led to decreased perinatal risks for ART offspring and improved overall health.

References

1. Elder K, Johnson MH. The Oldham Notebooks: an analysis of the development of IVF 1969–1978. II. The treatment cycles and their outcomes. *Reprod Biomed Soc.* 2015;1:9–18.

2. Fishel S. First in vitro fertilization baby – this is how it happened. *Fertil Steril.* 2018;110:5–11.

3. Steptoe PC, Edwards RG. Birth after the reimplantation of a human embryo. *Lancet.* 1978 August 12:366.

4. Jones HW Jr, Jones GS, Andrews MC, Acosta A, Bundren C, Garcia J, et al. The program for in vitro fertilization at Norfolk. *Fertil Steril.* 1982;38:14–21.

5. Baerwald AR, Adams GP, Pierson RA. Ovarian antral folliculogenesis during the human menstrual cycle: a review. *Hum Reprod Update.* 2012;18:73–91.

6. Zuccotti M, Merico V, Cecconi S, Redi CA, Garagna S. What does it take to make a developmentally competent mammalian egg? *Hum Reprod Update.* 2011;17:525–40.

7. Hogden GD. The dominant follicle. *Fertil Steril.* 1982;38:281–300.

8. Gruhn JR, Zielinska AP, Shukla V, Blanshard R, Capalbo A, Cimadomo D, et al. Chromosome errors in human eggs shape natural fertility over reproductive life span. *Science.* 2019;365:1466–9.

9. Franasiak JM, Forman EJ, Hong KH, Werner MD, Upham KM, Treff NR, et al. The nature of aneuploidy with increasing age of the female partner: a review of 15,169 consecutive trophectoderm biopsies evaluated with comprehensive chromosomal screening. *Fertil Steril.* 2014;101(3):656–63.

10. Misell LM, Holochwost D, Boban D, Santi N, Shefi S, Hellerstein MK, Turek PJ. A stable isotope-mass spectrometric method for measuring human spermatogenesis kinetics in vivo. *J Urol.* 2006;175:242–6.

11. Colaco S, Sakkas D. Paternal factors contributing to embryo quality. *JARG.* 2018;35:1953–68.

12. Fragouli E, Alfarawati S, Spath K, Wells, D. Morphological and cytogenetic assessment of cleavage and blastocyst stage embryos. *Mol Hum Reprod.* 2014;20(2):117–26.

13. Fragouli E, Munne S, Wells D. The cytogenetic constitution of human blastocysts: insight from comprehensive chromosome screening strategies. *Hum Reprod Update.* 2019;25:15–33.

14. Lubinsky M. Evolutionary justification for human reproductive imitations. *JARG.* 2018;35;2133–9.

15. Wale PL, Gardner DK. The effect of chemical and physical factors on mammalian embryo culture and their importance for the practice of assisted human reproduction. *Hum Reprod Update.* 2016;22:2–22.

16. Kleikers SHN, Eijssen LMT, Coonen E, Derhaag JG, Mantikou E, Jonker MJ, et al. Difference in gene expression profiles between human preimplantation embryos cultured in two different IVF culture media. *Hum Reprod.* 2015;30:2303–11.

17. Sunde A, Brison D, Dumoulin J, Harper J, Lundin K, Ven den Abbeel E, Veiga A. Time to take human embryo culture seriously. *Hum Reprod.* 2016;31:2174–82.

18. Munné S, Alikani M, Ribustello L, Colls P, Martínez-Ortiz PA, Referring Physician Group, McCulloh DH. Euploidy rates in donor egg cycles significantly differ between fertility centers. *Human Reprod.* 2017;32(4):743–9.

19. Dumoulin JC, Land JA, Van Montfoort AP, Nelissen EC, Coonen E, Derhaag JG, et al. Effect of in vitro culture of human embryos on birthweight of newborns. *Human Reprod.* 2010;25(3):605–12.

20. Klejkers SHM, Mantikou E, Slappendel E, Consten D, van Echten-Arnds J, Wetzels AM, et al. Influence of embryo culture medium (G5 and HTF) on pregnancy and perinatal outcome after IVF: a multicenter RCT. *Hum Reprod.* 2016;31:2219–30.

21. Zandstra H, Brentjens LBPM, Spauwen B, Touwslager RNH, Bons JAP, Mulder AL, et al. Association of culture medium with growth, weight and cardiovascular development of IVF children at the age of 9 years. *Hum Reprod.* 2018;33:1645–56.

22. Wyns C, De Geyter C, Calhaz-Jorge C, Kupka MS, Motrenko T, Smeenk J, et al. ART in Europe, 2018: results generated from

European registries by ESHRE. *Hum Reprod Open.* 2022;Jul 5.

23. Sunderam S, Zhang Y, Jewett A, Kissin DM. State-specific assisted reproductive technology surveillance, United States: 2019 data brief. Centers for Disease Control and Prevention; 2021 Oct. Available from: www.cdc.gov/art/state-specific-surveillance/2019/pdf/state-specific-art-surveillance-u.s.-2019-data-brief-h.pdf

24. Bergh T, Ericson A, Hillensjö T, Nygren KG, Wennerholm UB. Deliveries and children born after in-vitro fertilisation in Sweden 1982–95: a retrospective cohort study. *Lancet.* 1999;354:1579–85.

25. Multiple gestation pregnancy. The ESHRE Capri Workshop Group. *Hum Reprod.* 2000;15:1856–64.

26. Helmerhorst FM, Perquin DA, Donker D, Keirse MJ. Perinatal outcome of singletons and twins after assisted conception: a systematic review of controlled studies. *BMJ.* 2004;328:261.

27. Wen SW, Demissie K, Yang Q, Walker MC. Maternal morbidity and obstetric complications in triplet pregnancies and quadruplet and higher-order multiple pregnancies. *Am J Obstet Gynecol.* 2004;191:254–8.

28. Pinborg A, Wennerholm UB, Romundstad LB, Loft A, Aittomaki K, Söderström-Anttila V, et al. Why do singletons conceived after assisted reproduction technology have adverse perinatal outcome? Systematic review and meta-analysis. *Hum Reprod Update.* 2013;19:87–104.

29. Sazonova A, Källen K, Thurin-Kjellberg A, Wennerholm UB, Bergh C. Neonatal and maternal outcomes comparing women undergoing two in vitro fertilization (IVF) singleton pregnancies and women undergoing one IVF twin pregnancy. *Fertil Steril.* 2013;99:731–7.

30. Karlström PO, Bergh C. Reducing the number of embryos transferred in Sweden – impact on delivery and multiple birth rates. *Hum Reprod.* 2007;22:2202–7.

31. Henningsen AA, Gissler M, Skjaerven R, Bergh C, Tiitinen A, Romundstad LB, et al. Trends in perinatal health after assisted reproduction: a Nordic study from the CoNARTaS group. *Hum Reprod.* 2015;30:710–16.

32. Thurin A, Hausken J, Hillensjö T, Jablonowska B, Pinborg A, Strandell A, Bergh C. Elective single-embryo transfer versus double-embryo transfer in in vitro fertilization. *N Engl J Med.* 2004;351:2392–402.

33. McLernon DJ, Harrild K, Bergh C, Davies MJ, de Neubourg D, Dumoulin JC, et al. Clinical effectiveness of elective single versus double embryo transfer: meta-analysis of individual patient data from randomised trials. *BMJ.* 2010;341:c6945.

34. Pandian Z, Marjoribanks J, Ozturk O, Serour G, Bhattacharya S. Number of embryos for transfer following in vitro fertilisation or intra-cytoplasmic sperm injection. *Cochrane Database Syst Rev.* 2013 Jul 29(7):CD003416.

35. Stone BA, March CM, Ringler GE, Baek KJ, Marrs RP. Casting for determinants of blastocyst yield and of rates of implantation and of pregnancy after blastocyst transfers. *Fertil Steril.* 2014;102:1055–64.

36. Poulain M, Hesters L, Sanglier T, de Bantel A, Fanchin R, Frydman N, Grynberg M. Is it acceptable to destroy or include human embryos before day 5 in research programmes? *Reprod Biomed Online.* 2014;28:522–9.

37. Sallem A, Santulli P, Barraud-Lange V, Le Foll N, Ferreux L, Maignien C, et al. Extended culture of poor-quality supernumerary embryos improves ART outcomes. *J Assist Reprod Genet.* 2018;35:311–19.

38. Li M, Wang Y, Shi J. Do day-3 embryo grade predict day-5 blastocyst transfer outcomes in patients with good prognosis? *Gynecol Endocrinol.* 2019;35:36–9.

39. Armstrong S, Bhide P, Jordan V, Pacey A, Farquhar C. Time-lapse systems for embryo incubation and assessment in assisted reproduction. *Cochrane Database Syst Rev.* 2019;May 29;5:CD011320.

40. Basile N, Elkhatib I, Meseguer M. A strength, weaknesses, opportunities and threats analysis on time lapse. *Curr Opin Obstet Gynecol.* 2019;31:148–55.

41. Rubio I, Kuhlmann R, Agerholm I, Kirk J, Herrero J, Escriba MJ, et al. Limited implantation success of direct-cleaved human zygotes: a time-lapse study. *Fertil Steril.* 2012;98:1458–63.

42. Athayde Wirka K, Chen AA, Conaghan J, Ivani K, Gvakharia M, Behr B, et al. Atypical embryo phenotypes identified by time-lapse microscopy: high prevalence and association with embryo development. *Fertil Steril.* 2014;101:1637–48.

43. Kuznyetsov V, Madjunkova S, Antes R, Abramov R, Motamedi G, Ibarrientos Z, et al. Evaluation of a novel non-invasive preimplantation genetic screening approach. *PLoS ONE* 2018;13:e0197262.

44. Huang L, Bogale B, Tang Y, Lu S, Xie XS, Racowsky C. Noninvasive preimplantation genetic testing for aneuploidy in spent medium may be more reliable than trophectoderm biopsy. *Proc Nat Acad Sci.* 2019; 116(28):14105–12.

45. Chen J, Jia L, Tingting L, Yingchun G, He S, Zhang Z, et al. Diagnostic efficiency of blastocyst culture medium in noninvasive preimplantation genetic testing

(niPGT-A). *Fertil Steril Reports.* 2021;2(1):88–94.

46. Magli MC, Albanese C, Crippa A, Tabanelli C, Ferraretti AP, Gianaroli L. Deoxyribonucleic acid detection in blastocoelic fluid: a new predictor of embryo ploidy and viable pregnancy. *Fertil Steril.* 2019;111:77–85.

47. Khosravi P, Kazemi E, Zhan Q, Malmsten JE, Toschi M, Zisimopoulos P, et al. Deep learning enables robust assessment and selection of human blastocysts after in vitro fertilization. *NPJ Digit Med.* 2019;2:21.

48. Tran D, Cooke S, Illingworth PJ, Gardner DK. Deep learning as a predictive tool for fetal heart pregnancy following time-lapse incubation and blastocyst transfer. *Hum Reprod.* 2019;34:1011–18.

49. Berntsen J, Rimestad J, Lassen JT, Tran D, Kragh MF. Robust and generalizable embryo selection based on artificial intelligence and time-lapse image sequences. *PLoS ONE* 2022 17(2).

Embryo Developmental Programming

Virginia N. Bolton

2.1 Introduction

It is over 40 years since the successful fertilization of a human egg in vitro and development of the resulting human preimplantation embryo led to the birth of a healthy baby. In the intervening years, assisted reproduction technology (ART) has become routine treatment for infertility worldwide with the birth of over 8 million babies to date [1] yet gaps remain in our understanding of the earliest stages of human embryogenesis. We know that human embryos vary in their potential to implant and lead to a healthy pregnancy, but are we confident that exposure to in vitro culture conditions does not compromise their inherent viability? Can we be certain that the embryo's intrinsic developmental program is sufficiently robust to withstand environmental insults imposed during ART, or does in vitro culture lead to genetic or epigenetic changes in the more vulnerable embryos, contributing to the known high rate of implantation failure and early pregnancy loss? May there even be long-term consequences for offspring? These questions underline the importance of detailed knowledge and understanding of the developmental program of the human embryo, and emphasize the vital need for continued study of the human preimplantation embryo in a research setting.

For obvious reasons, the human preimplantation embryo as the subject of pure research is a precious and limited resource. Consequently, while there is a wealth of knowledge derived from direct observations of human preimplantation embryos developing in vitro in a clinical setting, much of our perceived understanding of the cellular and molecular mechanisms underlying this early phase of human development is extrapolated from studies of other mammalian species, formerly the rabbit, and latterly the mouse. However, recent advances in molecular, genomic, and noninvasive imaging technologies have begun to lead to significant advances in the direct investigation, and as a result our understanding, of human development.

In the clinical setting, the varying developmental potential of individual human embryos presents clinical scientists with the challenge of developing methods for embryo selection, to enable distinction between those embryos destined to fail and those that have the potential to lead to a viable pregnancy. This chapter will summarize what is currently understood about the developmental program of the human embryo, setting the scene for an evaluation of the different approaches to embryo selection for use in ART treatment that will be considered in subsequent chapters.

2.2 Preimplantation Embryo Development

2.2.1 Fertilization

Penetration of the oocyte by a spermatozoon triggers the complex series of fertilization events that culminate in the formation of a diploid zygote from two haploid gametes. This series of events includes the establishment of the block to polyspermy, establishment of diploidy, securing the cytoplasmic constitution of the oocyte, syngamy, initiation of the developmental program, and culminates in the first cleavage division.

2.2.2 Cleavage

During the cleavage stages of development, the embryo remains the same size within the glycoprotein matrix, the zona pellucida, that forms its outer coating while its component spherical cells (totipotent blastomeres) halve in size at each division. Cleavage of the blastomeres is asynchronous, so that embryos with intermediate blastomere numbers (3-cell, and 5- to 7-cell stages) are seen before completion of the second and third cleavage divisions. During each cleavage division, the maternal cytoplasm inherited from the oocyte is divided between progressively smaller blastomeres.

2.2.3 Blastocyst Formation

The 8- to 16-cell embryo begins to undergo the process of compaction, where individual blastomeres of the cleavage stage embryo become indistinct, as they maximize intercellular contact through tight junction formation, and adhere to and flatten against each other to form a ball of indistinct cells (the morula). Subsequent cell divisions within the embryo are less easily discernible using conventional microscopy than during cleavage stages.

During compaction, the phenotype of the cells within the embryo changes for the first time during embryogenesis, as the cells become polarized and lay down the basis for the differential inheritance in subsequent cell divisions that leads ultimately to differentiation of the different cell types within the blastocyst.

By day 5–6L, a fluid-filled cavity forms and expands within the embryo and the blastocyst is formed. The blastocyst is comprised of an outer layer of trophectoderm (TE) cells that surround a blastcoelic cavity and an inner cell mass (ICM). While TE cells are destined for an extra-embryonic lineage, giving rise to placental tissues, early ICM cells remain pluripotent, and can give rise to all the cell types of the fetus. Around the time of implantation, cells of the ICM differentiate into pluripotent epiblast cells, and into primitive endoderm, whose cells will not contribute to the fetus, but instead give rise to extra-embryonic endoderm cells that will form the yolk sac.

2.2.4 Implantation

Implantation takes place at around day 7 of development. As the blastocoelic cavity continues to expand, TE cells emerge from the thinned zona pellucida, the blastocyst hatches and attaches to the uterine lining. Pregnancy is established and further development of the embryo proper can begin.

2.3 Developmental Programming and Control

Human embryogenesis begins in the near complete absence of transcriptional activity, and the first three days of development are directed by the maternally inherited program that has been laid down in the oocyte. The maternal program for development directs fusion of the egg and sperm, migration and fusion of the male and female pronuclei, genetic and epigenetic reprogramming within the cytoplasm of the blastomeres, and three cleavage divisions (reviewed by [2, 3]).

2.3.1 The Maternal Program for Development

2.3.1.1 Oocyte Maturation and Laying Down the Maternal Inheritance

Gene expression remains relatively inactive during maturation of the oocyte from the germinal vesicle stage, through germinal vesicle breakdown, metaphase I (MI), anaphase I (AI), and telophase I (TI), and then through the brief transition of prophase II (PII) prior to becoming the mature ovulatory oocyte that is arrested in second meiotic metaphase (MII). When at MII, the oocyte has the capacity to achieve fertilization. Within the cytoplasm of the MII oocyte resides the maternal inheritance of organelles and macromolecules that will direct the program for embryo development until the embryonic genome is activated. This includes ribosomes and a broad spectrum of mRNAs along with the full protein biosynthetic apparatus; mitochondria and an ATP-generating system; a Golgi system for synthesis and modification of glycoproteins; and a cytoskeletal system of microfilaments and microtubules for the organization of cytokinesis and karyokinesis.

Maintenance of arrest at MII depends on the balance of the cytoplasmic maturation-promoting factor (MPF) that stabilizes the meiotic MII phase, and cytostatic factor (CSF) that stabilizes MPF.

2.3.1.2 Fertilization and the Establishment of Diploidy

Fusion of the sperm and oocyte triggers a dramatic increase in the level of free calcium in the egg, due largely to the release of calcium from internal stores mediated through the action of a sperm enzyme, phospholipase-zeta (PLCZ), that passes into the oocyte after fusion. The first rise, lasting 2–3 minutes, sweeps in a wave across the oocyte from the point of sperm entry, and is followed by a series of calcium spikes that can last for several hours.

The calcium pulsations play a critical role in achieving successful fertilization and the establishment of diploidy. Calcium-binding proteins are activated, which in turn phosphorylate or dephosphorylate several target proteins, and penetration by additional spermatozoa is blocked. The block to polyspermy is achieved through the cortical reaction, where peripheral cortical granules in the oocyte cytoplasm fuse with the oocyte membrane and release their contents into the perivitelline space between the oocyte membrane and the zona pellucida. The contents of cortical granules include enzymes that act on the zona pellucida to prevent further sperm binding. Through a mechanism that remains unexplained, the oocyte membrane also undergoes changes that reduce its sperm-binding properties.

The calcium pulses also lead to resumption of meiosis by the arrested MII oocyte, through the inhibition of CSF and the consequent destabilization of MPF. The second polar body is extruded and meiosis II is complete resulting in a haploid oocyte.

2.3.1.3 Syngamy

Once the sperm and oocyte have fused, the contents of the sperm, including the nucleus and centriole, are incorporated into the oocyte cytoplasm. The sperm nuclear membrane breaks down and, under the influence of maternally inherited cytoplasmic factors in the oocyte, the chromatin begins to decondense. Membranes form around each set of haploid chromosomes from the male and female gametes, and two pronuclei are formed. Both pronuclei are clearly visible at the level of the light microscope (Figure 2.1), with the male pronucleus usually the larger of the two, and contain multiple nucleoli. The pronuclei, in which DNA synthesis is underway in preparation for the first mitotic division, migrate from the periphery to the center of the oocyte, where they meet, the pronuclear membranes break down, and syngamy is achieved as the two sets of chromosomes come together, resulting in diploidy. As the first mitosis of the developing embryo commences the cytoskeleton of the fertilized zygote is reorganized, and a cleavage furrow forms in preparation for cytokinesis and the first cleavage division.

2.3.1.4 Initiation of Embryo Development

The maternal program for development persists in the human embryo until day 3 of development, when the second cleavage division has been completed in embryos displaying a normal rate of development. Even if transcription is blocked using the transcriptional inhibitor α-amanitin, human embryos nonetheless undergo cleavage to the 4-cell stage and display normal patterns of protein synthesis until day 3 of development. Although some paternal transcripts have been identified in the embryo before the 4-cell stage, it is now accepted that these represent the products of minor transcriptional activity, and their detection may be a reflection of their preferential stability in an environment where maternal transcripts are being degraded rapidly through subsequent rounds of cell division.

2.3.2 Activation of the Embryonic Genome

Morphological changes such as compaction as the morula forms, or cavitation as blastulation proceeds, take place according to a temporal program for development. These changes are a function of the interval (s) following trigger events such as the ovulatory luteinizing hormone surge, or specific events associated with fertilization, rather than of the number of cycles of cell division.

It is not until around day 3 of development that the developmental program of the human embryo switches from maternal to embryonic control, with activation of a wave of transcription from the embryonic genome (Figure 2.2). In embryos undergoing cleavage at the normal rate, this coincides with genome activation taking place between the 4- and 8-cell stages, as shown when the distinct, novel patterns of proteins synthesized between those stages is blocked in embryos exposed to the transcription inhibitor α-amanitin.

The timing of embryonic genome activation is independent of cell number, or number of cleavage divisions, and occurs on day 3 of development even in embryos that have undergone developmental arrest

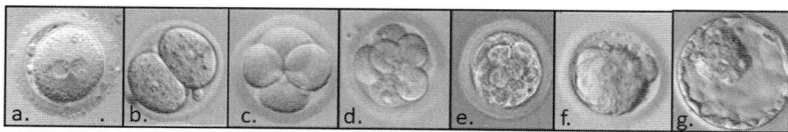

Figure 2.1 Preimplantation stages of human embryo development
a. Normally fertilized oocyte 18–20 hours post insemination, day 1; b–d. cleavage stages, days 2–3; e. compacting, day 4; f. compacted morula, day 4; g. expanded blastocyst, day 5

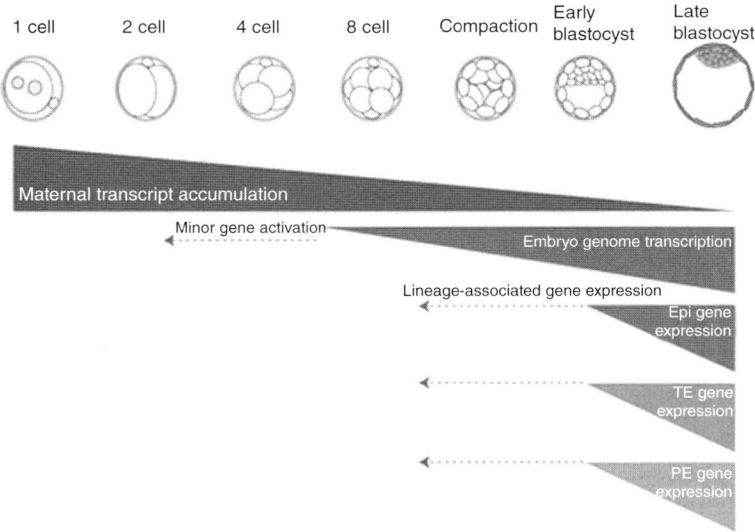

1 cell | 2 cell | 4 cell | 8 cell | Compaction | Early blastocyst | Late blastocyst

Maternal transcript accumulation

Minor gene activation

Embryo genome transcription

Lineage-associated gene expression

Epi gene expression

TE gene expression

PE gene expression

Figure 2.2 Programs for human preimplantation development
Maternal transcripts inherited from the oocyte are degraded through subsequent rounds of cell division. Human genome activation principally occurs between the 4- and 8-cell stages. It is unclear when genes associated with the restriction of the TE or ICM cell lineage are expressed in human embryos, but data suggest that it is around the early blastocyst stage. Human embryos implant around day 7. The dashed arrows indicate the possibility of earlier minor gene activation and lineage-associated gene expression. Epi, epiblast; TE, trophectoderm; PE, primitive endoderm. Note: This figure is a copy of Figure 4 from [2]. Verbal permission has been granted by Kathy Niakan for its use.

by that time. It remains the subject of debate as to how, and precisely when, on day 3 embryonic transcription is initiated.

Activation of the embryonic genome coincides with the downregulation or degradation of maternally inherited transcripts. In the mouse, it has been shown that the widespread wave of embryonic gene activation is accompanied by major changes in chromatin modeling and accessibility, and in DNA demethylation (reviewed by [4]). This presumably serves to reset the genome toward the state required for totipotency and pluripotency. While it is possible that similar mechanisms for enabling widespread transcription may apply across mammalian species, in the human it is unlikely that demethylation is a direct initiator of embryonic genome activation, as progressive demethylation of both paternal and maternal genomes begins at the 2-cell stage, well before its onset [5].

Analysis of transcription products of whole embryos, and of individual cells within the embryo, has enabled identification of the range of genes expressed when the human embryonic genome is activated. These include the dynamic expression of genes encoding transcription factors, epigenetic modifiers, and chromatin remodeling factors, but as yet, the function of many more upregulated genes is unknown. Further investigations are beginning to lead to an understanding of the complexity of transcriptional activation of the embryonic genome but, currently, our understanding of the mechanisms for generation of cell diversity, and for the establishment of distinct cell lineages from pluripotent cells in the human embryo, is far from complete. Interembryo variability means that further extensive investigation of individual embryos, and of individual blastomeres or cells from embryos at different stages of preimplantation development, is needed to understand the full nature and mechanism of regulation of transcriptional activity and embryonic genome activation.

After embryonic gene activation, the vast majority of newly synthesized proteins are no longer maternally coded. However, many of the proteins already synthesized from maternal mRNA templates persist, and therefore the maternal program continues to influence development until the blastocyst stage and beyond. Meanwhile, from the 8-cell stage onward the embryo shows a marked increase in protein and RNA synthesis, in amino acid and nucleotide transport, and in synthesis and modification of phospholipids and cholesterol.

2.3.3 Lineage Commitment

Identifying and understanding the molecular differences between ICM and TE cell lineages, the mechanisms that underlie them, and whether they cause or are an effect of lineage commitment is important in understanding how the ICM and TE form. It is unclear precisely when genes associated with lineage decisions toward cell fate are expressed in human embryos, but it would appear to be later than in the mouse embryo, at around the early blastocyst stage. Although some TE-associated gene expression has been reported to occur as early as the 4-cell stage, before major activation of the embryonic genome takes place, there is some dispute over this. There is a considerable body of evidence to suggest that, prior to compaction, blastomeres in the human embryo remain uncommitted regarding lineage (reviewed by [6, 7]). Differences in transcriptomes and their products have been observed between individual 8-cell stage blastomeres, some of which have characteristics of the maternal, and others the paternal molecular program. Perhaps individual blastomeres within the 8-cell embryo acquire molecular readiness to differentiate into either ICM or TE cell lineage asynchronously, in a cell-autonomous manner, around the time of compaction. This seems plausible, given the asynchronous cleavage of individual blastomeres between the 4- and 8-cell stages.

Several lineage-defining transcription factors (notably OCT4 and CDX2) have been identified that are common to embryos of a number of mammalian species including the human, and which show species-specific differences in their patterns of expression. Further direct studies of the temporal and spatial expression of these and similar proteins throughout human preimplantation embryogenesis is needed to increase understanding of the molecular mechanisms of lineage restriction.

Experimental separation of ICM and TE from early human blastocysts has shown that both cell types are able to regenerate a complete blastocyst, indicating that irreversible commitment to the respective cell lineages has not yet occurred. Although there is, as yet, no direct evidence, differences between mouse and human embryos in this respect suggest that different signaling pathways may operate in the human embryo with respect to establishing the two cell lineages, compared with the mouse. Indeed, there is some evidence to suggest that, in the human, the three cell lineages for epiblast, primitive endoderm, and TE are established in the same time frame. If correct, this differs from the progressive segregation of these three lineages seen in the mouse and implies that novel mechanisms may be involved. It seems clear that full understanding of the mechanisms for human embryo cell pluripotency and cell lineage decisions cannot simply be extrapolated from findings in the mouse. To achieve this, further direct analysis of human embryos is required.

2.4 Kinetics of Preimplantation Development

The timings of each cleavage division, of compaction, morula, and blastocyst formation have been monitored and documented since the earliest days of IVF, providing a temporal framework for the accepted "norms" for each event. Initially, when ART treatment first became routine, embryo morphology was assessed at discrete, relatively infrequent intervals until day 2 or day 3 of development, only extending to day 5 when improved culture conditions led to the practice of in vitro culture to the blastocyst stage, in the early 2000s. A consensus for optimal rates of embryo development has been agreed, derived from conventional morphology assessment data [8]. More recently still, with the introduction of time-lapse imaging technology, detailed information has become available concerning dynamic changes throughout preimplantation embryo development (reviewed by [9]; see this volume, Chapter 11).

2.4.1 Timing of Cleavage Divisions

In embryos considered to be developing at a "normal" rate in vitro, cleavage divisions take place every 18–20 hours (Figure 2.3). Embryos undergoing cleavage more slowly or quickly may have lower viability and may be manifesting inherent metabolic and/or chromosomal defects, or display compromised viability exacerbated by suboptimal culture conditions. The consensus for optimum times by which embryos are expected to have completed each cleavage division, derived from conventional morphology assessment, are: 2-cell stage: day 1 (26±1h post intracytoplasmic sperm injection [ICSI], 28±1 h post-IVF); 4-cell stage: day 2 (44±1 h post IVF/ICSI); and 8-cell stage: day 3 (68±1 h post IVF/ICSI).

2.4.2 Morula Formation

The consensus derived from conventional morphology assessment for the optimum time by which the embryo should have commenced compaction and morula formation, and undergone the fourth cycle of cell division, is on day 4 (by 92±2 h post IVF/ICSI).

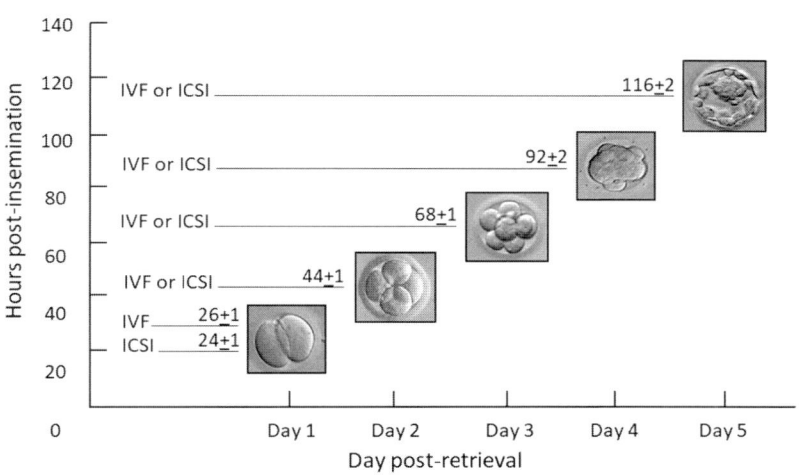

Figure 2.3 Normal developmental timeline of human preimplantation embryos

2.4.3 Blastulation

The consensus for the optimum time by which the embryo should have developed to the fully expanded blastocyst stage, derived from conventional morphology assessment, is on day 5 (116±2 h post IVF/ICSI).

2.5 Embryo Metabolism

Meeting the needs of the human preimplantation embryo in vitro requires more than the simple provision of adequate conditions for sustenance to maintaining stable physiological pH and osmolarity, and provision of adequate levels of the appropriate energy substrate. Similarly, evaluating the quality of culture conditions requires more than the assessment of the rate of successful blastocyst formation, or even the rate of successful live birth following ART treatment. It has become increasingly clear that the environment to which the embryo is exposed, whether in vivo or in vitro, influences the complex interplay of molecular processes that regulate development. Perturbation of the environment may lead to disruption of these processes, or trigger adaptive compensatory responses in the embryo that may contribute either to its demise before successful implantation or persist beyond implantation and affect the phenotype of offspring across their lifespan. Understanding details of the metabolic needs of the preimplantation embryo is important if optimum conditions for development in vitro are to be developed and maintained. The potential consequences of suboptimal culture conditions for the embryo, and for the long-term welfare of the offspring born after ART treatment, cannot be ignored (reviewed by [10, 11]).

ART entails manipulation of events related to ovulation, fertilization, and embryo development. Animal studies have shown effects of different in vitro microenvironments, including constituents of culture media such as hormones (insulin), amino acids, pyruvate, lactate, glucose, and growth factors, on birth weight, growth rate, and cardiovascular function. In humans, differences in the composition of culture medium are thought to be associated with effects on birth weight, and on body weight and BMI examined in ART children at the age of 9 years. Some of these effects have been shown to be reversed in animal models through modification of culture media.

The effects of ART on offspring health are widely considered to be epigenetic in origin. As described earlier, the mechanism for regulation of gene expression is associated with DNA methylation and demethylation. The observation that methylation of certain imprinted genes in ART-derived human preimplantation embryos is perturbed supports this conclusion. Altered DNA methylation has also been reported in the placenta, cord blood, and blood spots from newborn ART offspring. The increased methylation of a paternal imprinted gene observed in the buccal cells of children aged 2 years conceived following ICSI, but not through conventional IVF, led to the suggestion that this change is associated with the extended manipulation in vitro that is necessary for ICSI [12].

That epigenetic changes may be influenced by the microenvironment in which embryos are cultured has been shown in numerous animal and human studies with respect to culture media composition and DNA methylation, and oxygen tension during culture [13, 14]. There is evidence to suggest that ART-induced changes in DNA methylation could be gene- and/or tissue-specific, and/or that subtle changes in DNA methylation induced by ART may be compensated or masked by the postnatal environment. Wide variations among and between populations and lifestyles means that epigenetic studies in humans are inevitably complex, and useful epigenetic data difficult to extract. There is an urgent need for greater emphasis on establishing databases for surveillance of ART offspring, which have been implemented to date in relatively few countries.

2.5.1 Metabolism Pre–Genomic Activation

2.5.1.1 Energy Substrate

Metabolic activity and substrate preferences of the human preimplantation embryo alter between early cleavage stages when pyruvate is the primary substrate, to increased glucose and oxygen consumption during later cleavage as embryos approach cavitation (reviewed by [15]). Data from studies of nutrient consumption by the embryo vary according to medium composition and culture conditions, and their interpretation is further complicated by the existence of endogenous maternally inherited stores. Nonetheless, the temporal association in the human between the change in energy substrate utilization and activation of the embryonic genome suggests a functional relationship between the two, with significant potential consequences for any perturbation of substrate availability in vitro.

2.5.1.2 Hyperglycemia and Metabolic Stress

The implications of impaired metabolic activity in the embryo is potentially serious. Direct consequences for the cleavage stage human embryo must be inferred from animal studies and understanding of cell physiology, which suggest impacts on cell proliferation and later development. Thus, elevated glucose levels can result in suppression of insulin and glucokinase expression, decreased mitochondrial function, and accelerated apoptosis. Increased formation of reactive oxygen species can lead to activation of common stress-activated signaling pathways.

2.5.1.3 Reactive Oxygen Species

Reactive oxygen species (ROS) represent a source of stress for the embryo during in vitro culture, causing an increase in hydrogen peroxide production and possible DNA damage [16]. In response to ROS exposure, homeostatic control is maintained through increased activity of antioxidant enzymes, which may itself compromise development. In bovine embryos, vitamin E supplementation of culture medium has been shown to suppress ROS damage.

2.5.1.4 Amino Acids

The many roles amino acids play in embryo developmental programming, in addition to protein synthesis, include energy production, regulation of osmolarity and pH, homeostasis, and signal transduction [17]. Although animal studies have shown enhanced embryo development when cultured in the presence of certain amino acids, the optimum amino acid supplementation for human embryo culture media has yet to be identified; surplus or inappropriate amino acids in the culture medium may spontaneously break down to produce ammonium ions, which can cause short- and long-term damage during development. The potential consequences of unphysiological amino acids in culture media on metabolic pathways in the developing embryo are widespread.

Intracellular amino acid content in the embryo, which is regulated through sodium-dependent and -independent transporter systems, has been shown to differ between mouse embryos in vivo and in vitro, and its turnover to differ between human embryos in vitro. Extensive in vivo studies in animal models have demonstrated that the amino acid profile of uterine fluid is influenced by manipulation of the maternal diet, with consequences for abnormal programming of preimplantation embryo development. Altered levels of amino acids such as leucine, which is known to play important roles in signaling and regulation of protein synthesis, were identified. It is not difficult to extrapolate these findings to conclude that there is significant potential for effects on human preimplantation embryos of exposure to altered amino acid environments in vitro (reviewed by [10]).

2.5.2 The Metabolism Post–Genome Activation

The level of metabolic activity in the 8-cell embryo post activation of the embryonic genome increases significantly compared with earlier cleavage stages, reflecting the major increase in levels of protein and lipid biosynthesis and in transport of macromolecules.

2.5.2.1 Energy Substrate

Glucose consumption increases in late cleavage, but oxidative phosphorylation is the primary source of energy production in blastocysts, rather than glycolysis, due to the corresponding elevation in oxygen consumption. However, hyper-elevated glucose metabolism, particularly via glycolysis, may be a stress response in the developing embryo.

2.5.2.2 Hyperglycemia and Metabolic Stress

Although information from direct investigation of the human embryo is limited, using animal models (rodent and bovine), where the extent of glucose uptake in the late cleavage stage embryo shows a positive association with developmental potential, studies have shown that significant elevation of glucose utilization is associated with reduced embryo potential [18]. Hyperglycemia is known to affect the expression of at least one transcription factor (NF-$_k$B), which regulates the expression of certain growth factors, cytokines, and adhesion molecules with roles in embryo developmental programming. Exposure to excess external levels of glucose leads to depleted glucose transporter expression, at both transcriptional and translational levels, with consequences for activation of the embryonic genome, apoptotic pathways, chromatin degradation, and nuclear fragmentation. Reduced cell number in resulting blastocysts exposed to these conditions in vitro may disturb later morphogenesis and events associated with implantation, through disruption of interactions between the ICM and TE required for maintaining trophectoderm proliferation.

2.5.2.3 Amino Acids

Again, our limited understanding of the specific amino acid requirements, and their roles in human preimplantation embryo development in vitro, is derived almost exclusively by extrapolation from animal models, so must be interpreted with caution. Any direct role in activation of the embryonic genome has yet to be demonstrated, but there is sufficient knowledge of cellular physiology and the metabolic pathways for amino acid turnover and protein biosynthesis to indicate that activation of the

embryonic genome and blastocyst formation and hatching will all be influenced by the in vitro amino acid environment. In the mouse, a critical role in blastocyst formation and expansion in vitro is suggested for specific amino acids, notably isoleucine and valine, by their significant uptake during these phases of development. The overall pattern of amino acid turnover and exchange observed in the mouse embryo correlates with the capacity for blastocyst formation, and the observation that embryos with lower turnover exhibit greater developmental potential has led to formulation of the "Quiet Embryo" hypothesis [19, 20].

2.6 Concluding Comments

The direct study of human embryos in a research setting has revealed that preimplantation development is characterized by reprogramming and programming, triggered by sperm penetration, directing the formation and fusion of the male and female pronuclei and initiation of cleavage divisions. Epigenetic reprogramming and modification direct activation of transcription from the embryonic genome between the 4- and 8-cell stages, degradation of maternally inherited transcripts, and the differentiation of and commitment to different cell lineages.

If parameters are identified during the cleavage stages of human embryo development that predict accurately the success or failure of a given embryo to develop into a viable blastocyst, implant, and lead to a viable pregnancy, it follows that the success or failure of the embryo is predetermined in early embryonic cells, even as early as the oocyte.

Key Messages

- A maternal program directs development almost exclusively for the first three days of development, from fertilization through to the 4- to 8-cell stage, utilizing macromolecules and organelles laid down in the oocyte.
- In response to sperm penetration, calcium pulsations in the oocyte trigger the cortical reaction and resumption of meiosis.
- The sperm centriole is essential for mitosis in the embryo.
- The first cycles of cell division in the embryo are cleavage divisions with no net growth in embryo size; cells halve in size at each division and the

oocyte cytoplasm is divided between pluripotent blastomeres.

- The embryonic program directs development beyond the 8-cell stage, with major activation of transcription from the embryonic program during the third cleavage division.
- Maternal transcripts are degraded by this time, although some functional maternal proteins persist after the embryonic program assumes overall direction of further development.
- Compaction, resulting in morula formation on day 4 of development, is characterized by increased cell–cell adhesion and intracellular polarization, laying down the basis for differentiation during subsequent cell divisions, and the generation of cell lineages in the embryo.

- The blastocyst forms on day 5 of development, within which different cell types with different fates are evident for the first time: the pluripotent inner cell mass (ICM) and the outer trophectoderm (TE).
- The primary energy substrate for the embryo changes from pyruvate during cleavage to glucose after embryonic genome activation, which coincides with a major increase in metabolic and biosynthetic activity.
- The environment of developing gametes and embryos, whether in vivo or in vitro, influences the complex interplay of molecular processes that regulate development; full understanding of these processes and influences is essential if embryo development in vitro during ART is to be optimized.

References

1. Fauser BCJM. Towards the global coverage of a unified registry of IVF outcomes. *Reprod Biomed Online.* 2019;38:133–7.

2. Niakan KK, Han JH, Pederson RA, Simon C, Reijo Pera RA. *Human pre-implantation development. Dev.* 2012;139:829–41.

3. Rossant J, Tam PL. New insights into early human development: lessons for stem cell derivation and differentiation. *Cell Stem Cell.* 2017;20:18–28.

4. Eckersley-Maslin MA, Alda-Catalinas C, Reik W. Dynamics of the epigenetic landscape during the maternal-to-zygotic transition. *Nat Rev Mol Cell Biol.* 2018;19:436–50.

5. Guo H, Zhu P, Yan L, Li R, Hu B, Lian Y, et al. The DNA methylation landscape of human early embryos. *Nature.* 2014;31:606–61.

6. De Paepe C, Krivega M, Cauffman G, Geens M, Van de Velde H. Totipotency and lineage segregation in the human embryo. *Mol Hum Reprod.* 2014;20:599–618.

7. Smith HL, Stevens A, Minogue B, Sneddon S, Shaw L, Wood L, et al. Systems based analysis of human embryos and gene networks involved in cell lineage allocation. *BMC Genomics.* 2019;20:171.

8. Alpha Scientists in Reproductive Medicine and ESHRE Special Interest Group of Embryology. The Istanbul consensus workshop on embryo assessment: proceedings of an expert meeting. *Hum Reprod.* 2011;26:1270–83.

9. Wong C, Chen AA, Behr B, Shen S. Time-lapse microscopy and image analysis in basic and clinical embryo development research. *RBMO.* 2013;26:120–9.

10. Fleming TP, Watkins A, Velazquez MA, Mathers JC, Prentice AM, Stephenson J, et al. Origins of lifetime health around the time of conception: causes and consequences. *Lancet.* 2018;391:1842–52.

11. Velasquez MA, Fleming TP, Watkins AJ. Periconceptional environment and the developmental origins of disease. *J Endocrinol.* 2019;242:T33–T49.

12. Whitelaw N, Bhattacharya S, Hoad G, Horgan GW, Hamilton M, Haggarty P. Epigenetic status in the offspring of spontaneous and assisted conception. *Hum Reprod.* 2014;29:1452–8.

13. Market-Velker BA, Fernandes AD, Mann MR. Side-by-side comparison of five commercial media systems in a mouse model: suboptimal in vitro culture interferes with imprint maintenance. *Biol Reprod.* 2010;83:938–50.

14. Canovas S, Ivanova E, Romar R, Garcia-Martinez S, Soriano-Ubeda C, Garcia-Vazquez FA, et al. DNA methylation and gene expression changes derived from assisted reproductive technologies can be decreased by reproductive fluids. *eLife* 2017;6: e23670.

15. Leese HJ. What does an embryo need? *Hum Fertil.* 2003;6:180–5.

16. Johnson MH, Nasr-Esfahani MH. Radical solutions and cultural problems: could free oxygen radicals be responsible for the impaired development of preimplantation mammalian embryos in vitro? *Bioessays.* 1994;16:31–8.

17. Van Winkle LJ. Amino acid transport regulation and early

embryo development. *Biol Reprod.* 2001;64:1–12.

18. Scott R, Zhang M, Seli E. Metabolism of the oocyte and the preimplantation embryo: implications for assisted reproduction. *Crr Opin Obstet Gynecol.* 2018;30:163–70.

19. Leese HJ. Quiet please, do not disturb: a hypothesis of embryo metabolism and viability. *Bioessays.* 2002;24:845–9.

20. Baumann CG, Morris DG, Sreenan JM, Leese HJ. The quiet embryo hypothesis: molecular characteristics favoring viability. *Mol Reprod Dev.* 2007; 74:1345–53.

Chapter 3

Embryo–Maternal Interactions

Lois A. Salamonsen, Tracey A. Edgell, Guiying Nie, and Jemma Evans

3.1 Introduction

Following a natural conception, the embryo undergoes preimplantation development sequentially within the fallopian tube and the uterus. In the fallopian tube, the ovum is fertilized and the resultant embryo undergoes serial divisions to morula stage; it enters the uterine cavity as a morula or unhatched blastocyst (Figure 3.1). Here it is nurtured by endometrial secretions and other critical uterine fluid components to complete its final preimplantation development before attaching to and invading the endometrium. Subsequently, the placenta will develop to sustain fetal growth and development until birth. Both the fallopian tubes and the endometrium undergo cyclical morphological and molecular changes driven predominantly by ovarian hormones during each menstrual cycle. In the macaque, which undergoes menstrual cycles similar to the human, estradiol-17β (E) is the critical hormone for preparation of the fallopian tubes whereas progesterone (P) (in the presence of E) is critical for endometrial differentiation. The fallopian tubes provide the milieu to support sperm transport, fertilization, and very early embryo development, while the endometrium undergoes its major progesterone-driven differentiative changes in preparation for implantation, which typically occurs some 7–10 days after ovulation. Importantly the embryo is relatively "quiet" during its time in the tubes (see Chapter 12 in this volume)

although there are some influences of tubal fluid contents on embryo development. The embryo becomes highly active at a molecular level once it enters the uterine environment as a blastocyst. In infertile couples, after tubal patency is proven during early workup, artificial reproductive technologies are generally applied to fertilize and culture the embryo in vitro to the morula or early blastocyst stage and then transfer it directly into the uterine cavity, thus bypassing tubal influence.

Embryo transfer studies in a range of animals and subsequent human data from early IVF clinics [1] unequivocally demonstrate the necessity for developmental synchrony between the preimplantation embryo and the cyclically changing endometrium. Indeed, in women there is only a brief period of ~4 days in each menstrual cycle, termed the window of implantation (WOI), when the endometrium is receptive to implantation. This coincides with the blastocyst entering the uterine cavity, undergoing final development, and attaching to the endometrial surface.

3.2 Endometrial Cyclicity and the Development of Receptivity

The endometrium undergoes remarkable remodeling during each menstrual cycle [2], with the functionalis layer being shed at menstruation, followed by regeneration (proliferation of all cell types) under the influence of rising estrogen during the proliferative phase. Following ovulation and largely driven by rising progesterone and estrogen levels, all cells then differentiate to achieve endometrial receptivity for embryo implantation in the mid-secretory phase. If no conception occurs in that cycle, progesterone levels fall with the demise of the corpus luteum, inducing menstruation (Figure 3.2). Differentiative processes in each of the endometrial cell types are required for receptivity and implantation.

Work in the author's laboratory is largely funded by NHMRC of Australia (project and fellowship grants) and by the Victorian State Government's Infrastructure Support to the Hudson Institute. Thanks to designers Kim-Vu Salamonsen (kDesignandthings.com) for Figure 3.1 and Sue Panckridge at the Hudson Institute for Figure 3.2 and Figure 3.3.

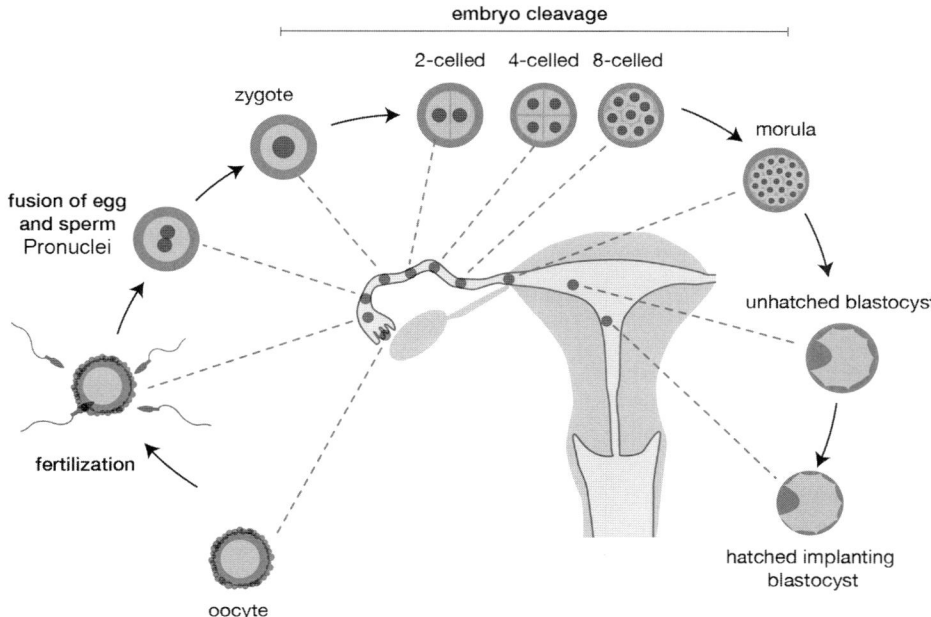

Figure 3.1 The pathway of normal embryo development
The oocyte released from the dominant ovarian follicle enters the fallopian tube, where it is fertilized to form a zygote, then undergoes a series of cell divisions to form 2-, 4-, and 8-cell embryos. A morula/early blastocyst is the embryonic stage of entry into the uterine cavity. It is within this microenvironment that the blastocyst hatches and prepares for attachment to and invasion between the endometrial epithelial cells, in the process of implantation.

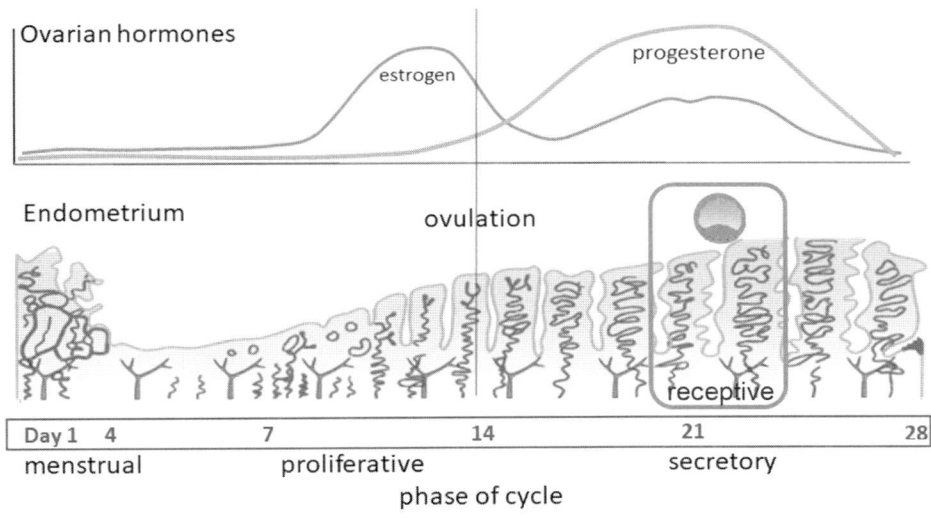

Figure 3.2 Cyclical endometrial changes are normally driven by hormones
Following endometrial shedding at menstruation, the tissue is restored during the proliferative phase of the cycle under the stimulus of rising estrogen from the dominant follicle. Following ovulation, all the cells undergo differentiation under the influence of progesterone in the presence of estrogen. This results in the endometrium becoming "receptive" to embryo implantation. In the absence of an embryo, falling estrogen and progesterone levels result in menstruation.

3.2.1 Luminal Epithelium

The endometrial surface facing the uterine cavity is covered by a tightly packed layer of epithelial cells, the luminal epithelial cells, which form a barricade guarding and protecting the endometrium from chemical injury and microbial infection. These cells, being the first endometrial contact by an embryo for implantation, must "weaken" their barrier function to allow embryo attachment and penetration. Indeed, the process of embryo implantation presents a paradox in cellular biology. To maintain their epithelial characteristics, epithelial cells are generally polarized. Both the outer layer of the embryo (the trophectoderm) and the luminal epithelial layer of the endometrium typically present with a polarized phenotype. Naturally two polarized epithelial surfaces will repel each other. As an analogy, imagine the similar poles of two magnets when introduced to each other will be mutually repulsive. So too are two polarized epithelial surfaces. Polarity also maintains tight junctional complexes between the epithelial cells, providing an impenetrable layer. The polarity of the luminal epithelium must therefore change in preparation for embryo implantation. This is demonstrated by a decrease in electronegativity (shown in marmosets) and a downregulation in factors controlling epithelial polarity. Thus, the luminal epithelium undergoes a partial epithelial-to-mesenchymal transition. In laboratory assays, downregulation of polarity molecules in human endometrial epithelial cells decreases tight junctions for implantation, reinforcing the importance for receptivity of polarity changes in the luminal epithelium [3].

The luminal epithelial surface must also become adhesive for attachment of the trophectoderm. Some of the molecules adapted for this purpose include those that are important for leukocytes to adhere to a vessel wall, such as the lectin-like protein L-selectin (present on the trophectoderm) that can bind to specific carbohydrate structures on the endometrium. Other candidate adhesion systems present at this interface include integrins, heparin-like EGF-like growth factor (HB-EGF), and its receptor Erb4. In addition, the cells remodel their plasma membrane through a process called the "plasma membrane transformation" (reviewed in [4]). For instance, they lose long and regular microvilli and flatten their apical plasma membrane, presumably to allow a closer physical contact with the implanting blastocyst.

The membrane–cytoskeleton interactions inside the cell also alter substantially, and in the meantime special apical protrusions termed uterodomes or pinopodes develop on the cell surface, likely to assist the immobilization of the blastocyst. These structural alterations are achieved through molecular changes, one of which is the enzymatic cleavage of the scaffolding protein EBP50 and membrane protein dystroglycan by proprotein convertase (PC) 5/6 [5, 6]. Another significant remodeling is the thinning of glycocalyx, a layer of gel-like substance on the external surface that lubricates epithelial cells but poses a steric hindrance for blastocyst attachment. An example of glycocalyx thinning for receptivity is the dramatic downregulation of mucin-1 in mouse uterine epithelial cells. However, mucin-1 is increased rather than decreased at receptivity in the human endometrium, signifying that the mechanisms of endometrial epithelial glycocalyx remodeling for receptivity differ between species.

3.2.2 Glandular Epithelium

The glandular epithelium plays a different role from the luminal epithelium, being the primary source of secretions into the uterine cavity. Accordingly, their expression of polarity markers does not change considerably throughout the menstrual cycle, likely reflecting the need for the glandular epithelial cells to maintain apico-basal polarity to facilitate secretion of key factors into the glandular lumen [3]. Indeed, while proteins released or "secreted" from the endometrial glands can be identified within the uterine cavity during the proliferative phase of the cycle, the diversity of these secretions increases during the secretory phase under the combined influence of E and P. During this time these factors released by the endometrial epithelium can enter into a "dialogue" with the preimplantation embryo to facilitate implantation [7]. Furthermore, alterations in such endometrial factors within the uterine cavity may underpin infertility in some women. Subsequent to implantation and during the first trimester, secretions from the endometrial glands supply the histotrophic nutrition to the developing conceptus while the placenta is being formed [8].

3.2.3 Stromal Cell Decidualization

While the endometrial luminal epithelial cells undergo a partial epithelial-to-mesenchymal transition in preparation for receptivity, the endometrial stromal cells undergo the opposite process; a partial mesenchymal-to-epithelial transition known as decidualization [2]. Menstruating species alone spontaneously undergo this hormone-mediated terminal differentiation of the endometrial stroma as P levels rise. During decidualization, polarity markers are upregulated in stromal cells, highlighting that they become more epithelial-like. Indeed, they fail to decidualize when polarity marker expression is prevented by genetic manipulation, suggesting that the development of epithelial-like characteristics is a key component in stromal cell decidualization. Together with infiltrating leukocytes and cells of the vasculature, these differentiated stromal cells will subsequently form the decidua, the maternal component of the placenta. Rising levels of P, acting at least in part through the mediator cyclic AMP, induce decidualization initially in the stromal cells close to the spiral arteries. Its progression is enhanced by a number of paracrine factors that create a "wave of decidualization" throughout the endometrial stromal compartment. Decidualization alters cellular cytoskeletal organization, extracellular matrix composition, and secretion of cytokines and chemokines. Cell responsiveness to external stimuli is also altered and indeed this leads to their "sensing of embryo quality" [9] and restraint of trophoblast cell invasion after implantation. Other steroid hormones (E, glucocorticoids, mineralocorticoids, and androgens) acting through their receptors in the endometrium may help confer specificity of hormone action during decidualization. In a nonconception cycle, as P levels fall, the decidualized stromal cells secrete degradative enzymes contributing to the tissue breakdown at menstruation.

3.2.4 Changes in Blood Vessels

Spiral arterioles, unique to the endometrium, are small vessels that temporarily supply blood to the endometrium in the secretory phase. These are subsequently converted for uteroplacental blood flow during the first trimester of pregnancy, when invasive trophoblasts colonize the vessels, transforming the elastic lamina and enabling the vessels to become flaccid sacs, ideal for gas and nutrient exchange. Histologically, spiral arterioles are useful for defining cycle stage.

3.2.5 Leukocyte Infiltration

Leukocytes are present in the endometrium in varying numbers across the menstrual cycle and contribute to its constant remodeling. These include uterine natural killer cells (uNK), mast cells, T cells, and dendritic cells. Many of these are quiescent and nonfunctional until their activation. During the prereceptive phase (early secretory) uNK cells proliferate and macrophages influx into the endometrium. There is no evidence that uNK cells initiate or promote decidualization. These leukocytes have specific phenotypes, expressing different markers of differentiation and function compared with peripheral leukocytes. Decidualized stromal cells secrete mediators including chemokines and chemokines that can influence the function and differentiation of these leukocytes. In a nonconception cycle, the falling P and E levels in the late secretory phase result in a massive influx of leukocytes, mainly neutrophils, that create a highly inflammatory milieu, critical for menstrual breakdown.

3.3 Events of Implantation

Within the uterine cavity in vivo, the blastocyst first hatches from the surrounding zona pellucida, presumably by mechanical forces and/or enzymatic lysis using species-specific proteases of uterine origin (currently not characterized in the human). At this stage, the outer layer of the blastocyst (that surrounds the inner cell mass (ICM) and the blastocoele), the trophectoderm, a layer of epithelial cells, participates in implantation and will eventually form the maternal component of the placenta. The polar trophectoderm (that adjacent to the ICM) becomes apposed to and attaches to the endometrial luminal epithelium. As discussed in Section 3.2.2, since epithelial cells are mutually repulsive by nature, there must be changes in one or both surfaces to permit adhesion. The endometrial epithelial cells also must reduce their polarity, and decrease their lateral and basal junctional complexes, to enable the blastocyst cells to penetrate between the epithelial cells and their basal lamina (Figure 3.3) to form a syncytium beneath the epithelial layer, from which invasive trophoblast cells arise. Simultaneously, the stroma has been undergoing decidualization (as detailed in Section 3.2.3), with formation of decidual cells and influx of immune cells, particularly macrophages and uterine natural killer cells, that together comprise the decidua. The invasive trophoblasts traffic through the decidua (which exerts constraint by secretion of antiproteases), until by the end of the first trimester, they reach and invade the spiral arterioles, transforming them into large conduits

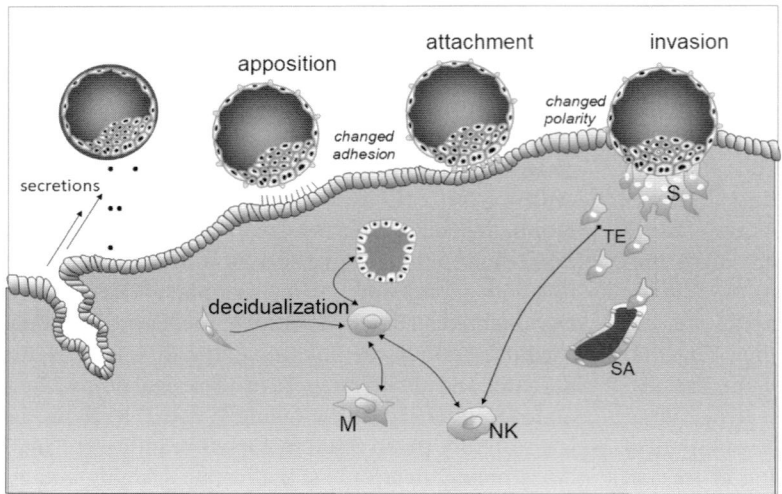

Figure 3.3 Processes leading to successful implantation and early placentation

The embryo as a blastocyst undergoes preimplantation development within the microenvironment of the uterine cavity. This enables it to become apposed to, then attach to the receptive luminal epithelium of the endometrium. The trophectodermal cells then penetrate between the epithelial cells that transiently lose their polarity. The trophectoderm forms a syncytium (S) beneath the epithelium, from which invasive trophoblast cells (TE) invade through the decidual compartment to reach the spiral arterioles (SA). Simultaneously, endometrial stromal fibroblasts undergo decidualization. The resultant decidual cells release chemokines and other factors that attract macrophages (M) and uterine natural killer cells (NK) into the decidua. Straight arrows represent soluble secretions. • represent extracellular vesicles.

of low resistance to provide the flaccid sacs of the placenta, needed for gas and nutrient exchange for the remainder of pregnancy (Figure 3.3).

3.3.1 The Uterine Tract Microenvironment: Why Is It Important?

Since preimplantation embryo development occurs within the uterine cavity, the components of uterine fluid are of considerable importance. They comprise a complex molecular soup (the histiotroph) that includes the nutrients required to nurture the final blastocyst development, along with bioactive factors that promote changes necessary for implantation on both the endometrial and blastocyst surfaces. It is these factors that provide a local embryo-maternal dialogue essential for implantation. Some are soluble, while others are contained within extracellular vesicles (EV) that protect them from degradation, and include proteins, lipids, and miRNA. Both soluble and EV-contained mediators are controlled by steroid hormone action on their cell of origin, with changes between proliferative (E-regulated) and secretory (E +P regulated) phases clearly identified. While uterine fluid contents can be derived from serum (selective transudation) and the fallopian tubes, most are secreted from the endometrial glands, particularly in the mid-secretory phase when these are at their most active, and also in conception cycles, from the blastocyst (these include the hormone human chorionic gonadotrophin [hCG]) [7]. Most factors are at concentrations differing from those in the serum. For many of the secreted factors, the corresponding receptor can be found; for example, for the secreted chemokines CXCL3, CCL14, and CCL4 of endometrial epithelial origin, specific receptors have been identified on trophoblast cells and these chemokines can regulate trophoblast migration. Likewise, secreted proteolytic enzymes such as PC 5/6 can cleave epithelial cell surface proteins, which act as a barrier for embryo attachment.

3.3.2 Effects of an Elevated BMI

While a "cause" for infertility remains unknown in many women, an elevated body mass index (BMI) is significantly associated with infertility and an increased time to pregnancy. A large oocyte donation study linked an altered uterine environment/altered endometrium with reduced pregnancy success in women with BMI > 30. To underpin this finding, an adverse environment within the uterus of women with BMI > 30, characterized by ~4-fold elevated levels of advanced glycation end products (AGEs) has recently been identified [10]. AGES are derivatives of fat- and sugar-related molecules, that can cause "toxic" inflammation within the body. Such AGEs can detrimentally impact both the developing embryo (particularly the ratio of trophectodermal/ICM cells, and embryo outgrowth ex vivo), the endometrial epithelium (adhesive and proliferative capacity), and stromal cell decidualization. Thus, reduction of AGEs prior to treatment for infertility in obese women is likely to enhance success rates.

3.4 Changes Induced in the Infertility Clinic

3.4.1 Effects of Ovarian Stimulation

Controlled ovarian hyperstimulation, a key step in IVF treatment, aims to stimulate production and maturation of multiple follicles, rather than as occurs in normal cycles, when only one follicle reaches maturation and ovulation, with the remainder undergoing atresia. Stimulation is usually with GnRH agonists or antagonists, the latter most commonly used, with dosages and protocols differing between clinics. However, such stimulation affects hormonal levels and can be detrimental to development of endometrial receptivity. It can also result in ovarian hyperstimulation stimulation syndrome (OHSS, not discussed here).

3.4.1.1 Hormonal Levels

In a stimulated cycle, the multiple follicular growth results in supraphysiological serum E levels during the follicular phase, and daily injections with follicle-stimulating hormone (FSH) are necessary to prevent FSH levels falling below the threshold needed for follicle stimulation. Elevation of serum P levels during the late follicular phase in stimulated IVF cycles is frequent, probably due to the action of the injected FSH on granulosa cells, even in the absence of luteinization. Since P is the major driver of endometrial differentiation, these prematurely rising serum P levels detrimentally affect the endometrium and lead to asynchrony between embryo and endometrium [11]. Thus, many clinics now adopt a "freeze-all" strategy when P levels are >1.5 ng/ml on the day of hCG administration. It is also likely that in "high responders" the P threshold to induce detrimental effects is higher than in low and normal responders. A freeze-all strategy or personalized stimulation could overcome this problem, and the former is now widely applied.

3.4.1.2 Effects on Endometrial Development

Despite the availability of high-quality embryos, fresh embryo transfer cycles regularly fail to result in a positive pregnancy outcome. Many studies have demonstrated a detrimental impact of ovarian hyperstimulation protocols on endometrial receptivity and gene expression. A careful histological comparison of endometrium from fertile women on LH+2, fertile oocyte donors on hCG+2, and infertile women (either GnRH agonist or GnRH antagonist protocols followed by fresh embryo transfer) showed clearly that, histologically, the endometrium was altered at hCG+2 in all women who had undergone ovarian hyperstimulation compared with the natural cycle at LH+2. These changes encompassed advanced glandular development, precocious downregulation of the progesterone receptor, altered blood vessel development, and increased infiltration of inflammatory leukocytes. Importantly, those women who became pregnant after fresh embryo transfer had a more "normal" endometrial histology (more similar to that on LH+2 of a natural cycle) than those who did not become pregnant, highlighting the critical role of appropriate endometrial preparation in pregnancy outcomes [12].

3.4.1.3 Effects of Ovulation Induction with hCG on Endometrial Receptivity

The role of hCG in endometrial receptivity is controversial. In natural cycles, release of hCG by the developing embryo acts on the maternal endometrium to enhance expression/production of proimplantation factors. However, precocious exposure to hCG as experienced in IVF cycles in which hCG has been used for ovulation induction appears to be detrimental to endometrial receptivity. This likely relates to hCG downregulating its own receptor. Thus, when the embryo is transferred back into the uterine cavity 5–7 days after an hCG bolus, the endometrium can no longer respond appropriately to hCG released by the embryo [12]. Indeed, a recent Cochrane review found insufficient evidence to support the use of adjuvant hCG in IVF cycles to improve pregnancy success [13]. Further, two prospective and one retrospective clinical studies found a negative effect of intrauterine hCG administration on pregnancy outcomes, reinforcing the need for "physiological" rather than "supraphysiological" communication between endometrium and embryo in achieving a pregnancy.

3.4.2 Freeze–Thaw Cycles

The recent increase in the proportion of frozen embryo transfers (FET) can be ascribed to the factors detailed in Table 3.1. While transfer in either modified natural cycles (mNC-FET) or in artificial cycles (AC-FET) are both widely practiced, the best method of endometrial preparation before thawing and transfer remains under debate. Embryo transfer must be within the endometrial "window of implantation" or

Table 3.1. Reasons for increased frozen embryo transfers

Increased number of oocytes generating viable embryos

Widespread move to single blastocyst transfer

Vitrification replacing slow freeze cryopreservation

Understanding that ovarian stimulation protocols adversely impact endometrial function

receptive period, which starts 5–7 days after ovulation and remains for 4–5 days. Despite numerous trials including "ANTARCTICA," no endometrial preparation method has been shown as superior in terms of live births (review in [14]).

3.5 Testing for Endometrial Receptivity

Endometrial receptivity should not be considered a single event but rather a period of orchestrated multifactorial change, during which the endometrium becomes able to interact with an embryo to a greater or lesser extent. This complexity of "receptivity," combined with a variety of fertility-impacting etiologies and a range of patient outcomes (e.g. recurrent implantation failure, pregnancy loss, and pregnancy complications), has meant that progress toward an endometrial receptivity test has been slow. While many individual markers (proteins, genes, or miRNAs) have been proposed, few have reached the clinic because proofing studies are either absent or inadequate, with likely useful markers abandoned due to unrealistic performance expectations that failed to account for the complex nature of receptivity, etiologies, and outcomes [15].

Histological analysis to define the timing of the endometrial cycle, either conventional Noyes criteria or more recently integrin analysis, has been displaced in favor of gene expression analysis of endometrial biopsy, in the form of the "Endometrial Receptivity Array" (ERA) and the new ERPeak (for which no data are published). The ERA combines expression of 238 genes to optimize the synchrony of the endometrium and embryo. Endometrial biopsy is collected in a prior cycle raising concern of potential intercycle variation. To date published intercycle comparisons have demonstrated consistency but results are limited to women with dysregulated endometrium in whom greater cycle variation might reasonably be anticipated. More recently, the ReceptivaDx test measuring BCL6 as a marker of progesterone resistance, typically associated with endometriosis, has

become available. Thus far mixed results are published from small cohorts and retrospective studies comprising a mix of patient subgroups and patient outcomes. Effectiveness and applicability of all these assays are not evaluated supportively [16], and better assays are still required along with multicenter randomized clinical trials of well-defined patient cohorts with pregnancy outcome as an endpoint.

It is anticipated that in the future a single yes/no receptivity test will be abandoned in favor of patient stratification and multivariate testing combining many biomarkers. Expanded knowledge is hoped to deliver a broadly useful and reliable test.

3.6 Adjuvant Therapies

A large number of adjuvant therapies have been introduced into clinics in recent years. Many of these are suggested to improve endometrial receptivity. However, evidence for benefit is largely absent and some are shown to be even somewhat detrimental. A summary derived from a number of excellent reviews of the topic is provided in Table 3.2.

3.6.1 The Endometrial Scratch: Myth or Reality

The first report that an endometrial "injury" in the cycle preceding embryo transfer could double the chance of pregnancy success spurred the assisted reproductive technology world to routinely offer this intervention. The original study examined women defined as "good responders to hormone stimulation" who had failed to conceive in at least one previous IVF-ET cycle. Pipelle biopsy was performed on days 8, 12, 21, and 26 of the spontaneous menstrual cycle prior to the IVF-ET cycle. This resulted in a live birth rate of 48.9% versus 22.5% in the control group. Subsequently, multiple global studies were performed in a variety of patient groups, with some supporting the original findings while some did not. A recent international randomized trial examining 1 364 women did not support endometrial scratching to improve pregnancy outcomes [21]. However, the timing of endometrial injury occurred over a large time span, day 3 of preceding cycle to day 3 of embryo transfer, and did not focus on women with recurrent implantation failure. Thus, there is potential for this intervention to benefit some women, but how to define such women remains to be determined.

Table 3.2. Adjuvant therapies: what is the evidence?

Treatment	Proposed mechanism of action	Overall outcomes – pregnancy rates in nonselected IVF populations	Any detrimental effects
Hormonal			
Prolonged progesterone	Luteal phase supplementation in downregulated cycle	No significant benefit[1]	
Luteal estradiol supplementation	Luteal phase supplementation in downregulated cycle	Still controversial[1]	
Aromatase inhibitors	Reduced estrogen synthesis reducing endometrial receptivity	No significant benefit[1]	
Insulin-sensitizing drugs	Minimizing insulin resistance	No significant benefit. May reduce miscarriage and OHSS rate in women with PCOS[1]	
GnRH agonist	LH-releasing properties	No significant benefit[1]	
DHEA (dehydro-epiandrostenedione)	Helps in production of testosterone and estrogen	No significant benefit[2,3]	Minor androgenic side effects
Growth hormone	Indirect via follicular insulin-like growth factor stimulating estradiol production	Inconclusive – may be effective but only in GnRH agonist cycles[2,3]	May negatively affect endometrial receptivity
Testosterone	Modulation of decidualization and decidual-trophoblast interactions	No significant benefit[3]	
Human chorionic gonadotropin infusion	May affect implantation through angiogenesis, increased endometrial receptivity, and reduction in NK cells	No significant benefit, but new Cochrane trial suggested significant improvement[3]	Its use in stimulating ovulation reduces subsequent endometrial receptivity[4]
CSF3 (G-CSF) as Filgrastim	Affects endometrium via its receptors on endometrial epithelium	Inconclusive – new evidence indicates no effect on implantation but possibly positive for recurrent miscarriage postimplantation[3]	There may be a fine balance between too little and too much[4]
Immune therapies			
Ascorbic acid	Anti-inflammatory and immunostimulant	No significant benefit[1]	
Glucocorticoids	Immunomodulatory, suppress NK cells	No significant benefit[1]	

Table 3.2. (cont.)

Treatment	Proposed mechanism of action	Overall outcomes – pregnancy rates in nonselected IVF populations	Any detrimental effects
Immune therapies including IV immunoglobulins, TNFα inhibitors, GCSF, PIF, LIF PBMCs, intralipids vitamin D supplementation	Manipulating peripheral NK cells	No significant benefit, no randomized control trials[2,3]	Many have side effects including anaphylaxis (ivlg), lymphoma, heart failure, infections, induction of autoantibodies (anti-TNFα)
Antibiotics	May reduce infection in upper genital tract	No significant benefit[3]	
Steroids	Alter immunological uterine environment	No significant benefit[1] Significant benefit[3]	
Melatonin	Antioxidant	No proven benefit	
Antioxidants including CQ-10	No known action in implantation	No significant benefit[2,3]	
Vasoactive drugs			
Aspirin	Improving uterine blood flow, reducing platelet aggregation and vasoconstriction	No significant benefit in 4/5 meta-analyses[1,3]	
Heparin	Antiplatelet aggregation	No significant benefit[2,3]	May increase bleeding
Combined aspirin and heparin		No significant benefit[2]	May increase bleeding including vaginally; thrombophilia
Nitric oxide donors and nitric oxide (as sildenafil)	Uterine vasodilatation	No significant benefit[1,2]	Possibly detrimental to embryo development

Note: Data derived from 1. [17]; 2. [18]; 3. [19]; 4. [20].

3.7 Conclusions

The importance of the endometrium in achieving a pregnancy within an infertility clinic setting can no longer be ignored. The evidence is clear. Preparation of the endometrium to be receptive at the appropriate time must be considered in clinical protocols – often this will not require any external treatment other than a high-quality embryo transfer into a fully natural cycle. Most of the adjunct treatments offered to couples provide no advantage, and indeed some can be detrimental. A good test for endometrial receptivity in the cycle of transfer is still not available but, once it is, will provide considerable benefit to

outcomes of medical fertility treatment. Emerging technologies, including new genomic techniques, and those using organoids and blastoids, are rapidly expanding our knowledge in this field [22] and are providing solid support for these conclusions.

> **Key Messages**
> - The endometrium undergoes shedding, restoration, and differentiation in each menstrual cycle.
> - This is driven predominantly by the ovarian steroid hormones estradiol 17β and progesterone. In the proliferative phase the

tissue is restored while after ovulation the endometrial cells differentiate in preparation for implantation.

- The endometrium is receptive for an embryo to implant for only ~4 days in the mid-secretory phase of the cycle, known as the "receptive phase" or "window of implantation."
- The embryo undergoes its final development (blastocyst hatching, preparation for implantation) in the uterine cavity, which is rich in nutrients and regulatory factors that support this development.
- The blastocyst comprises two cell types, the inner cell mass and the outer trophectoderm. It is the trophectoderm that must attach to, and penetrate the outer epithelial layer of the endometrium and then further passage through the tissue to form the placenta.
- The blastocyst and the endometrial epithelium set up an embryo–endometrial dialogue, mediated largely by their secretions into the uterine cavity. This enhances implantation potential.
- In an IVF cycle, the hormones used for ovarian stimulation disturb endometrial development. The more disturbance, the less likely it is that an embryo will implant.
- The hCG given to stimulate ovulation downregulates its own receptors on the endometrium, making it unresponsive to the subsequent hCG originating from the blastocyst.
- There is little evidence to support any of the currently available adjuvant therapies. Indeed, there is evidence of some harm.
- Evidence for the "endometrial scratch" is indecisive with methodological issues in trials indicating bias.
- The move toward "freeze all" transfers into modified natural cycles is promising, but protocols for optimal endometrial preparation remain under debate.

References

1. Wilcox AJ, Baird DD, Weinberg CR. Time of implantation of the conceptus and loss of pregnancy. *N Engl J Med.* 1999;340 (23):1796–9.

2. Evans J, Salamonsen LA, Winship A, Menkhorst E, Nie G, Gargett CE, Dimitriadis E. Fertile ground: human endometrial programming and lessons in health and disease. *Nat Rev Endocrinol.* 2016;12 (11):654–67.

3. Whitby S, Salamonsen LA, Evans J. The endometrial polarity paradox: differential regulation of polarity within secretory-phase human endometrium. *Endocrinology.* 2018;159 (1):506–18.

4. Aplin JD, Ruane PT. Embryo-epithelium interactions during implantation at a glance. *J Cell Sci.* 2017;130(1):15–22.

5. Heng S, Cervero A, Simon C, Stephens AN, Li Y, Zhang J, et al. Proprotein convertase 5/6 is critical for embryo implantation in women: regulating receptivity by cleaving EBP50, modulating ezrin binding, and membrane-cytoskeletal interactions. *Endocrinology.* 2011;152(12):5041–52.

6. Heng S, Paule SG, Li Y, Rombauts LJ, Vollenhoven B, Salamonsen LA, Nie G. Posttranslational removal of α-dystroglycan N terminus by PC5/6 cleavage is important for uterine preparation for embryo implantation in women. *FASEB J.* 2015;29 (9):4011–22.

7. Salamonsen LA., Evans J, Nguyen HPT, Edgellet TA. The microenvironment of human implantation: determinant of reproductive success. *Am J Reprod Immunol.* 2016;75(3):218–25.

8. Burton GJ, Watson AL, Hempstock J, Skepper JN, Jauniaux E. Uterine glands provide histiotrophic nutrition for the human fetus during the first trimester of pregnancy. *J Clin Endocrinol Metab.* 2002;87 (6):2954–9.

9. Teklenburg G, Salker M, Molokhia M, Lavery S, Trew G, Aojanepong T, et al. Natural selection of human embryos: decidualizing endometrial stromal cells serve as sensors of embryo quality upon implantation. *PLoS ONE*, 2010;5(4):e10258.

10. Antoniotti GS, Coughlan M, Salamonsen LA, Evans J. Obesity associated advanced glycation end products within the human uterine cavity adversely impact endometrial function and embryo implantation competence. *Hum Reprod.* 2018;33(4):654–65.

11. Drakopoulos P, Racca A, Errázuriz J, De Vos M, Tournaye H, Blockeel C, et al. The role of progesterone elevation in IVF. *Reprod Biol.* 2019;19(1):1–5.

12. Evans J, Hannan NJ, Edgell TA, Vollenhoven BJ, Lutjen PJ, Osianlis T, et al. Fresh versus frozen embryo transfer: backing clinical decisions with scientific and clinical evidence. *Hum Reprod Update.* 2014;20(6):808–21.

13. Craciunas L, Tsampras N, Raine-Fenning N, Coomarasamy A. Intrauterine administration of human chorionic gonadotropin (hCG) for subfertile women

undergoing assisted reproduction. *Cochrane Database Syst Rev.* 2016;5:Cd011537.

14. Groenewoud ER, Cohlen BJ, Macklon NS. Programming the endometrium for deferred transfer of cryopreserved embryos: hormone replacement versus modified natural cycles. *Fertil Steril.* 2018;109(5):768–74.

15. Altmäe S, Esteban FJ, Stavreus-Evers A, Simón C, Giudice L, Lessey BA, et al. Guidelines for the design, analysis and interpretation of 'omics' data: focus on human endometrium. *Hum Reprod Update.* 2014;20(1):12–28.

16. Craciunas L, Gallos I, Chu J, Bourne T, Quenby S, Brosens JJ, Coomarasamy A. Conventional and modern markers of endometrial receptivity: a systematic review and meta-analysis. *Hum Reprod Update.* 2019;25(2):202–23.

17. Boomsma CM, Macklon NS. What can the clinician do to improve implantation? *Reprod Biomed Online.* 2006;13 (6):845–55.

18. Datta AK, Campbell S, Deval B, Nargund G. Add-ons in IVF programme – hype or hope? *Facts Views Vis Obgyn.* 2015;7 (4):241–50.

19. Shirlow R, Healey M, Volovsky M, MacLachlan V, Vollenhoven B. The effects of adjuvant therapies on embryo transfer success. *J Reprod Infertil.* 2017;18 (4):368–78.

20. Kovacs G, Salamonsen L, editors. *How to prepare the endometrium to maximize implantation rates and IVF success.* Cambridge, UK: Cambridge University Press; 2019.

21. Lensen S, Osavlyuk D, Armstrong S, Stadelmann C, Hennes A, Napier E, et al. A randomized trial of endometrial scratching before in vitro fertilization. *N Engl J Med.* 2019;380(4):325–34.

22. Salamonsen LA, Dimitriadis E. Infertility and the endometrium. *Clin Exp Obstet Gynecol.* 2022;14 (9):195–206.

Chapter 4

The Sperm's Role in Embryo Development

Nahid Punjani, Russell P. Hayden, and Peter N. Schlegel

4.1 Introduction

It is commonly stated that a male factor is involved in up to 50% of couples presenting with infertility. With the advent of IVF, intracytoplasmic sperm injection (ICSI), and testicular sperm extraction (TESE), the most severe forms of male infertility became treatable. This apparent ability to bypass significant sperm dysfunction drove much of the early research of embryo development to focus on the oocyte. With direct observation of oocyte and sperm interaction, the role of sperm contributions to fertilization, early embryo quality, and subsequent development of a successful pregnancy became possible. Evidence is now mounting concerning the importance of DNA integrity, chromatin organization, epigenetics, and prepackaged RNA that the sperm passes to the zygote.

The optimization of IVF and IVF-ICSI outcomes has been hindered by several ongoing obstacles regarding the male gamete. Nearly all of the current assays used to judge sperm quality are destructive in nature, precluding the rational selection and eventual use of sperm following these tests. In addition, sperm DNA integrity tests likely only detect the most severely damaged spermatozoa, so the proportion of damaged or defective sperm is underestimated by such evaluations. Inferences are usually made about a given semen sample based upon the analysis of previously procured sperm. For instance, all currently available methods to measure sperm DNA fragmentation destroy the cell. Ideally, when spermatozoa are selected for use in ICSI, the embryologist would choose the cells with the best DNA integrity. Such technology does not yet exist, and so judgments are made based upon prior testing, and the motility and morphology of the current sample at hand. Unfortunately, traditional semen parameters such as morphology have proven poor predictors of reproductive outcomes. Additionally, it is now appreciated that even favorable appearing sperm assessed by microscopy may harbor significant DNA fragmentation [1].

Assessment of sperm quality beyond traditional semen parameters has been hindered by limited evaluation of sperm quality and the lack of standardization for sperm quality testing. Much of the data generated for newer forms of male assessment have relied upon retrospective and or highly heterogenous cohorts. For instance, it is well known that without strict control of female factors, which are often strong predictors of reproductive outcome, the signal from even significant sperm dysfunction may be easily obscured [2]. The resulting multitude of contradictory studies have discouraged investment into advanced semen assays and obscured the importance of a secondary reproductive factor such as sperm quality. Currently, the sperm chromatin structure assay (SCSA™) remains the only primary test that has been clinically standardized with established thresholds.

Nevertheless, the initially underappreciated role of the sperm, and how it may be manipulated to improve the outcomes of advanced reproductive technology, remains a promising territory for embryologists. In this chapter we will highlight the sperm's influence on embryo development. Firstly, the current understanding of sperm physiology will be discussed, as emerging clinical technology will hinge upon this knowledge. Lastly, the currently available techniques for sperm assessment and selection will be reviewed. Special attention will be paid to sperm DNA integrity, as this topic carries the broadest data and is already being used for specific clinical scenarios.

Salary support provided by Frederick J. and Theresa Dow Wallace Fund of the New York Community Trust, Mr. Robert S. Dow Foundation, and the Irena and Howard Laks Foundation. The authors would also like to thank Vanessa Dudley for her outstanding illustrations.

4.2 Implications of Sperm Physiology for the Embryo

Spermatozoa are remarkably specialized cells adapted to deliver their genetic payload across two distinct reproductive tracts, all the while evading an immune response. Once deposited in the lower female reproductive tract, motility and chemotaxis are both employed to hone to an oocyte. The process of capacitation in the female reproductive tract further enhances sperm functionality. Successfully engaged with its target, both sperm and oocyte begin a coordinated species-specific fusion event that leads to fertilization. Considerable effort has been spent in exploring the mechanics of these processes. As stated, the advent of IVF-ICSI has deemphasized much of the importance of reproductive physiology's "front end." Beyond the necessary contribution of the sperm-derived centrosome and sperm-based oocyte activation factors, the male's role in early embryogenesis has remained understudied [3]. We will detail the current understanding of the sperm's contribution to a developing embryo following fusion, an emerging field that will potentially alter clinical embryology.

4.2.1 DNA Packaging and Delivery

The male gamete is equipped with a unique chromatin structure that prepares it for safe transport, while also carrying implications for the embryo. Spermatozoa are uniquely prone to oxidative damage because of a lack of cytoplasm and cytoplasm-derived antioxidant enzymes. When considering DNA organization, three elements currently appear relevant to embryo development: nuclear matrix attachments, protamination, and regions of preserved histone backing (Figure 4.1).

4.2.1.1 Nuclear Matrix Attachments

Appropriate chromatin organization requires attachments of the sperm DNA to the nuclear matrix approximately every 50 kb. These matrix attachment regions appear necessary and sufficient to promote pronuclear formation and for the initiation of DNA replication within the zygote [4]. Animal studies have shown that even with significant removal of up to 50% of the sperm's DNA with endonucleases, preserving the matrix attachment regions will still permit the initiation of DNA replication within the oocyte. On the other hand, injecting intact DNA without attachment to the nuclear matrix did not result in either formation of the male pronucleus or initiation of DNA replication [4]. The matrix attachment regions remain an underappreciated, and understudied, aspect of sperm physiology.

4.2.1.2 Protamine

The replacement of histones for protamines is a sperm-unique process that imparts a significant decrease in size and increases resistance to exogenous insults such as reactive oxygen species (ROS) [5]. The importance of protamination beyond its protective role has been debated for several decades [6]. Multiple groups have purported that incomplete protamination may lead to impaired decondensation of the male genome, delayed cleavage, and impaired embryo development overall. Much of the initial data that demonstrated an association with chromatin maturity and reproductive outcomes have been refuted by more contemporary studies with higher power, which have also been substantiated by findings in mouse models [4, 6].

Nevertheless, the repeated observation that infertile males are more likely to have incomplete or aberrant DNA condensation continues to fuel further attempts to establish a causal relationship between protamination and embryogenesis [7]. Particular interest has been paid to the ratio of protamine 1 to protamine 2, in addition to the protamine to histone proportion. Stronger evidence has been presented that altered ratios of either variety may deter normal fertilization and impair subsequent progression to the blastocyst stage [6].

Proponents that improper DNA packaging leads to poor reproductive outcomes, independent of DNA damage that may accrue due to incomplete protamination, point to two proposed mechanisms. Firstly, DNA wrapped into protamine toroids will undergo demethylation in the zygote, an epigenetic process that is further discussed in Section 4.2.2. The second mechanism involves desynchronization of the oocyte and sperm genomes. Adequate protamine content within the sperm imparts resistance to meiosis-promoting factors, allowing the male's contribution to remain in G1 of the cell cycle as the oocyte progresses through the remainder of meiosis from metaphase II. It is theorized that an inappropriately histone-rich male nucleus would be responsive to these meiosis-promoting factors, prematurely leading to condensation of the sperm's DNA prior to the oocyte reaching G1 [8]. Premature chromosomal

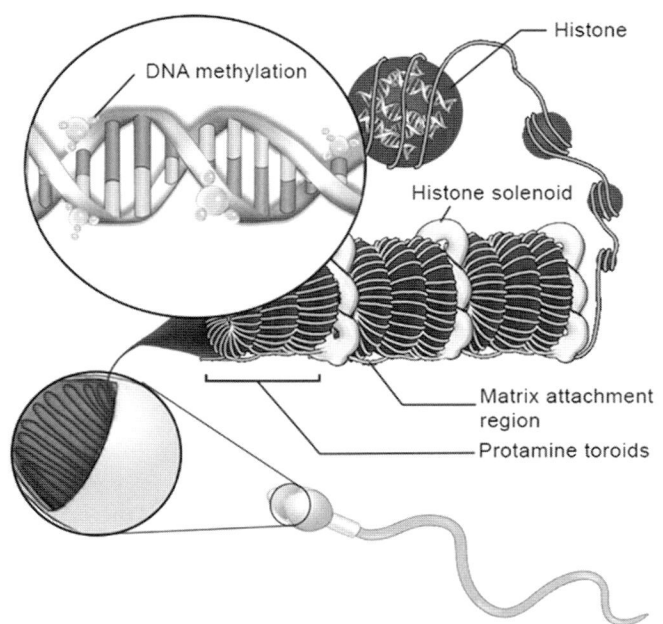

Figure 4.1 DNA chromatin remodeling and packaging
Schematic depicting chromatin remodeling and DNA packaging including histone modifications, protamine toroid structure, and connection with the matrix attachment regions.

condensation will lead to fertilization failure, limiting outcomes for IVF and ICSI cycles. However, abnormal sperm protamination appears to be a relatively rare cause of reproductive failure.

4.2.1.3 Sperm Histones

A small percentage of sperm DNA will remain bound to histone-based nucleosomes. The amount of DNA remaining in this chromatin structure is species dependent, and is approximately 15% in humans [3]. The properties of the histones that remain in the cell nucleus are significant, as they partially determine early gene expression in the developing embryo. Multiple groups have now established that the remaining histone residues in the male genome are not randomly distributed but appear to be concentrated in predictable locations [4]. As protamine-bound regions will initially be silent in the zygote, these histone-bound regions that are open for transcription are thought to be linked to genes important in early embryogenesis.

The evidence supporting the putative action of these genes within the male genome is supported by three pieces of evidence. Efforts to localize the loci in which histone backing is preserved have revealed that these locations are often rich in gene-promoter regions, suggesting they will become influential in transcription once fusion with the oocyte is achieved

[3, 4]. Additionally, genes known to partake in embryogenesis have been linked, either directly or indirectly through their promotors, to these regions, including the HOX family of transcripts [3]. Lastly, it has been demonstrated that the histones within the sperm nucleus are heavily acetylated, a property linked to upregulation of gene expression. These histones are not replaced by maternal proteins during sperm chromatin remodeling, and so maintain these epigenetic marks that will promote expression in the period of early transcription [3, 4].

4.2.2 Understudied and Evolving Topics in Epigenetics

4.2.2.1 Imprinting

As discussed in Section 4.2.1.3, the histone residues that remain within the sperm nucleus retain their epigenetic marks during chromatin remodeling in the early embryo [4]. However, the epigenetic modification of the male genome involves several other mechanisms that may be relevant to embryogenesis. Beyond histone modification, imprinted genes will often carry differential methylation of cytosines between the paternal and maternal alleles. It was initially assumed that much of these paternal epigenetic marks were erased during genome reprogramming in the developing gamete, in addition to the round of reprogramming shortly after fertilization in the zygote [3, 9]. However, multiple groups have now pointed to significant morbidity in the offspring of men with epigenetic derangements [3]. Relevant to the embryologist, it has also been posited that advanced reproduction techniques may result in global hypomethylation of the embryo's DNA, perhaps potentially explaining the slight increase of imprinting disorders in children stemming from assisted reproductive technology (ART) [10].

In terms of early embryo development, imprinting becomes particularly relevant when considering impaired protamination within the sperm genome. During the early phases following fertilization, genes originating in protamine toroids will undergo significant demethylation, whereas methylation may be preserved in those segments of DNA wrapped around paternal histones. As a result, imprinted genes are often found in the locations where nucleohistones remain after spermiogenesis [8]. However, inappropriately high histone content within the sperm's chromatin, which is often observed in subfertile males, may preserve methylation of key genes involved in early embryogenesis [8]. In normal fertilization, it has been observed that the male pronucleus is considerably hypomethylated compared to the female's, resulting in an apparent several-fold increase in transcription of paternal genes. Additionally, several key developmental promoters are hypomethylated in healthy mature sperm, including most of the Yamanaka factors [3]. Theoretically, if hypomethylation failed at these loci due to impaired histone-to-protamine exchange, embryogenesis may be irreparably altered.

4.2.2.2 Sperm RNA

During the later stages of spermatogenesis, much of the cytosol is shed, along with the majority of RNA transcripts carried from earlier stages of development. However, it has long been appreciated that a subset of RNAs remain with the mature sperm, protected by RNA-binding proteins. Initially, these were thought to be relics of prior transcription during spermatogenesis [3, 10]. However, newer evidence is demonstrating that these transcripts may be necessary for embryo development and may also carry epigenetic information to influence phenotype.

Rodent models have been helpful in elucidating the importance of sperm RNAs. As these transcripts are carried into the oocyte, they may undergo translation (messenger RNAs), or modulate gene expression (small RNAs and long noncoding RNAs). Removal of the sperm's RNA content in a murine model, via RNase treatment, resulted in a significant decrease in the progression to the blastocyst stage [10]. With the advent of next-generation sequencing and single-cell sequencing, more than 4 000 different RNA species have been found in mature sperm [10]. The significance of nearly all of these transcripts is not yet understood, though mounting evidence suggests that they are influential in altering offspring phenotypes based upon environmental exposure of the father [9]. As of yet, sperm RNAs remain an understudied but promising paradigm for embryology.

4.2.3 DNA Integrity

Sperm DNA integrity has become an increasingly popular area of study over the last decade. It has become apparent that all sperm accrue some level of damage to their genome, whether during spermatogenesis or during storage and transit. A multitude of conditions have been reported to initiate DNA damage in sperm, ranging from varicocele to xenobiotic exposure, and even lifestyle factors such as cigarette smoking. Observations of ejaculated sperm, when compared to testicular sperm from the same men, strongly suggest that the majority of the identifiable sperm DNA damage occurs during sperm transit through the reproductive tract (Figure 4.2) [11]. Early work by Aitken and colleagues has convincingly argued that nearly all of these etiologies share oxidative stress within their mechanistic pathways [1]. The inevitable insult to the male genome can result in a variety of modifications to the DNA molecule, although most assays used for sperm DNA integrity are designed to detect only DNA strand breaks.

Interestingly, the sperm requires a small amount of oxidative activity for capacitation during natural conception [1]. Additionally, low levels of oxidative stress may provide a protective effect on sperm has been hypothesized, thought to occur from increased cross-linking of sperm chromatin secondary to glutathione peroxidase, an enzyme that normally protects DNA from ROS [12]. However, at high concentrations, ROS may cause a multitude of direct or indirect changes to the DNA, as well as to effect endogenous ROS production by the sperm's mitochondria. In the latter case, a positive feedback loop is established where a cell exposed to too much oxidative stress begins to produce a surge of ROS from its midpiece.

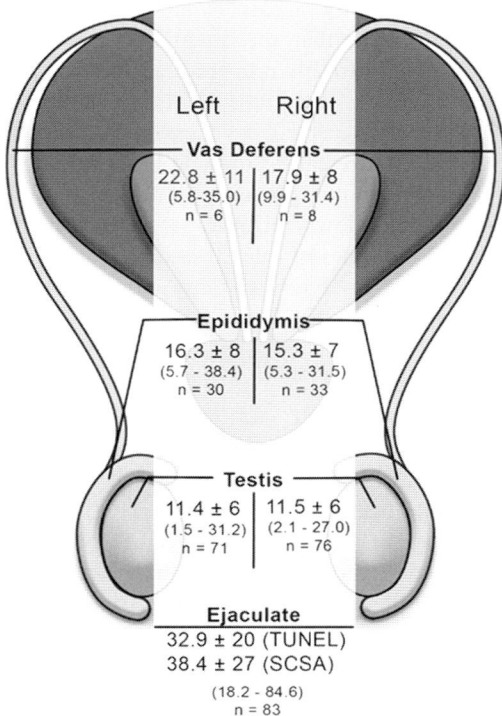

Figure 4.2 DNA fragmentation throughout the male reproductive tract
Schematic showing measurements of DNA fragmentation in the male reproductive tract, from the lowest levels in the testis, followed by the epididymis and then vas deferens, with the highest levels in the ejaculate. Measurement data are adapted from Xie et al. [11].

This altered and unique form of apoptosis is necessary in sperm secondary to their unique morphology, as much of the nucleus and its contents are not readily accessible to the traditional pathways of programmed cell death [1]. The process results in a spectrum of cell states, ranging from a healthy but uncapacitated spermatozoon to a moribund cell with complete fragmentation of its genome. Abortive apoptosis has been used to describe the situation in the middle of this spectrum, in which significantly damaged sperm can still fertilize an egg, or in cases of ART, be selected for ICSI [2]. Under normal circumstances, the oocyte has some capacity to repair the genetic defects within the male genome prior to the first cleavage event [1].

Returning to chromatin organization within the sperm, it is well known that the exchange of histones for protamines imparts significant sperm resistance to ROS. Some authors have postulated that the poor performance of sperm that have impaired protamination is mainly a reflection of the resulting DNA damage that accrues due to increased sensitivity to oxidative stress [3, 6]. Ni et al. conducted a meta-analysis evaluating the correlation of DNA fragmentation and protamine content [13]. Combining the data of 12 studies, they confirmed the initial suspicions that deficient protamination resulted in significantly worse DNA fragmentation, especially when chromomycin A3 (CMA3) staining was used as the methodology for quantifying protamine content.

However, it has been more difficult to establish a relationship between sperm DNA damage and early reproductive outcomes. Simon et al. reviewed the clinical data from a single high-volume institution in an attempt to connect poor sperm DNA integrity to deficient embryo development [14]. In their cohort, in which they attempted to correct for female factors, DNA fragmentation in the male genome predicted worse embryo quality and lower implantation rates. Of note, female factors dominated the fertilization rates, whereas a damaged paternal genome was not as influential. In a follow-up meta-analysis, which suffered from significant study heterogeneity, male DNA integrity had a less convincing impact on fertilization and embryogenesis, although an adverse effect on pregnancy outcomes was seen [15]. However, when examining studies that utilized the alkaline comet test as in the Simon et al. cohort, a more convincing relationship was found between sperm DNA damage and embryo quality. The authors attribute this finding to the sensitivity of the comet test when compared to competing methods. Unfortunately, clean clinical data in which female factors are well controlled have yet to be published, and so it is difficult to make strong inferences from these observations.

Many have argued that the effects of a compromised male genome are not manifested in the early embryonic period, but later in pregnancy. This "late paternal effect" has stronger clinical evidence than that connecting DNA fragmentation and preimplantation rubrics [2]. Zhao and colleagues conducted a meta-analysis comparing ART technique and miscarriage rates [16]. They found an approximately 2.5-fold increase in pregnancy loss for those couples who underwent IVF-ICSI as opposed to IVF alone. Presumably, the ICSI process allows for successful fertilization by sperm that may have accrued significant DNA damage. Conversely, those undergoing traditional IVF preserved the competitive nature of fertilization, in which sperm may be less likely to have damage, or less damaged sperm may outperform their impaired counterparts. These data bolster prior work conducted by Zini et al. [17]. With current embryo-grading practice, it appears that the late paternal effect could not be anticipated based upon clinical criteria at the time of embryo selection for transfer.

Nevertheless, sperm DNA integrity remains at the forefront of much of the research in male factor infertility. As a result, many of the evolving techniques in sperm assessment and manipulation involve either quantification of DNA fragmentation or methods to select for sperm with the least genomic damage. As a result, much of the remaining content of this review will focus on the practical techniques and methods relevant to sperm DNA integrity that may be employed by clinical embryologists.

4.3 Techniques for Sperm Assessment and Manipulation

In this section, we will present a detailed discussion of the many techniques for the quantification of sperm DNA damage, as this serves as one of the paradigms to assess male fertility potential beyond the basic semen analysis.

Finally, as ART outcomes can be dependent upon sperm quality, techniques for sperm separation and selection will be addressed (Table 4.1). Commonly utilized techniques include the swim-up method, migration-sedimentation method, density gradient centrifugation, and glass wool filtration [18]. We will present a detailed discussion of each technique, including emerging microfluidic methods that may become more commonplace.

4.3.1 Techniques for Assessing DNA Fragmentation

4.3.1.1 Terminal Deoxynucleotidyl Transferase dUTP Nick End Labeling (TUNEL)

TUNEL works via the utilization of a labeled deoxyuridine triphosphate (dUTP) that is incorporated at single- and double-strand breaks. This labeled molecule can then be identified and further quantified utilizing flow cytometry, fluorescence, or light microscopy [15].

Advantages

This technique is able to capture both single- and double-stranded DNA breaks, with relatively little intrasubject variability across time [15]. Another benefit of TUNEL is that specimens may be frozen or be completed on freshly prepared samples with no impact on the results of the assay. This allows significant use, ease, and cost effectiveness in the clinical setting as well as in research studying DNA fragmentation. This technique prevents issues related to fading dyes that allows technicians more time to analyze higher volumes of cells. It also has low interobserver and intraobserver variability and therefore is a reliable diagnostic tool [15].

Disadvantages

Unfortunately, the TUNEL assay is expensive in terms of reagents and labor. The assay does not quantify the magnitude of DNA damage within a cell, rather it counts the number of cells within a subset with a threshold level of DNA damage. In TUNEL, no nuclear decondensation technique is used and therefore labeling of the DNA fragments is restricted to the sperm nucleus periphery [15]. Universal clinical norms have not been set, although many studies report an effect on reproductive outcomes when more than 25–30% of sperm are TUNEL positive [15].

4.3.1.2 Comet

The comet assay works by analyzing single-sperm nuclear DNA that is separated based on charge and fragment size in an electric field, which can then be stained and assessed by fluorescence microscopy either qualitatively or quantitatively. The images then resemble comets with a head- and tail-like configuration depending on the extent of DNA damage. The double-stranded DNA tends to remain in the head and single DNA strands and shorter DNA fragments migrate to the tail [15].

Advantages

The assay is simple to complete and affordable. It measures both single- and double-stranded DNA breaks. The assay may be performed in a neutral environment where only double-strand DNA damage is measured, or an alkaline environment where both single- and double-stranded defects are appreciated due to DNA strand unwinding. This technique has the benefit of qualitatively measuring levels of DNA damage within a cell, which other techniques are not able to do. The assay may also be used in other cell types and not just sperm [15].

Table 4.1. Comparison of techniques for assessing DNA fragmentation

	TUNEL	Comet	SCSA™	In situ nick translation	Sperm chromatin dispersion assay
Commercially available	No	No	Yes	No	No
Cost	High for labor and supplies	Affordable	Equipment is expensive	Inexpensive	Inexpensive (no complex equipment needed)
Double- or single-stranded DNA damage	Both	Both	Both	Single	Both
Ease of use	Relatively easy	Time consuming and laborious	Standardized and fast protocol	Simple and only requires fluorescence microscope	Simple and rapid
Variability and reproducibility	Low inter- and intra-observer variability	High variation and accuracy impacted by overlapping tails	DNA damage constant over freeze-thaw Multiple lab factors that may increase variation	Low inter- and intra-observer variability	Reproducible
Other	Labeling restricted to nucleus No clinical norms	Applicable to other cell types Qualitatively measures DNA damage Standardization is difficult	Measures large number of sperm but cannot be used with very low counts Needs flow cytometer	Associated with protamine deficiency Low sensitivity	Halo assessment can be challenging; Sperm tails are not preserved

Notes: TUNEL: terminal deoxynucleotidyl transferase dUTP nick end labeling; SCSA™: sperm chromatin structure assay.

Disadvantages

The technique, although affordable and simple, has a much higher rate of interlaboratory (and intralaboratory) variation due to the lack of standardized protocols for the technique. Since alkaline reagents are used, they mark alkali-labile sites that may make it difficult to discriminate between endogenous and induced DNA breaks. This technique may also underestimate the amount of DNA damage due to DNA strand entanglement in instances of incomplete chromatin decondensation, in which all DNA breaks will not be revealed. Overlapping tails also decrease accuracy and therefore small tails can be difficult to see, or lost. The assay is also very time consuming and laborious [15].

4.3.1.3 Sperm Chromatin Structure Assay (SCSA™)

This technique utilizes flow cytometry to determine abnormal sperm chromatin. DNA is denatured using heat or acid, and then labeled using acridine orange to intercalate with DNA. This allows for a metachromatic shift from green (double-stranded DNA bounded by dye) to red fluorescence (single-stranded DNA bounded by dye). The flow cytometry separation process identifies the number of cells with DNA damage as well as the percentage of those sperm with high DNA stainability [15].

Advantages

It is the only commercially available test, and so benefits from established norms and protocols. It may be used to measure large numbers of spermatozoa per sample. The DNA damage measured by SCSA™ is constant over long periods, is reproducible, and can be conducted after a freeze–thaw cycle. This test may also determine the actual total percentage of sperm with damaged DNA [15].

Disadvantages

As with TUNEL, this technique does not report the extent of DNA damage in each individual sperm. While the test is easy to complete, the equipment required for analysis is expensive. There have also been reported laboratory factors that may affect the test creating potential for result variation [15]. Large numbers of cells are required, and so this test cannot be conducted on patients with cryptozoospermia or on testicular samples.

4.3.1.4 In Situ Nick Translation

This technique is a modified version of TUNEL that quantifies the incorporation of dUTP at single-stranded DNA breaks in a reaction that is catalyzed by DNA polymerase I [15].

Advantages

The test can identify sperm with low and variable levels of endogenous DNA damage and is positively associated with protamine deficiency [15].

Disadvantages

It can only be utilized for single-strand breaks, precluding any assessment of double-strand breaks. There are no correlated studies to reproductive outcomes and the test lacks sensitivity. Very low levels of fluorescence can be seen with this assay, which introduces background noise, thereby making interpretation difficult [15].

4.3.1.5 Sperm Chromatin Dispersion Assay

This test utilizes the concept that fragmented DNA fails to produce a characteristic halo when mixed with agarose, followed by acid denaturation and removal of nuclear proteins. Removal of sperm nuclear proteins leaves a nucleoid with a central core and a peripheral halo of dispersed DNA loops. Fluorescent staining is then used to examine the sperm with elevated DNA fragmentation as they produce very small or no halos of DNA dispersion, while low DNA fragmentation sperm have large halos [15].

Advantages

The assay is simple and inexpensive. The assay is reproducible and rapid. It does not rely on fluorescence intensity, which certainly makes it easier to analyze. No complex instrumentation is needed [15].

Disadvantages

Unfortunately, the assay can result in low-density nucleoids that are fainter, and therefore the limit of the halo where the chromatin is less dense may not be accurately seen on the background. The halos may also be in different planes, which makes focusing challenging. Finally, the sperm tails are not preserved and therefore it can be difficult to differentiate a sperm from another cell type [15].

4.3.2 Methods for Sperm Manipulation and Selection for ART

The selection of sperm has been proposed to identify gametes with less DNA damage and hence to abrogate the effects of sperm DNA damage on reproductive outcomes (Table 4.2). Since only neat sample DNA integrity testing predicts outcomes (not processed sample testing), it is quite possible that high DNA fragmentation in the neat sample predicts a significant level of "subclinical" damage in the other sperm, limiting the value of sperm selection for ART.

4.3.2.1 Swim-Up Method

The swim-up method, which was originally described by Mahadevan and Baker, is commonly used for couples with limited male factor infertility and abnormal semen parameters. The technique relies on intrinsic sperm motility and active sperm movement [18]. Typically, semen is taken and combined with appropriate media and is subsequently centrifuged to form a pellet. The supernatant is discarded and new media is added to the pellet. This is then incubated for up to 60 minutes at 37°C. This step permits separation of both cellular debris and other cells as the motile sperm swim up away from the pellet [18].

Advantages

This technique is very simple to perform, and inexpensive compared to other methods. Swim-up generally produces a clean sample to be used for ART [18].

Table 4.2. Comparison of methods for sperm manipulation and selection for assisted reproductive technologies

	Swim-up	Migration-sedimentation	Density gradient centrifugation	Glass wool filtration	Microfluidics
Clean sample	Clean samples	Very clean samples	Clean fraction	Has debris remnants, not as clean	Clean sample
Cost	Inexpensive	Higher cost for collection cones	Expensive due to gradient supplies	Expensive	Higher equipment cost, but limited reagent requirement due to small volumes
Ease to perform	Simple to perform	Requires caution and gentle handling	Easy to perform	Easy to perform	Easy to use
Reactive oxygen species	Yes from contact with debris and leukocytes	Limited as no direct contact	Eliminates the majority of leukocytes	Reduced	Reduced
Sperm yield	Low	Low	Good yield	Good yield	Low
Other	Relies on favorable semen parameters	Removes need for centrifugation	May be either continuous or discontinuous	Can be used for retrograde samples	Works with small volume

Disadvantages

The technique relies on patients with favorable semen parameters such as good motility and high counts. The actual yield of sperm may be low due to the reliance on the surface of the centrifuged pellet and the actual quality of the patient sample. There have been reported decreases in in the proportion of sperm obtained with normally condensed chromatin. Also, due to the pelleting method, there is increased cellular contact with sperm to other cell types including debris and leukocytes that are capable of producing high levels of oxidative damage, inducing sperm DNA damage and potentially impacting sperm motility [18].

Suggested methods to overcome the significant impact of reactive oxygen species damage may be to perform the technique on liquified semen rather than a pellet, but this typically requires multiple tubes to maximize surface area and contact between the media and the liquified semen [18].

4.3.2.2 Migration-Sedimentation

This technique developed by Tea et al. builds upon the swim-up technique by utilizing sedimentation [18]. As opposed to the swim-up technique, in migration-sedimentation, the sperm swim up directly from semen into a supernatant medium, in which an additional inner cone or container is present, which serves as the location where the sperm will sediment. There is no centrifugation step in this technique [18].

Advantages

The technique provides a very clean fraction of sperm. Without the centrifugation step in the swim-up method, there is no increased risk of direct contact with cells that may cause reactive oxygen species [18].

Disadvantages

Given the absence of a centrifugation step, this technique requires caution and gentle handling. The technique also has a lower yield, and therefore also requires high-quality ejaculated semen. This technique does require additional collection cones or tubes that may add cost [18].

Some groups have shown this method to be helpful in cases of oligospermia and asthenozoospermia with a sperm yield enough for some ART methods such as ICSI [19].

4.3.2.3 Density Gradient Centrifugation

In this technique, previously created polymer gradients are used, and the ejaculated semen is placed on

39

top of the lowest-density media. It is then centrifuged for up to 30 minutes [18]. Highly motile sperm move more efficiently and effectively in the direction of the gradient providing a pellet of the most motile sperm at the bottom of the gradient.

Advantages

Similar to the previous methods, a clean fraction of motile sperm is typically obtained. The yield is more reasonable than some of the other methods, has limited reactive oxygen species created, and is easy to perform. Given the density gradient method, leukocytes and cellular debris are usually limited [18].

Disadvantages

Since the procedure requires a gradient, the technique is more expensive and may require more time to perform in order to produce high-quality interphases. The technique is also known to potentially increase the risk of endotoxins, cause membrane alteration, and create inflammatory responses [18].

In general, this technique provides an opportunity for modification and optimization for different sperm parameters given the ability to modify the various levels of density gradients.

4.3.2.4 Glass Wool Filtration

This method was first described by Paulson et al. [20]. The method permits separation of motile sperm using glass wool fibers that are densely packed [18]. As glass wool has natural filtration effects, the technique is linked to the type of glass wool used (chemical composition, surface area, charge, thickness, pore size) [18]. Of course, the outcomes are also related to the initial quality of the sperm.

Advantages

This technique generally provides a good yield of motile sperm since it uses the entire volume of the ejaculate. The technique is generally considered easy to perform. Similar to the density gradient method, leukocytes are often eliminated, and reactive oxygen species are therefore minimized. The procedure may also select for sperm without chromatin-condensation abnormalities. This technique may also be used for patients with retrograde ejaculation but does require centrifugation of the postejaculate urine specimen and resuspension in media before use [18].

Disadvantages

This method is more expensive and may include remnants of debris with the final product, which may not be as clean as the other methods listed above [18].

Given its ease and use of whole-volume ejaculate, this technique may be ideal for the oligospermic or asthenozoospermic patient.

4.3.2.5 Microfluidics

This may carry the greatest potential for sperm selection, but the effect of this sperm preparation technique (based on sperm motility and microfluidics) on reproductive outcomes has not been demonstrated to date [22].

Another novel and promising technique involves microfluidics, which is the manipulation of fluid on a microscopic level by way of microchannels and their physical properties. This allows fluid mixing but also fluid separation and isolation of particles, including cells such as sperm (Figure 4.3) [21]. These devices have been able to analyze sperm count, motility, and morphology. The technology is simple, accurate, and rapid [22]. In addition to recognition of sperm, the technology has been successfully used for sperm sorting, in which sperm with the best motility and morphology are selected [11]. Sperm populations selected with microfluidics can also be dramatically enriched for cells with significantly lower DNA fragmentation and appears to confer improved ICSI and clinical outcomes [11, 23].

4.3.2.6 Other Techniques

Other techniques have been described but are much less commonly used. Glass beads have been studied previously but have not been adopted due to spillover of the beads [18]. Sephadex columns have produced high yields but lower counts and poorer morphology than other gradient and centrifugation methods [18]. Transmembrane migration uses a Nucleopore membrane filter, but due to issues with the cross-sectional area of the pores, the yield has been very low [18].

4.4 Conclusions

The role of the male gamete in embryo development has been underappreciated until recent years. The early embryo is influenced by the sperm's unique arrangement for genome delivery and the physiologic processes that result in DNA oxidative damage. Although our current understanding is limited, it is

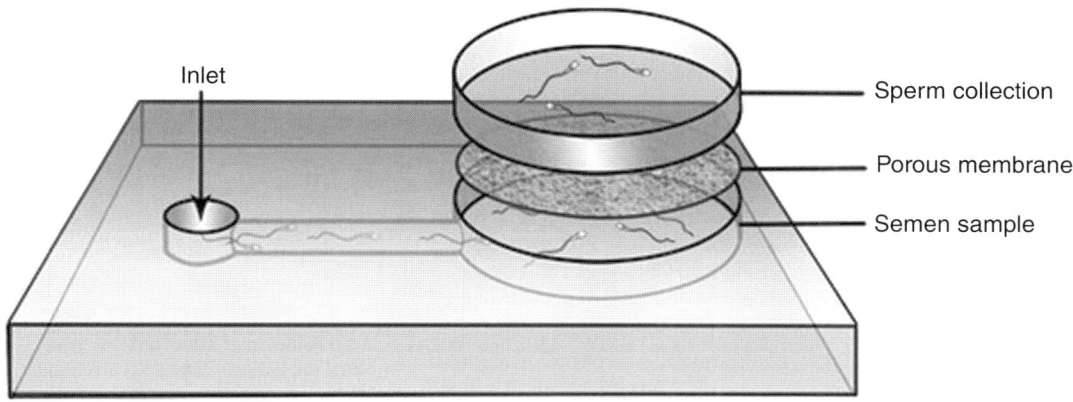

Figure 4.3 A microfluidic technique for isolating the highest-quality sperm
Schematic of a microfluidic technique demonstrating that the highest-quality sperm (high motility and low DNA fragmentation levels) are able to traverse through the porous membrane into the upper chamber.

already apparent that important epigenetic processes are at play, the understanding of which may ultimately prove useful to optimize ART outcomes. As our knowledge evolves, it is clear that more emphasis will be placed on the impact of oxidative damage and DNA fragmentation within the sperm. In the above review we presented the current state-of-the-art for assessment of sperm DNA integrity. We also outlined the laboratory techniques that may help enrich a sperm population for higher quality. A critical understanding of these subjects is necessary for the embryologist to optimize current protocols, as well as to judge and interpret new studies and technology that may influence ART in the future.

Key Messages

- Necessary components of embryogenesis contributed by sperm include oocyte-activating factors and the sperm-derived centrosome.

- Epigenetics inherited from the male include histone modifications, DNA methylation, and prepackaged RNA transcripts. Alternations in each of these have been linked to adverse reproductive outcomes in early studies.
- Sperm chromatin organization results from a coordinated exchange of histones for protamines, which has implications regarding genome stability, epigenetic reprogramming, and chromatin accessibility within the early embryo.
- Nearly all sperm will have some level of DNA damage that the oocyte must repair. The majority of damage accrues due to oxidative stress. The majority of the effects of a damaged male genome appear to manifest following implantation.
- Abnormal sperm DNA integrity may reflect multiple types of genetic insults, although most current testing methods for sperm DNA only assess for DNA strand breaks.

References

1. Aitken RJ, Baker MA, Nixon B. Are sperm capacitation and apoptosis the opposite ends of a continuum driven by oxidative stress? *Asian J Androl*, 2015;17(4): 633–9.

2. Bach PV, Schlegel PN. Sperm DNA damage and its role in IVF and ICSI. *Basic Clin Androl*. 2016;26:15.

3. Steger K, Cavalcanti MC, Schuppe HC. Prognostic markers for competent human spermatozoa: fertilizing capacity and contribution to the embryo. *Int J Androl*. 2011;34(6 Pt 1):513–27.

4. Ward WS. Function of sperm chromatin structural elements in fertilization and development. *Mol Hum Reprod*. 2010;16 (1):30–6.

5. Aitken RJ, De Iuliis GN. On the possible origins of DNA damage in human spermatozoa. *Mol Hum Reprod*. 2010;16 (1):3–13.

6. Colaco S, Sakkas D. Paternal factors contributing to embryo

quality. *J Assist Reprod Genet.* 2018;35(11):1953–68.

7. Van Voorhis BJ, Barnett M, Sparks AE, Syrop CH, Rosenthal G, Dawson J. Effect of the total motile sperm count on the efficacy and cost-effectiveness of intrauterine insemination and in vitro fertilization. *Fertil Steril.* 2001;75(4):661–8.

8. Depa-Martynow M, Kempisty B, Jagodziński PP, Pawelczyk L, Jedrzejczak P. Impact of protamine transcripts and their proteins on the quality and fertilization ability of sperm and the development of preimplantation embryos. *Reprod Biol.* 2012;12(1):57–72.

9. Sharma U. Paternal contributions to offspring health: role of sperm small RNAs in intergenerational transmission of epigenetic information. *Front Cell Dev Biol.* 2019;7:215.

10. Giacone F, Cannarella R, Mongioì LM, Alamo A, Condorelli RA, Calogero AE, La Vignera S. Epigenetics of male fertility: effects on assisted reproductive techniques. *World J Mens Health.* 2019;37(2):148–56.

11. Xie P, Keating D, Parrella A, Cheung S, Rosenwaks Z, Goldstein M, Palermo GD. Sperm genomic integrity by TUNEL varies throughout the male genital tract. *J Urol.* 2020;203(4):802–8.

12. Aitken RJ, Smith TB, Jobling MS, Baker MA, De Iuliis GN. Oxidative stress and male reproductive health. *Asian J Androl.* 2014;16(1):31–8.

13. Ni K, Spiess A-N, Schuppe H-C, Steger K. The impact of sperm protamine deficiency and sperm DNA damage on human male fertility: a systematic review and meta-analysis. *Andrology.* 2016;4 (5):789–99.

14. Simon L, Murphy K, Shamsi MB, Liu L, Emery B, Aston KI, et al. Paternal influence of sperm DNA integrity on early embryonic development. *Hum Reprod.* 2014;29(11):2402–12.

15. Simon L, Emery BR, Carrell DT. Review: diagnosis and impact of sperm DNA alterations in assisted reproduction. *Best Pract Res Clin Obstet Gynaecol.* 2017;44:38–56.

16. Zhao J, Zhang Q, Wang Y, Li Y. Whether sperm deoxyribonucleic acid fragmentation has an effect on pregnancy and miscarriage after in vitro fertilization/ intracytoplasmic sperm injection: a systematic review and meta-analysis. *Fertil Steril.* 2014;102 (4):998–1005.e8.

17. Zini A, Boman JM, Belzile E, Ciampi A. Sperm DNA damage is associated with an increased risk of pregnancy loss after IVF and ICSI: systematic review and meta-analysis. *Hum Reprod.* 2008;23(12):2663–8.

18. Henkel RR, Schill WB. Sperm preparation for ART. *Reprod Biol Endocrinol.* 2003;1:108.

19. Hinting A, Lunardhi H. Better sperm selection for intracytoplasmic sperm injection with the side migration technique. *Andrologia.* 2001;33(6):343–6.

20. Paulson JD, Polakoski KL, Leto S. Further characterization of glass wool column filtration of human semen. *Fertil Steril.* 1979;32(1):125–6.

21. Parrella A, Keating D, Cheung S, Xie P, Stewart JD, Rosenwaks Z, Palermo GD. A treatment approach for couples with disrupted sperm DNA integrity and recurrent ART failure. *J Assist Reprod Genet.* 2019;36 (10):2057–66.

22. Samuel R, Feng H, Jafek A, Despain D, Jenkins T, Gale B. Microfluidic-based sperm sorting & analysis for treatment of male infertility. *Transl Androl Urol.* 2018;7(Suppl 3):S336–47.

23. Quinn MM, Jalalian L, Ribeiro S, Ona K, Demirci U, Cedars MI, Rosen MP. Microfluidic sorting selects sperm for clinical use with reduced DNA damage compared to density gradient centrifugation with swim-up in split semen samples. *Hum Reprod.* 2018;33(8):1388–93.

The Oocyte's Role in Embryo Development

David F. Albertini

5.1 Introduction

The adage that "embryogenesis begins with oogenesis," conceptualized and experimentally established decades ago for animal models, has withstood the test of time within the purview of contemporary human assisted reproductive technology (ART). While broadly applicable to the practice of human embryology, evaluating oocyte quality as a predictor of embryo quality has remained a challenge despite the improvements in technology and the efforts of both clinical- and embryologic-oriented specialists. This chapter will take the reader through two parallel areas of interest for the student of human embryology: (a) an updated understanding of how the differentiation of the ovarian oocyte contributes directly to the developmental competence exhibited from the zygote to blastocyst stages of the early development (up to implantation) and (b) what current practical and future considerations are anticipated in the embryology laboratory setting that will contribute to evaluation of human oocyte quality for use in embryo selection for transfer or cryopreservation.

Current efforts to evaluate oocytes for embryo selection rely primarily upon morphological criteria. Even though the evaluation of high-quality mature human oocytes has followed standards adopted over 40 years ago, it remains a fact that despite the vast majority of oocytes undergoing fertilization and cleavage, only about 50% form blastocysts, and embryos selected for transfer on day 5 or 6 yield term live births in, at best, 50–60% of cases.

The reasons for failure to implant and sustain term gestations are manifold and extend well beyond attempts to deselect embryos harboring abnormal chromosomal composition. Patient age, health status, and methods of controlled ovarian hyperstimulation and ovulation triggering, while not visibly altering the appearance of mature oocytes, contribute to variations in the extent of development evident during culture. Moreover, cryopreservation and endometrial preparation prior to transfer also contribute to loss of developmental competence of normal-appearing mature oocytes and their associated embryos. It is against this clinical backdrop that we review the female gamete's contribution to embryo development. In many ways, the ability to culture zygotes produced by IVF or intracytoplasmic sperm injection (ICSI) up to the blastocyst stage yields testimony to the developmental fitness or competence in at least a fraction of retrieved oocytes. However, what it is at a cellular and molecular level that distinguishes oocytes capable of yielding a term pregnancy, or not, remains an elusive question.

Until recently, our knowledge base for understanding how the mammalian oocyte contributes to and directs early embryonic development has relied upon a vast literature on ART in laboratory and domesticated animals. One attempt to combine assessments and biology between mammalian species and human biology is the book by Coticchio and colleagues [1]. Classical, and largely invasive analyses, or those deploying genetic or pharmacological manipulations have been reviewed and provide a template for future exploration into the link between oogenesis and embryogenesis [2].

In the end, the qualities acquired by the oocyte while it grows, differentiates, and matures establish a platform for the remarkable ability to generate a complete organism. Estimates for the duration of oogenesis in humans encompass 90–100 days from activation of the primordial follicle to being able to ovulate in response to the luteinizing hormone (LH) surge. Some 34–38 hours following the LH surge maturation is completed with maintenance of a fertilizable state limited to a period of 12–24 hours. However, when are these qualities – or competencies – acquired? How is the manifestation of competencies regulated during ovulation and after fertilization? And how will our understanding of the human oocyte in future years contribute to the advancement of human ART?

5.2 Maternal Determinants of Embryogenesis

5.2.1 Current Clinical Standards

Over 40 years of experience have established criteria for oocyte selection that have become accepted and put into practice. Organizations like the European Society of Human Reproduction and Embryology provide regularly updated guidelines for evaluating oocyte and embryo quality [3]. Practice patterns worldwide rely heavily on oocyte morphology seeking to define the stages of maturity using conventional optics or polarization microscopy – evaluations always occurring after the removal of cumulus cells. Figure 5.1 illustrates variance in oocyte maturity as well as variations in the appearance of intact cumulus oocyte complexes suggestive of oocyte maturity status. Many other parameters are considered when evaluating oocytes including distortions in oocyte and/or zona shape, size of the polar body, morphological qualities of the oocyte cytoplasm (granularity, vacuoles), blebs at the cell surface, and extent and contents of the perivitelline space) [4].

Despite these rather obvious signs of maturity and morphological abnormalities recognized as signs of degeneration, prematurity, or follicular atresia, reliable quantifiable biomarkers that directly predict developmental potential have eluded critical demonstration thus far.

5.2.2 Monitoring Developmental Competence

The oocyte acquires numerous developmental competencies at specific stages of oogenesis, each of which is associated with key developmental events and outcome failures when disrupted (Table 5.1). The

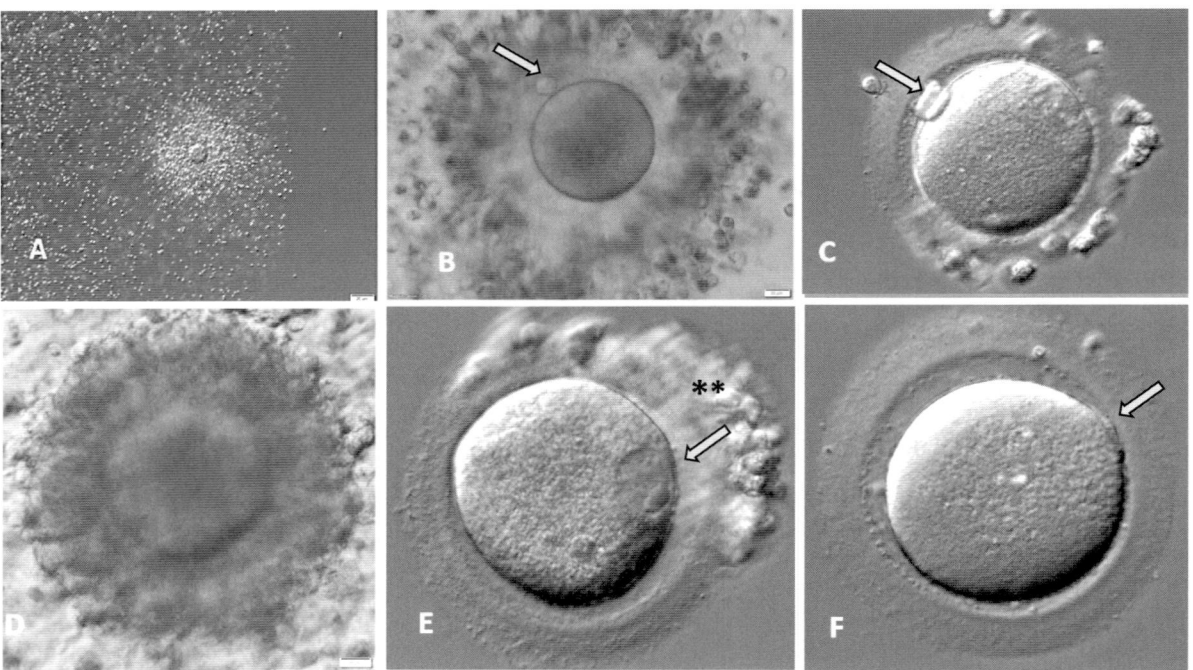

Figure 5.1 Human oocyte morphology following controlled ovarian stimulation
A: low-magnification image of cumulus–oocyte complex shortly after retrieval illustrating monodispersed nature of expanded cumulus and disposition of corona cells surrounding the oocyte. B: intact corona with enclosed metaphase-2 oocyte with polar body (arrow); note radially oriented striations formed by corona cell transzonal projections. C: metaphase-2 stage oocyte with polar body (arrow) following removal of cumulus corona; note abundance of vesicles within perivitelline space. D: compact, unexpanded corona enclosing immature, germinal vesicle (GV) stage oocyte; GV (arrow) shown in E following hyaluronidase and mechanical stripping, although some corona radiata cells remain (**). F: presumed aged metaphase-2 oocyte with flattened first polar body at 2 o'clock (arrow); cytoplasm lacks homogeneity. Hoffmann modulation optics (A, C, E, and F); polarization optics (B, D).

Table 5.1. Developmental competencies acquired during stages of oogenesis

Competency	Cell cycle stage acquired	Role in development	Outcome failure
Meiosis	Growth (late)	Cell cycle resumption and completion	Arrest at GV or M1, failed fertilization
Genomic imprinting	Growth (late)	Methylation of imprinted genes	Inappropriate lineage assignment
Cortical reaction	M-phase	Establish block to polyspermy	Polyspermy, multiple pronuclei
Calcium oscillations	M-phase	Egg activation	Failed fertilization
Male pronuclear development	M-phase	Protamine disulfide bond reduction	Failed fertilization
Subcortical maternal complex assembly	M-phase	Blastomere cytokinesis	Blastomere fragmentation
Compaction	PM/M-phase	Cell polarization and lineage assignment	Embryonic arrest
Derivation of totipotent stem cells	G/PM/M-phases	Propagate stem cells from inner cell mass	Embryonic arrest
Implantation	G/PM/M-phases	Correct lineage assignment	Failed implantation
Term birth	G/PM/M-phases	Sustained gestation	Miscarriage

Source: Modified from Albertini, Table 2.1, reference [2]. Based on sequential stages of oogenesis from early growth (G), prematuration (PM, oocyte arrested in Graafian following awaiting LH surge), and maturation (M) stage involving events elicited following reception of LH.

sequential and visible signs of competency are evident initially during the period encompassing meiotic maturation (meiotic competence), and then in corresponding embryos, through fertilization (competence to undergo cortical reaction, egg activation, completion of meiosis 2 upon second polar body extrusion), cleavage, compaction, and blastocyst formation.

The concept of competency took hold in studies on mouse and bovine, two of the best-studied animal models [5]. One of the many advantages established in these studies was the ability to evaluate competence to fertilize and beyond. In mouse studies this meant tracking through culture to blastocyst and importantly following embryo transfer. In bovine, evaluation includes in most cases the ability to reach blastocyst stage. This body of work established important physiological aspects of oocyte quality that in the case of the human has yet to receive adequate attention.

5.2.3 Reliance of Development on Metabolic Loading during Ovulation

There is mounting evidence to suggest that many of the processes driving early development depend on the procurement of metabolic substrates from cells of the cumulus during ovulation. This concept is referred to as metabolic loading [2]. The larger principle at hand pertains to the influence of cumulus cell metabolism on proximate bioenergetic requirements, such as those needed to drive nuclear and cytoplasmic maturation during ovulation, and those demands placed on the nascent zygote and early cleavage stage embryo. An example of the former applies to sourcing of ATP, the hydrolysis of which is tightly coupled to both cell cycle progression and cytoskeletal remodeling associated with meiotic spindle assembley and function as well as the cytokinesis that controls formation and emission of the first (and second) polar body. For these purposes, which very likely extend into the first few cell cycles of development, the oocyte, and subsequent embryo, does not rely on glycolysis or oxidative phosphorylation, but rather utilizes the adenosine salvage pathway to regenerate ATP from AMP, and in so doing avoids the costly consequences of free radical generation were mitochondrial metabolism called into play. A second classical example of how metabolic loading at the time of oocyte maturation ensures developmental progress relates to a mechanism that protects the oocyte, and zygote, from damage due to oxidative stress.

In this instance, it is important to bear in mind that cells deploy the tripeptide glutathione in its reduced form (GSH) as a potent and physiological antioxidant capable of neutralizing free radical oxidants generated from internal (e.g. mitochondrial) or external sources such as follicular fluid. For the oocyte, besides defending against protein or nucleic acid damage before and after fertilization, there is a crucial role served by GSH at the time of fertilization. The male genome as introduced into the oocyte cytoplasm consists of nonnucleosomal DNA complexed with disulfide-bonded protamines. For syngamy to occur, and development to proceed, the male genome must be quickly and efficiently converted into nucleosomes, a process catalyzed by the reducing activity of GSH on sperm protamine. As is already known, variations in the timing of sperm head decondensation after IVF or ICSI can lead to a loss of cell cycle synchrony offsetting DNA replication and chromosome formation, thus compromising syngamy. While not well understood, it is widely believed that inadequate stores of GSH could delay this fundamental modification in chromatin. So, where does the GSH come from that mediates this key event in development?

With transcriptional expression patterns well established in both cumulus cells and oocytes, it is now clear that the enzymatic pathway components responsible for the synthesis of GSH are within cumulus cells and not the oocyte. And as was discovered in the bovine system more than two decades ago, the upregulation of GSH pathway genes occurs within hours of the LH surge, giving sufficient time for robust synthesis and transport of GSH into the oocyte via gap junctions formed at the ends of transzonal projections at the oocyte cell surface. This fundamental and well-documented example of metabolic cooperation between the cumulus and oocyte emphasizes how critical this enduring relationship is in establishing a vital link between oogenesis and embryogenesis.

The role of metabolic cooperation between the somatic and germ cell lineages of the follicle begins with the activation of primordial follicles. Figure 5.2 illustrates the sequence of cell interactions that have been documented in mammals including those responsible for preventing the activation of dormant follicles, such as receptor-mediated tyrosine kinases and direct cell contact.

Following activation of follicle development, various ligands and their cognate receptors mediate information exchange during the growth phase of oogenesis, as well as the prematuration and maturation phases prior to and following the LH surge. Thus, the oocyte–cumulus relationship is truly enduring and complex drawing upon a variety of cell signaling modalities to assure that follicle quality is translated into oocyte quality well before fertilization.

5.2.4 Patient Health Status and Oocyte Quality in Clinical Settings

A large body of evidence now exists relating oocyte properties described above with documentation of developmental progress in culture or after embryo transfer when pregnancy outcomes are tracked. In general, this work has confirmed what was long expected from earlier studies monitoring morphology – that development during extended culture itself reflects oocyte competence. Further confirmation of the utility of morphological scoring as being predictive has derived from the growing use of oocyte donors in IVF centers offering treatment to older patients, or those exhibiting low antral follicle counts and/or low anti-Mullerian hormone levels.

Important variables that enter into the determination of oocyte quality based upon traditional criteria are a reflection of health status with respect to age, type of controlled ovarian stimulation (COS) used, or preconditions known to affect clinical outcomes. Obesity and BMI are examples where an influence of oocyte size has been noted. And recent studies have reinforced the relationship between oocyte size and ART outcomes in polycystic ovarian syndrome (PCOS) patients [6]. Why preexisting health

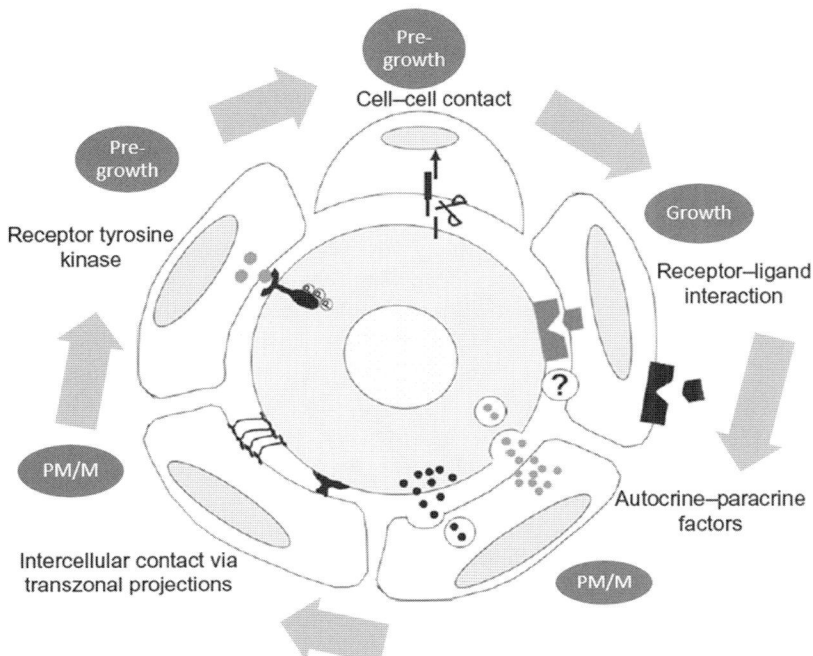

Figure 5.2 Schematic illustrating the sequence of signaling interactions known to occur between granulosa/cumulus cells and the oocyte during the course of folliculogenesis

In dormant primordial follicles (top), cell contact and receptor tyrosine kinases maintain oocytes in an arrested state. Upon follicle activation, a series of signaling systems develops at the cumulus–oocyte interface that regulate the growth phase of oogenesis (G) and the pre and maturation phases (PM/M). Image redrawn from reference [2].

conditions result in altered oocyte characteristics, in this case size, is not fully understood. However, evidence from animal studies strongly suggests that systemic metabolism alters the follicular environment in which the oocyte grows and matures possibly as a result of altered communication between oocyte and granulosa cells [2, 3].

To summarize, while some degree of variation in oocyte properties has been shown to be linked to poorer clinical outcomes, mounting evidence suggests that deficiencies are not generally manifest under typical laboratory evaluation of mature oocytes currently being practiced. Moreover, attention is increasingly being focused on the immediate environment in which the oocyte completes its development and the role of communication between oocyte and somatic cells whereby metabolic cooperation successfully, or pathologically, mediates the vital link between host metabolic status and oocyte quality [1].

5.3 Molecular and Physiological Correlates Linking Oogenesis and Embryogenesis

5.3.1 Molecular Determinants of Oocyte Developmental Competencies

The long road through oogenesis, culminating in the final stages of maturation, endows upon the oocyte multiple competencies. Most prominent among these are the ability to reinitiate and complete the meiotic cell cycle, the ability to mount and execute the block to polyspermy, the ability to support the remodeling of male chromatin, the ability to methylate and demethylate genomic DNA supporting progressive epigenetic modifications of chromatin, and the ability to compact and elicit the inner cell mass and trophectoderm lineages specified at the time of compaction.

From a molecular point of view, each of these competencies derives from precise changes in gene expression, translational and posttranslational protein modifications, proteostasis, and RNA stability [1, 2]. At the heart of this sequence of events lie the functions of gene products ranging from housekeeping genes, and genes responsible for some of the unique molecular signatures shown by mammalian oocytes, including those of the human. We now consider the molecular underpinnings of the transition from egg to embryo that define processes that in the final analysis determine the efficacy of developmental competencies.

Among the most substantive of reviews is that authored by Conti and Franciosi in 2018 [7]. While based primarily on studies done with the mouse, they take on the challenging task of describing how it is that maternally encoded gene products are subject to stage-specific alterations in RNA stability and turnover as the oocyte undergoes and completes the process of meiotic maturation. From first principles, it is known that critical cell cycle transitions constitute a series of starts and stops regulated by (a) the timely processing of mRNAs that support synthesis of key cell cycle factors, (b) the role of protein posttranslational modifications that either stabilize or destabilize components at key junctures in meiotic cell cycle progression, and (c) targeting mRNAs and proteins for rapid degradation or stabilization prior to or during the process of fertilization.

Among the more specialized targets for these cell cycle transitions are those of the cytoskeleton. As shown in Figure 5.3, remodeling of both the F-actin and microtubule cytoskeletons occur during the transition from the germinal vesicle stage (Figure 5.3A) to metaphase-2 (Figure 5.3B). Shifting from an interphase state in the germinal vesicle to that required to assemble the meiotic spindles involves precisely timed phosphorylation of key proteins that mediate the interaction of chromosomes with microtubules. Similarly, the assembly of actin filaments during meiotic maturation establishes the organization of the oocyte cortex that is polarized relative to the position of the meiotic spindle (compare Figure 5.2C with 5.2D). As will be noted in Section 5.3.2, superimposed upon these mechanisms resident within the oocyte are spatially proximal mediators of mRNA and protein homeostasis imposed by the surrounding cumulus granulosa cells and environmental conditions specified by the follicle itself.

5.3.2 Intrinsic and Extrinsic Mediators of Oocyte Developmental Competence

Oocyte intrinsic factors integrate nuclear and cytoplasmic events during the course of meiotic maturation and are the direct and indirect consequence of environmental signals processed within the ovarian follicle. Far from the original ideas implicating an uncoupling of physical interactions between oocyte and cumulus cells as the trigger for meiotic maturation, current evidence suggests a far more complicated system is at play involving granulosa cells and follicular fluid [8]. These extrinsic components participate by modulating the response of the follicle to ovulation-inducing ligands during natural LH-triggered cycles or triggering in the context of traditional ART [3, 4].

Follicular fluid is a serum transudate composed of blood-born factors required to assemble the hyaluronate-rich extracellular matrix, the formation of which is catalyzed by LH-induced changes in gene expression. The induction of enzymes like HAS-2 in granulosa cells initiate the assembly of the matrix that will come to encase not only the expanded cumulus mass but much of the mural granulosa cell population. Active cell motility coincident with matrix assembly is now believed to serve as a reservoir of factors retained within the zona pellucida that may have a role later in development. Central to eliciting the resumption of meiosis in the oocyte is the now-recognized synthesis and secretion of EGF-like molecules like AREG, whose role it is to effect changes in cAMP and cGMP metabolism in the oocyte that allow for the activation of the cell cycle. Coupling between corona cells persists for hours enabling the transport of small molecules synthesized in cumulus corona cells into the oocyte, the condition of metabolic loading referred to in Section 5.2.3. Thus, the timely transformation of matrix deposition with profound upregulation in granulosa cell gene expression and secretion serve to coordinate ovulation with the resumption of the meiotic cell cycle.

Besides modulating the metabolism and cell cycle status of the oocyte, the environment of the follicle serves to buffer potentially adverse outcomes associated with the inflammatory state established during ovulation. Oxidative stress introduced into this environment is not only a potential risk factor that the oocyte must somehow endure but the persistence of free radical generation during and after fertilization

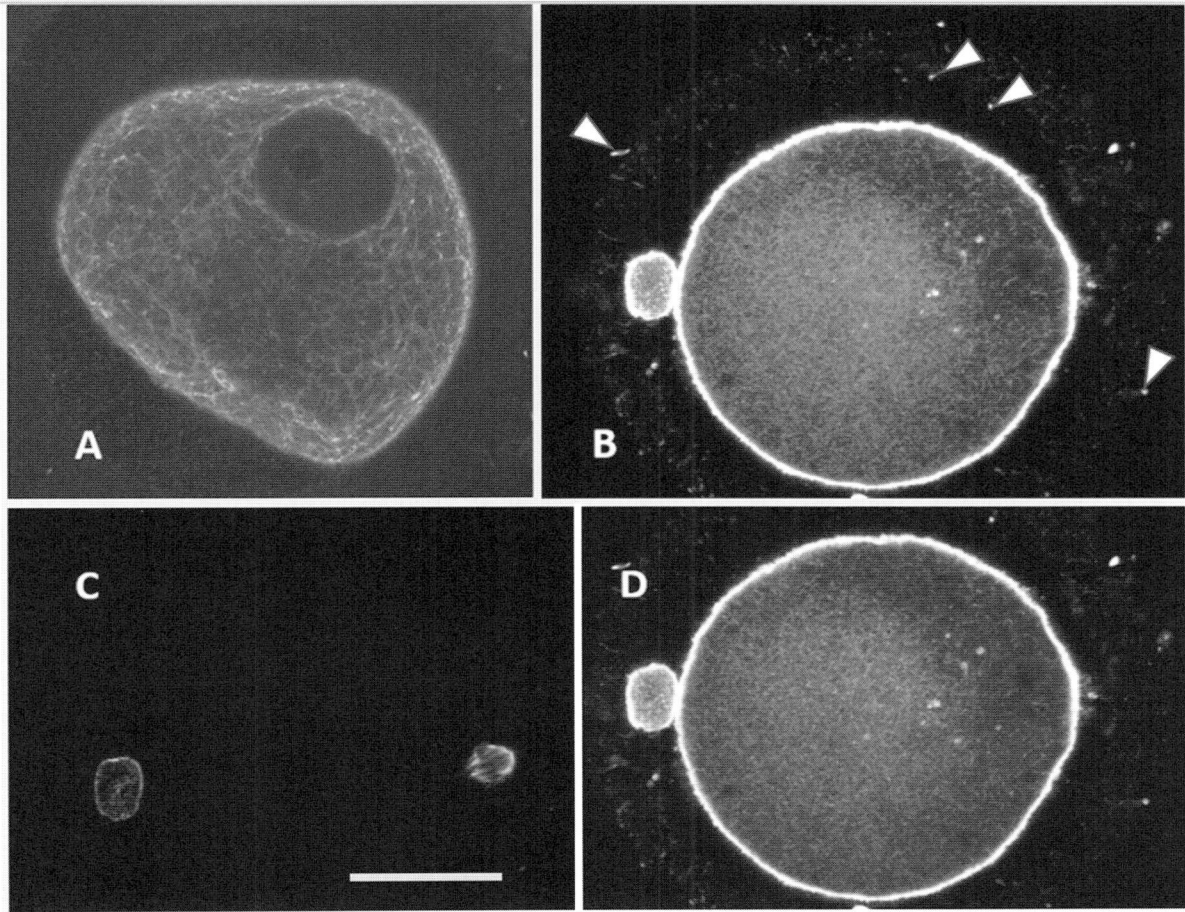

Figure 5.3 Comparison of immature GV stage oocyte (A) and mature metaphase-2 oocyte with spindle positioned 180 degrees opposite the first polar body (B, C, and D).
Note transzonal projection remnants within the zona pellucida (arrow heads, B), perpendicular orientation of metaphase-2 spindle with respect to the polar body (C), and gradient of filamentous actin from left to right, with lowest density apparent at pole demarcated by meiotic spindle (B, D). All images are single optical planes obtained with laser scanning light microscope after labeling with antitubulin antibodies (A, green; C, white) or red phalloidin (B, D). Scale bar = 50 microns.

continues due to intrinsic and extrinsic sources [9]. It is interesting to note that conditions for culturing human embryos have yet to fully address this matter.

5.3.3 Oocyte Competence: Insights from Clinical Practice

The combination of the expanded use of human ART and the opportunities to detect, report, and in some cases rectify abnormalities in normal development, has yielded a growing body of data with which to understand the function and dysfunction of oocyte competencies. The spectrum of recognized abnormalities is large, extending from defects in oocyte maturation, failure to fertilize and, in corresponding embryos disorders in the first cell cycle, fragmentation, delayed compaction, and failure to complete blastocyst formation [10]. In some cases, evidence for penetrance for a specific phenotype has warranted, and sometimes uncovered, a genetic basis to the disorder (see Section 5.3.4). More often, the defects observed exhibit mixed phenotypes from the same patient or even the same ART cycle suggesting a more complicated origin of the aberrant behavior. One of the earlier defects reported by Combelles and colleagues was a case where oocytes exhibited spontaneous activation [11]. One of the key events required for the egg to embryo transition is the removal of factors responsible for maintaining meiotic arrest at the metaphase-2 stage. The cMOS protooncogene has long been recognized as the cell cycle brake whose removal at fertilization by mRNA and protein degradation would permit entry into the first mitotic cell cycle of development. Not surprisingly, cases like this and others have noted disruptions in the state of cytoskeleton organization and cell cycle progression, or lack thereof.

To date, the majority of instances linking abnormalities in human oocyte or embryo developmental competencies to problems in cytoskeletal organization have been confined to the oocyte and early cleavage stages. Importantly, few of these have shown a level of penetrance that would be indicative of an underlying genetic basis for the observed defects [12]. With exception to the cases referred to below, and the mounting evidence regarding epigenetic determinants in early development, direct links between genotype and phenotype seem unlikely to explain the range of variations emerging from laboratory reports. It seems more likely that the root cause of competency failures will reside in other areas of control including RNA diversity and proteostasis. Regarding the latter, posttranslational regulation of protein function and turnover has long been understood to be fundamental to the control of cell cycle progression. And in the case of protein phosphorylation and dephosphorylation, the concept was advanced some years ago, now confirmed, that such a control system operating at the oocyte cell surface would be critical to both polar body extrusion and early cleavage stages of development [13]. Should we add the notion of "cortical maturation" to our attempts to bridge the gap between oogenesis and embryogenesis?

5.3.4 From Form to Genetics: The Subcortical Membrane Complex

The process of oocyte maturation is much more than one designed to support the genetic transformation from meiosis to mitosis. Shifting the unique program in oogenesis that allows for asymmetric cell division during polar body extrusion to that of symmetric division after syngamy and beyond may constitute one of the major logistical issues the embryo must

deal with. Over and above the biomechanics is the matter of sorting the maternally inherited hardware (e.g. mitochondria) that each resultant blastomere must retain in order to contribute to the trophectoderm or inner cell mass lineages. The subcortical membrane complex (SCMC) fulfills an important role in localizing and stabilizing maternal and zygotic gene products to prevent errant degradation and ensure correct positioning at later stages in development [14].

What has made this structure relevant to early development in the human is the recent identification of mutations in core components of the SCMC that appear to be associated with defects, either during oocyte maturation or after fertilization. TUBB8 was among the first of these genes where a genotype–phenotype relationship was revealed but since those earlier studies, other SCMC components have been recognized [15]. In the end, it is likely that the role of genetics will continue to contribute to the genomic basis of how oogenesis drives embryogenesis. However, many of the practical principles exploited in conventional ARTs, such as COS, extended culture, and elimination of follicular support at retrieval, may introduce subtle forms of stress that will challenge the overall performance of embryos with respect to competence expression before or after embryo transfer [16].

5.4 Future Directions

A look back at trends in clinical practice over the past decades reveals several patterns emerging including the adoption of extended embryo culture, time-lapse imaging/morphokinetics, biopsy and genetic assessments, and spent culture media sampling for subsequent -omics analyses. The emphasis placed on the embryo and not the oocyte is obvious and understandably related to the greater duration in which the embryo is available for analysis. The introduction of multi-parametric testing offers greater depth for clinical decision-making and can be expected to expand on current and future technologies designed to enrich the deselection strategy especially in the context of single-embryo transfer. One example of this pertains to comparison of conventional morphological grading and morphokinetics. While the overall utility of morphokinetics analysis continues to be debated, its dominant adoption from some centers has proven useful and predictive of likelihood of pregnancy with encouraging signs of widespread utility evidenced in large-scale center comparisons [17]. At the time of this writing, several other technologies including but not restricted to noninvasive autofluorescence assays of metabolism and artificial intelligence are under development and will likely complement the tests mentioned above [18].

But what about the oocyte? Reliance on morphology is insufficient due to the inability to determine qualities of obvious importance to embryo development. Indirect and noninvasive measures of oocyte competence derived from monitoring cumulus cell function have to date failed to demonstrate clinical utility. However, we can expect that many of the above techniques will eventually be applied as their sensitivity, reliability, and reproducibility continue to mature. Returning to the subject of multiparametric analyses, past efforts to monitor oocyte morphology with the earliest events of development hold promise such that the transition from egg to embryo offers quantifiable milestones that together report on the likelihood that certain oocytes exhibit properties indicative of developmental potential.

Matziotis and colleagues recently demonstrated an example of how linking oocyte morphology to cortical properties deduced from fertilization by ICSI reflect what is likely to be an important determinant of oocyte competence [19]. A major feature of oocyte maturation is the assembly of a rigid cortex due to reorganization of the oocyte cytoskeleton (Figure 5.2). It has long been recognized that oocytes exhibit a wide range of penetrance properties, from extreme fragility to resistance to penetration by an ICSI needle. This study shows an association between cortical stiffness and future development and should serve as a point of departure for exploring and monitoring this crucial dimension of oocyte quality [13, 14].

Finally, the stage is set to investigate early and late stages of oogenesis in the human at systematic and analytical levels not previously possible. While widely recognized for benefits that among other things would limit traditional exposures and consequences to COS such as ovarian hyperstimulation syndrome, the field of oocyte in vitro maturation (IVM), is poised to become a mainstay in ART practices. Several reasons account for mounting interest in IVM not the least of which is the fact that a much more detailed understanding is emerging of how the LH surge triggers and effects the process of oocyte maturation. Clinical success rates in PCOS patients undergoing a novel two-step IVM protocol are a promising indication of both clinical utility and a deeper understanding of the complexities and consequences of this stage-setting dimension of human oogenesis [20].

Key Messages

- Current standards for gauging the developmental potential of human oocytes remain primarily based upon gross morphology.
- Nuclear maturity, in the absence of biomarkers for cytoplasmic or cortical maturity, is insufficient to predict development in corresponding embryos beyond the zygote stage, failure to cleave, compact, form blastocysts, or implant after transfer.
- Developmental failure is likely a consequence of genetic and/or epigenetic factors attributable to events taking place during growth and maturation stages of oogenesis and perifertilization.
- Many conditions embedded in conventional ART protocols influence the acquisition and expression of developmental competence in human oocytes including stimulation protocols, media composition, and status of cumulus cells.
- Meiotic cell cycle exit and entry into the first mitotic cell cycle are key control points that involve maternal effect genes and their translational products whose localization and stability dictate the kinetics of cleavage divisions.
- The subcortical maternal complex provides a protein scaffold that integrates cell cycle progression and compaction via maternally inherited components of the cytoskeleton
- Biomarkers for the detection and assessment of maternal effectors are required before useful assays for the developmental potential of human oocytes enter the embryology laboratory
- At present, progress in artificial intelligence and noninvasive screening using oocyte-secreted products and/or -omics assessments of cumulus cells are paving the way for more discriminating methods to evaluate oocyte properties and characteristics consistent with improved embryo quality

References

1. Coticchio G, Albertini DF, De Santis L, editors. *Oogenesis*. New York: Springer; 2013.

2. Albertini DF. The mammalian oocyte. In: Plant T, Zeleznik, A, editors. *Knobil and Neill's Physiology of Reproduction*. 4th ed. New York: Elsevier; 2015. p. 59–97.

3. Vassena R, members of the EBART group. Evidence-based medicine in ART. *Hum Reprod*. 2017;32(1):256.

4. De los Santos MJ, Apter S, Coticchio G, Debrock S, Lundin K, et al. Revised guidelines for good practice in IVF laboratories (2015). *Hum Reprod*. 2016;31(4):685–6.

5. Krisher RL. The effect of oocyte quality on development. *J Anim Sci*. 2004;82(E-Suppl.):E14–23.

6. Weghofer A, Kushnir VA, Darmon SK, Jafri H, Lazzaroni-Tealdi E, Zhang L, et al. Age, body weight and ovarian function affect oocyte size and morphology in non-PCOS patients undergoing intracytoplasmic sperm injection (ICSI). *PLoS ONE*. 2019;14(10):e0222390.

7. Conti M, Franciosi F. Acquisition of oocyte competence to develop as an embryo: integrated nuclear and cytoplasmic events. *Hum Reprod Update*. 2018;24(3):245–66.

8. Da Broi MG, Giorgi VSI, Wang F, Keefe DL, Albertini D, Navarro PA. Influence of follicular fluid and cumulus cells on oocyte quality: clinical implications. *J Assist Reprod Genet*. 2018;35(5):735–51.

9. Latham KE. Stress signaling in mammalian oocytes and embryos: a basis for intervention and improvement of outcomes. *Cell Tissue Res*. 2016;363(1):159–67.

10. Combelles CMH, Rawe VY. Determinants of oocyte quality: impact on in vitro fertilization failures. In: Coticchio G, Albertini DF, De Santis L, editors. *Oogenesis*. New York: Springer; 2013. p. 307–27.

11. Combelles CM, Kearns WG, Fox JH, Racowsky C. Cellular and genetic analysis of oocytes and embryos in a human case of spontaneous oocyte activation. *Hum Reprod*. 2011;26(3):545–52.

12. Dal Canto M, Guglielmo MC, Mignini Renzini M, Fadini R, Moutier C, Merola M, et al. Dysmorphic patterns are associated with cytoskeletal alterations in human oocytes. *Hum Reprod*. 2017;32(4):750–7.

13. McGinnis LK, Albertini DF. Dynamics of protein phosphorylation during meiotic maturation. *J Assist Reprod Genet*. 2010;27(4):169–82.

14. Bebbere D, Masala L, Albertini DF, Ledda S. The subcortical maternal complex: multiple functions for one biological structure? *J Assist Reprod Genet*. 2016;33(11):1431–8.

15. Feng R, Yan Z, Li B, Yu M, Sang Q, Tian G, et al. Mutations in TUBB8 cause a multiplicity of phenotypes in human oocytes and early embryos. *J Med Genet*. 2016;53(10):662–71.

16. Andersen CY, Kelsey T, Mamsen LS, Vuong LN. Shortcomings of an unphysiological triggering of oocyte maturation using human chorionic gonadotropin. *Fertil Steril*. 2020;114(2):200–8.

17. Zaninovic N, Nohales M, Zhan Q, de Los Santos ZMJ, Sierra J, Rosenwaks Z, et al. A comparison of morphokinetic markers predicting blastocyst formation and implantation potential from two large clinical data sets. *J Assist Reprod Genet*. 2019;36(4):637–46.

18. Simopoulou M, Sfakianoudis K, Maziotis E, Antoniou N, Rapani A, Anifandis G, et al. Are computational applications the "crystal ball" in the IVF laboratory? The evolution from mathematics to artificial intelligence. *J Assist Reprod Genet*. 2018;35(9):1545–57.

19. Maziotis E, Sfakianoudis K, Giannelou P, Grigoriadis S, Rapani A, Tsioulou P, et al. Evaluating the value of day 0 of an ICSI cycle on indicating laboratory outcome. *Sci Rep*. 2020;10(1):19325.

20. Vuong LN, Le AH, Ho VNA, Pham TD, Sanchez F, Romero S, et al. Live births after oocyte in vitro maturation with a prematuration step in women with polycystic ovary syndrome. *J Assist Reprod Genet*. 2020;37(2):347–57.

Chapter

6

The Laboratory's Role in Embryo Development

Dean Morbeck

6.1 Introduction

The laboratory plays a key role in an embryo's development and therefore is a critical element of embryology key performance indicators (KPIs) [1]. The primary goal of the IVF laboratory is to provide an optimal environment for successful embryo development, mimicking an optimal in vivo environment. When the laboratory environment, culture conditions, and embryology handling are optimized, the collective environment yields embryology KPIs that translate into maximal fertilized embryos, high-quality blastocysts, and ultimately healthy live births. Ongoing and rigorous quality control within the embryology laboratory ensures that each patient's cohort of embryos has the appropriate environment to reach developmental milestones, with the goal of ensuring safety and quality of care. This chapter describes the laboratory's role in embryo development and embryo selection, including the embryology KPI frameworks and quality control pathways utilized by the laboratory.

6.2 The Laboratory's Role in Embryo Development

The laboratory itself accounts for a large proportion of the entire IVF process (Figure 6.1) and is consequently a significant influencer of embryo development and ultimately IVF outcome [1]. When suboptimal, laboratory conditions may compromise the pregnancy potential of an otherwise competent oocyte or embryo. A complex network of laboratory factors culminates in optimal conditions for in vitro embryo growth, and within each laboratory step there are many known physical, chemical, and biological modifiers to consider. These laboratory factors have been well described over the past few decades through research dedicated to optimizing embryo development within the IVF laboratory, now resulting in the modern-day laboratory [2].

6.3 The Laboratory and Culture Environment

The embryo's direct culture environment is ultimately assembled through many different physical and chemical constructs within the IVF laboratory (Figure 6.2). Although knowledge of what constitutes the optimized IVF laboratory has progressed immensely over the last decades, it is important to consider that it might only approximate an optimal in vivo environment that by nature is extremely difficult to replicate [3], though extensive research and improvement on culture conditions likely provides a better environment than is present in many patients experiencing infertility.

Immediately surrounding the embryo, culture media provides essential constituents necessary for metabolism and growth [4, 5], and which is covered with oil to minimize osmotic changes in this micro-environment. The incubator housing the dish must maintain appropriate temperature, humidity, and gas concentrations, which ultimately lead to optimal medium pH. However, as the embryo moves through the IVF process and transitions to different dishes or positions within the laboratory, along with numerous manipulations (e.g. pipetting sheer stress or technical variation), changes to this exacting environment are inevitable. The wider laboratory and external environment also influence the quality of air within the working environment [6]. The IVF process may also involve several adjunctive micromanipulations such as intracytoplasmic sperm injection (ICSI), trophectoderm biopsy, and cryopreservation that, despite being invasive and deviating significantly from the in vivo environment, are well tolerated by gametes and embryos under optimized conditions. In summary, the goal of the IVF laboratory is to create an in vitro environment that promotes successful embryo growth while limiting environmental and physical interference where possible.

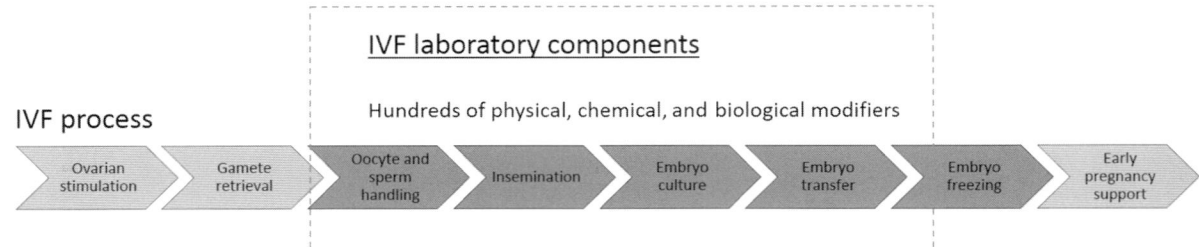

Figure 6.1 The laboratory's impact on the IVF process
The laboratory has a large impact on the IVF process, accounting for many steps that occur within the entire process. Each step within the laboratory process may be influenced by physical, chemical, and biological variation.

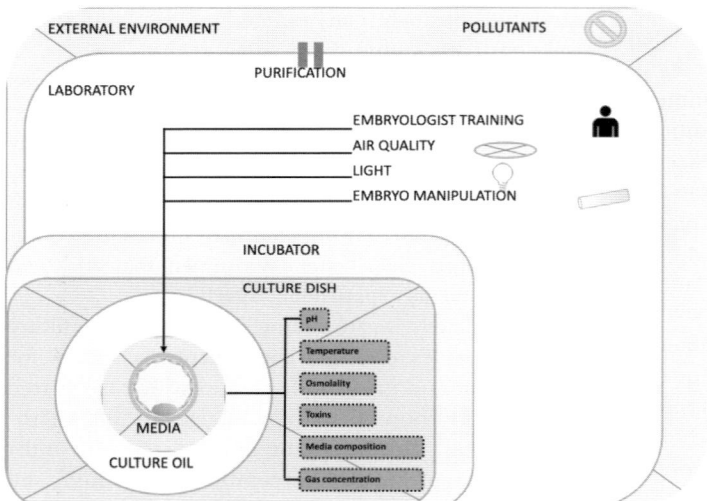

Figure 6.2 The laboratory and culture environment
The IVF culture environment is a result of complex interactions between hundreds of materials and physical settings. The microenvironment directly surrounding the embryo is a summation of the environment created by the embryo's direct (culture) and wider (laboratory) surroundings.

6.4 Biological Effects of an Environmental Stressor

If physical, chemical, or biological factors are not optimized for an embryo's developmental requirements, then biological effects on an embryo can arise (Figure 6.3; [1]). Translation of biological effects on embryos, however, is complex and not necessarily obvious or always detected at the time the insult occurs. Potential downstream effects of an environmental insult include, but are not limited to, slow speed of development, poor embryo quality, metabolic stress, and even epigenetic changes. Yet, the way a suboptimal culture environment acts on a developing embryo is poorly understood as it depends on the factors involved, including magnitude and duration, the stage of embryo development, and whether an embryo is adaptive to the environmental change. In terms of embryo stage, the oocyte and early embryo are the most sensitive to physical and chemical stress (Figure 6.4), and conversely the blastocyst, which has a more mature homeostatic regulatory system due to having more and differentiated cell types, is the least sensitive [3].

When performing troubleshooting in the IVF lab, we must acknowledge that our understanding of the causative biological effects following the presence of a laboratory stressor is usually speculative, and thus limited to observations inherent to the IVF process, such as embryo morphology, developmental timings, and ultimately pregnancy potential. At this intersection, embryology KPIs signal how the culture environment interacts with embryo biology as an indication of the overall health of the culture system.

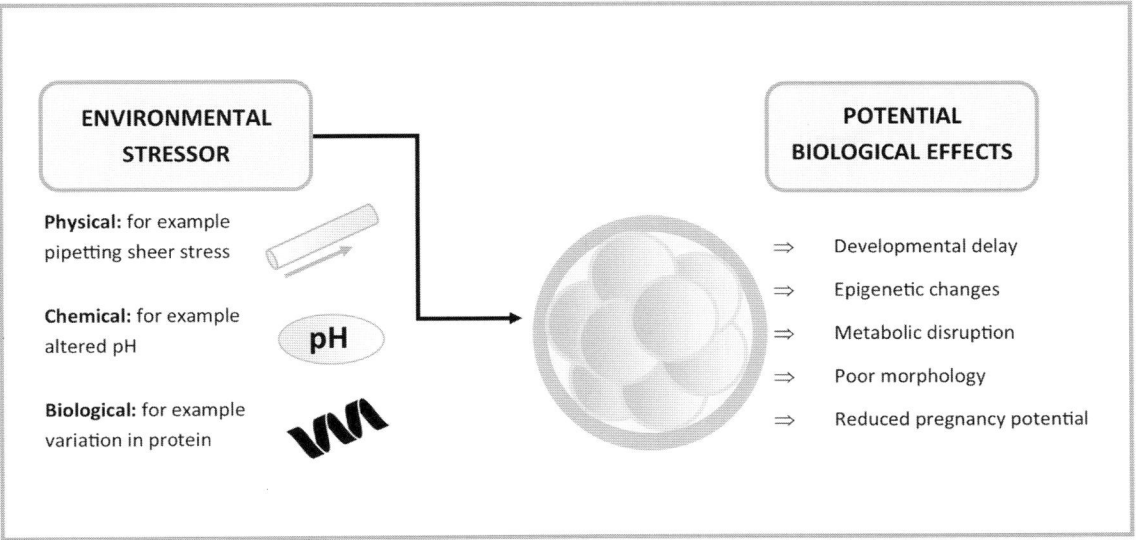

Figure 6.3 Potential biological effects of environmental stressors arising during embryo culture
Environmental stressors arising during embryo culture may perturb the embryo's microenvironment and result in an array of biological effects including developmental delay, epigenetic changes, metabolic disruption, poor morphology, and, ultimately, reduced implantation potential.

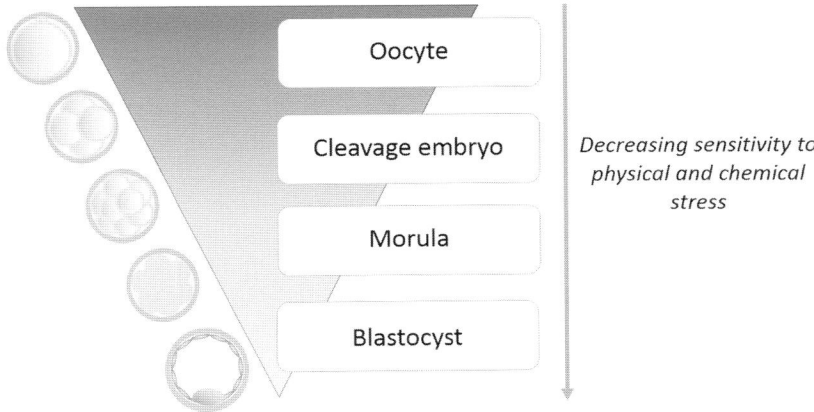

Figure 6.4 Impact of environmental stress by preimplantation stage of development
The gametes and early embryo have the highest sensitivity to physical and chemical stress. Conversely, the blastocyst, with a large number of differentiated cells, has the lowest sensitivity to environmental stress.

6.5 Embryology Key Performance Indicators

Embryology KPIs provide a measure of gamete competence and embryo development, for instance the rates at which successful fertilization, blastulation, and pregnancy occur [7]. They are a proxy or indicator of how the laboratory interacts with embryo development; if an embryology KPI is reduced across a sufficient number of cycles, then the laboratory environment is questioned, after ruling out known clinical or laboratory process changes or shifts in patient demographics. Monitoring embryology KPIs on a weekly and/or monthly basis is an important part of quality control within the IVF laboratory to ensure the absence of culture disruptors, and hence a stable culture environment [8]. The frequency of monitoring is influenced in part by the size of the laboratory. The timeline of embryology KPIs by developmental stage is shown in Figure 6.5.

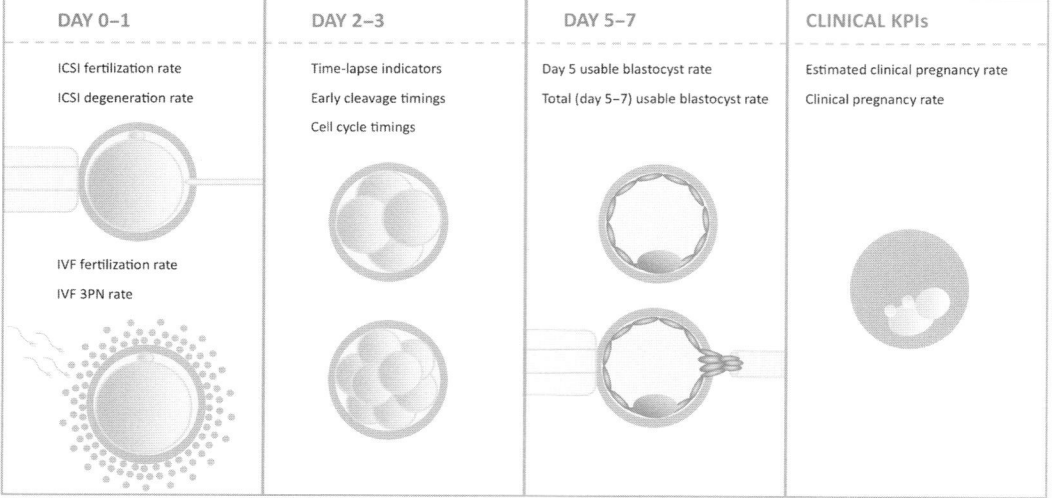

DAY 0–1	DAY 2–3	DAY 5–7	CLINICAL KPIs
ICSI fertilization rate	Time-lapse indicators	Day 5 usable blastocyst rate	Estimated clinical pregnancy rate
ICSI degeneration rate	Early cleavage timings	Total (day 5–7) usable blastocyst rate	Clinical pregnancy rate
	Cell cycle timings		
IVF fertilization rate			
IVF 3PN rate			

Figure 6.5 Embryology KPI timeline
Fertilization rate KPIs are assessed according to insemination type (IVF or ICSI). During the cleavage stage, time-lapse indicators identify delays in early development. During the postcompaction stage, the usable blastocyst rate assesses ability of the system to support blastocyst development as well as speed of blastocyst development. After embryo transfer, the estimated pregnancy rate based on serum βhCG level is used as a surrogate marker for implantation, and is later replaced by clinical pregnancy rate to confirm viability.

Embryology KPIs requiring frequent monitoring are described in Table 6.1, along with their calculations and competency and benchmark values (or aspirational goals) adapted from the Vienna consensus assisted reproductive technology laboratory performance indicators document [9].

Fertilization rates are calculated by insemination type (IVF or ICSI) and capture the number of normally fertilized oocytes (two distinct pronuclei [2PN]) from the number either injected (ICSI) or inseminated (IVF). Reduced fertilization rates may be caused by changes to oocyte quality, sperm preparation, culture conditions such as air quality or pH, or, in the case of ICSI, operator variation. The ICSI degeneration rate, reflecting the percentage of oocytes damaged following injection, can increase with operator variation or following changes to ICSI equipment and consumables [10]. Like all KPIs, degeneration rate can be influenced by patient characteristics and clinical factors, such as suction pressure at oocyte retrieval.

Time-lapse incubators have greatly increased the amount of data on pre-implantation development, enabling extension of the embryology KPIs described in Table 6.1. Cell cycle timings provide detailed information about early embryo development and are KPIs in their own right, a concept illustrated with mouse embryo quality control [11]. Time-lapse

reference values are either derived from the literature, or ideally established internally within each laboratory, in which timing differences have the potential to occur with respect to the ratio of IVF to ICSI insemination, utilization of thawed oocytes, culture media, and patient demographics.

Usable blastocyst rates reflect the proportion of embryos that progress past embryonic genome activation to become blastocysts of usable quality (transferred or frozen). Usable blastocyst rates are calculated for cycles that either have a blastocyst transfer or are "freeze all." Cycles that have cleavage stage transfer are not included in the usable blastocyst rate calculation as blastocyst development is not confirmed. Sites that mainly utilize day 3 transfer should develop an in-house validated KPI as a substitute to usable blastocyst rates, for example "good day 3 development rates" that take into account the proportion of embryos with 7–9 cells and less than 10% fragmentation on day 3. The day 5 usable blastocyst rate (D5BUR) measures speed of blastocyst development, whereas the total usable blastocyst rate (TBUR) measures the total proportion of embryos progressing to the blastocyst stage that are suitable for clinical use. We have observed that D5BUR was a more sensitive measure of a change in culture conditions than TBUR (Figure 6.6). In this example, a change to

Table 6.1. Definitions of several embryology key performance indicators with competency and benchmark values

Key performance indicator	Calculation	Competency	Benchmark
ICSI fertilization rate	$\dfrac{\text{number of oocytes with 2PN}}{\text{number of MII injected}} \times 100$	65%	80%
ICSI degeneration rate	$\dfrac{\text{number of degenerated oocytes}}{\text{number of MII injected}} \times 100$	10%	5%
IVF fertilization rate	$\dfrac{\text{number of oocytes with 2PN}}{\text{number of cumulus oocyte complexes (COCs) inseminated}} \times 100$	60%	75%
Day 5 usable blastocyst rate (D5BUR)	$\dfrac{\text{number of good quality blastocysts on day 5*}}{\text{number of oocytes with 2PN}} \times 100$	30%	40%
Total usable blastocyst rate (TBUR)	$\dfrac{\text{number of good quality blastocysts on day 5,6 or 7*}}{\text{number of oocytes with 2PN}} \times 100$	40%	50%
Estimated pregnancy rate (EPR)	$\dfrac{\text{number of embryo transfers resulting Beta human chorionic gonadotropin (}\beta\text{hCG)} \geq 50IU\backslash L \text{ on}\sim\text{day 14}}{\text{number of cycles with embryo transfer}} \times 100$	45% *blastocyst	75% *blastocyst
Clinical pregnancy rate (CPR)	$\dfrac{\text{number of embryo transfers resulting in fetal heart beat at weeks 7–9}}{\text{number of cycles with embryo transfer}} \times 100$	35% *blastocyst	60% *blastocyst

Note: *Blastocyst utilisation for transfer or vitrification (not calculated for cycles with cleavage stage utilisation).

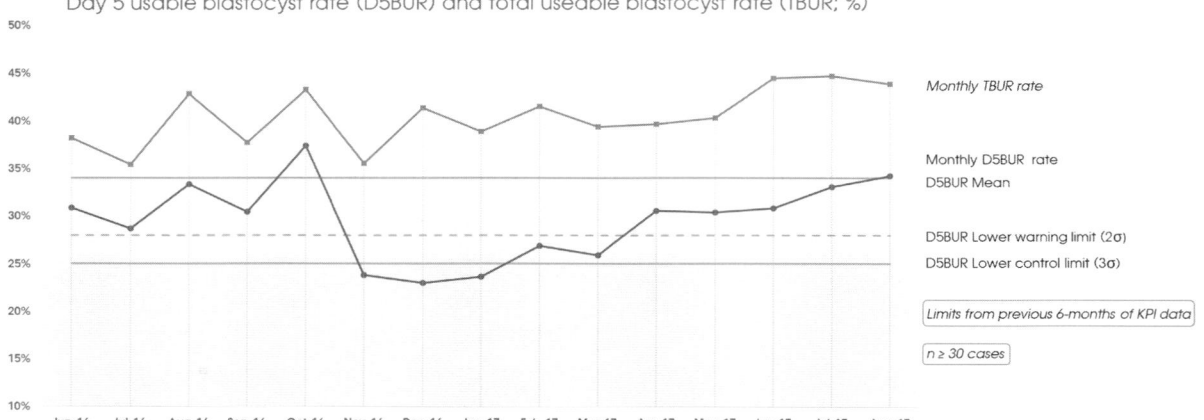

Figure 6.6 Illustration of time-series control chart for KPI tracking of monthly day 5 usable blastocyst rate (D5BUR) and total usable blastocyst rate (TBUR; %)

Lower warning (2σ) and control (3σ) limits are calculated retrospectively from the preceding six months of KPI data to distinguish meaningful changes from chance variation given an adequate sample size (30 cases or more). In this illustration, lower warning and control limits for D5BUR identified a shift in D5BUR, lasting for five months from November 2016 to March 2017 and corresponding to a change in embryo culture medium. During this time, TBUR remained within statistical process control and did not cross TBUR control limits (TBUR control limits not shown).

a new culture medium resulted in a significant shift in D5BUR that also coincided with a decrease in pregnancy rates [12], though the latter was only detected three months after the change. Had we been tracking D5BUR, we would have acknowledged the difference and changed back to our previous medium sooner. Note that TBUR is also influenced by other factors, such as changes to blastocyst grading protocols that occur following grading revision or gradual shifts to grading practices.

Clinical outcomes are determined by calculating the proportion of transfers resulting in a successful pregnancy. The pregnancy rate is tracked most accurately by determining those cycles resulting in fetal heartbeat at 7–9 weeks gestation (clinical pregnancy; CPR). The limitation associated with relying exclusively on clinical pregnancy, however, is the time delay following transfer, potentially delaying detection of effects on pregnancy rates. As an early surrogate marker for clinical pregnancy, serum beta human chorionic gonadotropin (βhCG) is used to calculate an estimated pregnancy rate (EPR). The cycle day of βhCG testing, the βhCG threshold level, and maternal age all influence the magnitude by which the calculated EPR correlates to CPR. Choosing a relatively high βhCG threshold (e.g. 50 IU/L) allows better correlation with CPR. For example, at day ~14 the CPR decreases by 29.6% and 19.4% for βhCG levels

of ≥10 IU/L and ≥50 IU/L, respectively, in women aged 37 years or younger. The relative difference is also more pronounced for those women aged 38 years and over. Table 6.1 uses a βhCG threshold of ≥50 IU/L at cycle day 14 (~) instead of βhCG levels of more than 0 or ≥10 IU/L because it has a higher degree of correlation to the eventual CPR.

The CPR varies by maternal age, number of embryos transferred, proportion of cleavage stage embryo transfer, and proportion of PGT-A cycles. Changes to clinical pregnancy rates relate to many clinical and embryology factors, as well as being heavily dependent on patient demographics, the most influential being maternal age [13]. CPRs are analyzed by maternal age subgroups, and while some groups use four or more subgroups, in the interest of sample size and simplicity, we find the most biologically relevant divide being 37 years or younger versus 38 and over, given the significantly higher aneuploidy rates for those over 38 years of age.

6.6 Tracking Key Performance Indicators

Tracking embryology KPIs is integral to the laboratory's quality management system. Electronic medical recording systems that promote timely and accurate access to cycle data are recommended for optimal and regular KPI tracking. Embryology KPIs are regularly tracked on a weekly and/or monthly basis, and frequency of tracking is modified according to cycle volume, patient demographics, and the KPI involved [8]. When a significant shift or drift is identified during these time frames, a root-cause analysis is performed to determine the source of the fluctuation (e.g. for a decrease in ICSI fertilization rates, a thorough review of technique, supplies, etc.).

Embryology KPIs are monitored using statistical process control with time-series control charts (Figure 6.6). Control charts have statistical control limits that aim to distinguish meaningful changes from chance variation when there are an adequate number of cases (e.g. n $\geq$ 30). Warning (2 sigma) and control limits (3 sigma) define the region of expected baseline variation determined by historical data, which can be derived from historical data, often corresponding to six months of performance during a stable period of performance. We use KPIs for two reasons – to compare to standards so we know we are doing well, and to track our performance over time. Analysis of data in relation to the laboratory's internal historical rates provides a measure of culture stability. When KPI changes are detected by control chart tracking, further root-cause analysis using appropriate statistical tests that account for confounding variables, such as patient age, are performed.

Control and warning limit thresholds as well as the clinic average should change over time as process improvement results in better outcomes. When a KPI consistently measures above the mean for several consecutive periods, the mean and limits should be recalculated to improve the sensitivity of the tracking process going forward. While control charts typically employ both upper and lower limits, for the purpose of tracking inadvertent deviations from good practice, it is acceptable to use a one-sided control chart, where either lower limits (e.g. fertilization rate) or upper limits (e.g. 3PN after IVF) are used.

6.7 Key Performance Indicators and Embryo Selection

The gradual increase in IVF success rates during the past three decades is in part attributed to enhancement of the laboratory environment and associated quality control operations, illustrating the laboratory's influence on embryo development and cycle outcome. Improvements in culture environment and stimulation protocols yield more embryos and thus better embryo selection. As one of the fundamentals of clinical embryology, more embryos enables choice about which embryo is selected for transfer to maximize success at single embryo transfer.

At the patient level, negative shifts in the culture environment and KPIs can directly influence embryo selection (Figure 6.7). The interaction between embryology KPIs and embryo selection occurs primarily by assuring development of suitable embryos available for transfer. When a negative KPI shift occurs (e.g. blastocyst use rate) selection of the best quality embryo within the patient cohort is compromised, especially if the number has been reduced

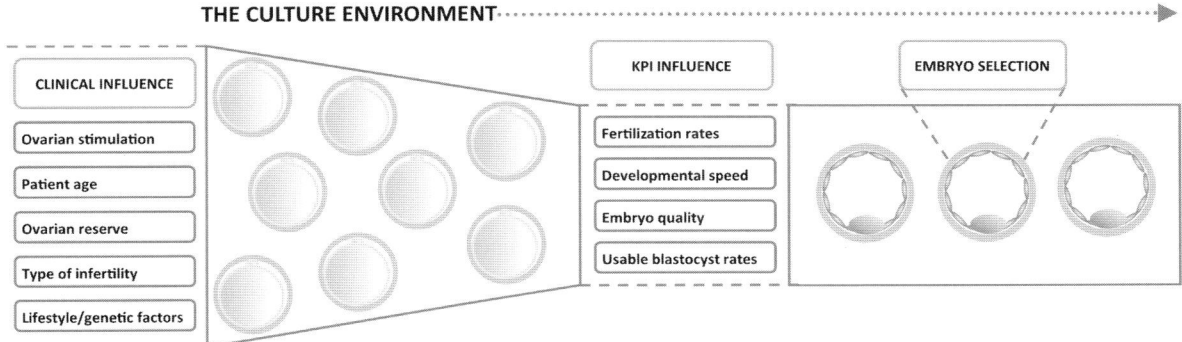

Figure 6.7 Influence of the culture environment and laboratory KPIs on embryo selection
Although the number and quality of gametes entering the laboratory are predetermined by clinical factors, the culture environment influences the development of each patient's cohort of embryos, which are thus captured by the respective KPIs. For example, lowered fertilization rates, reduced developmental speed and quality, as well as decreased usable blastocyst rates reduce the number of viable embryos suitable for transfer and ultimately prevent optimal embryo selection.

to one or none. Tracking embryology KPIs during a change in embryo culture media illustrates D5BUR as an important KPI that identifies reduced speed of blastocyst development by day 5, a change that has the potential to promote difficulty selecting the best quality embryo at day 5 fresh transfer. During the study, reduced D5BUR was also accompanied by reduced pregnancy rates, illustrating that in some cases D5BUR can act as an early indicator to changes in clinical outcomes [12].

6.8 Summary

Human embryos are sensitive to their culture environment and optimization and monitoring of this environment is critical to successful IVF outcomes. Culture stability is regularly monitored through embryology KPIs (including time-lapse indicators). Culture stability is key to ensuring that at each step of the IVF process, each patient's cohort of embryos is cultured in conditions that promote successful growth, thereby maximizing embryo quality and optimizing selection for increased odds of pregnancy after single embryo transfer. The laboratory role of ensuring safety and quality of care during the IVF process is critical. Deviation of embryology KPIs outside control limits may signal a shift within culture conditions, promoting further process investigation into settings, culture

environment, consumables, processes, and patient demographics.

Key Messages

- The laboratory covers a large number of steps and variations within the IVF process.
- The embryo's microenvironment is a summation of the physical, chemical, and biological settings of the culture and laboratory environment and the early oocyte/embryo is the most sensitive to culture disruptors.
- Environmental stressors arising within the culture environment have the potential to result in developmental delay, epigenetic changes, metabolic disruption, poor morphology, and ultimately reduced implantation potential.
- Stable culture conditions are monitored through embryology KPIs.
- Monitoring embryology KPIs is recommended weekly to monthly depending on clinic volumes.
- Tracking of KPIs using time-series control charts determines whether each KPI remains within statistical control limits.
- Deviation of a KPI outside control limits may signal an adverse event or shift within culture conditions, promoting further process and statistical investigation into patient demographics, laboratory processes, and the culture environment.

References

1. Cohen J, Consensus Group C. 'There is only one thing that is truly important in an IVF laboratory: everything' – Cairo Consensus guidelines on IVF culture conditions. *Reprod Biomed Online*. 2020;40:33–60.

2. Swain JE. Optimal human embryo culture. *Semin Reprod Med* 2015;33:103–17.

3. Wale P, Gardner D. The effects of chemical and physical factors on mammalian embryo culture and their importance for the practice of assisted human reproduction. *Hum Reprod Update*. 2016;22:2–22.

4. Morbeck DE, Baumann NA, Oglesbee D. Composition of single-step media used for human embryo culture. *Fertil Steril.* 2017;107:1055–60.

5. Tarahomi M, Vaz FM, van Straalen JP, et al. The composition of human preimplantation embryo culture media and their stability during storage and culture. *Hum Reprod.* 2019;34:1450–61.

6. Mortimer D, Cohen J, Mortimer ST, et al. Cairo consensus on the IVF laboratory environment and air quality: report of an expert meeting. *Reprod Biomed Online* 2018;36:658–74.

7. Mortimer ST, Mortimer D. *Quality and risk management in the IVF laboratory.* 2nd ed. Cambridge University Press; 2015.

8. ESHRE Guideline Group on Good Practice in IVF Labs, De los Santos MJ, Apter S, et al. Revised guidelines for good practice in IVF laboratories (2015). *Hum Reprod.* 2016;31:685–6.

9. ESHRE Special Interest Group of Embryology, Alpha Scientists in Reproductive Medicine. The Vienna consensus: report of an expert meeting on the development of art laboratory performance indicators. *Hum Reprod Open.* 2017;35:494–510.

10. Rubino P, Vigano P, Luddi A, Piomboni P. The ICSI procedure from past to future: a systematic review of the more controversial aspects. *Hum Reprod Update* 2016;22:194–227.

11. Wolff HS, Fredrickson JR, Walker DL, Morbeck DE. Advances in quality control: mouse embryo morphokinetics are sensitive markers of in vitro stress. *Hum Reprod.* 2013;28:1776–82.

12. Hammond ER, Morbeck DE. Tracking quality: can embryology key performance indicators be used to identify clinically relevant shifts in pregnancy rate? *Hum Reprod.* 2019;34:37–43.

13. Vaegter KK, Lakic TG, Olovsson M, Berglund L, Brodin T, Holte J. Which factors are most predictive for live birth after in vitro fertilization and intracytoplasmic sperm injection (IVF/ICSI) treatments? Analysis of 100 prospectively recorded variables in 8,400 IVF/ICSI single-embryo transfers. *Fertil Steril.* 2017;107:641–8.

Handling of Gametes and Embryos

Sharon T. Mortimer

7.1 Introduction

The underlying philosophy for assisted reproduction technology (ART) is to maximize the chances of pregnancy from a single oocyte retrieval cycle, by transferring an embryo with a high likelihood of implantation and cryopreserving the remaining embryos for transfer in later cycles. The ideal outcome would then be that all of the embryos required for the creation of the family would arise from that one oocyte retrieval. Following this philosophy means that it is the responsibility of the laboratory to maintain each gamete's and embryo's developmental potential. It is unlikely that the laboratory can increase this potential, as that is generally determined by patient-related factors such as age, health status, and gametogenesis, which are out of the laboratory's control. However, the conditions in the laboratory can certainly decrease this potential, if the gametes and/or embryos are exposed to environmental and culture conditions that are not optimal, as this requires them to expend energy in adapting to their environment, causing stress. As observed over the past 40 or so years, human gametes and embryos can adapt to the in-vitro environment, and still give rise to pregnancies and healthy live births. However, an improved understanding of the requirements of gametes and embryos in culture, and development of the technology to support these requirements, has increased the chance of pregnancy from around 10% per transfer (with up to four embryos per transfer) in the 1980s, to the current rates of around 35–60% per transfer (with only one or two embryos per transfer) depending on maternal age.

Although there have certainly been improvements in the ovarian stimulation protocols over this period, and improvements in embryo transfer catheters and transfer technique, which have all contributed to the increased chance of pregnancy, it has been the changes in the laboratory's handling methods that

have supported improved rates of embryo development, both in terms of speed and number. In the early days of clinical IVF, when the culture requirements were not as well understood, it was felt that embryos developed more slowly in vitro and so time in the lab should be minimized. To address this, day 2 (ideally 4-cell) embryos were transferred to the uterus based on the assumption that the uterine environment might provide better conditions to support embryo development than were available in vitro, even though in nature an embryo does not reach the uterus until the blastocyst stage. Although it was certainly possible to culture embryos to the blastocyst stage in the 1980s, the blastocyst development rates were often quite low, with low cell numbers. It was not until after significant changes in embryo culture systems were introduced in the 1990s that blastocyst development rates and blastocyst quality improved to the point that it became clinically feasible to move to the routine transfer of one or two blastocysts to the uterus on day 5. Further technological improvements since 2000, including the widespread use of time-lapse imaging of embryo development, are now increasing our knowledge and understanding of the requirements of gametes and embryos in vitro.

The aim of this chapter is to provide a general overview of the factors in gamete and embryo handling that can affect the cycle outcome, along with recommendations of approaches to support the control of variability in the culture system.

7.2 The Culture System

In nature, gametes and embryos exist within a dynamic environment that supports their functional and developmental requirements. While this cannot yet be replicated in vitro, there are several physical factors that can be maintained and controlled, specifically temperature, pH, oxygen, osmolarity, culture medium composition, contact materials, light exposure, and incubators, collectively termed the culture system. Gametes and embryos must also be protected against exposure to toxic substances, including volatile organic compounds (VOCs) such as aldehydes, which can cause significant damage to embryo development. VOCs can enter the laboratory from the outside air, or from materials in the fabric of the laboratory (e.g. offgassing of paints, adhesives, manufactured wood products, etc.), as well as in the day-to-day functioning of the laboratory (e.g. from sterilizing or sanitizing products). It is possible to manage the VOC load in the ART laboratory, but this is easier in a new facility, where various strategies can be incorporated into the lab design [1]. Further, the use of in-line filters in the gas supply lines to the incubators have been recommended to facilitate the removal of VOCs, bacteria, dust, etc. [2].

The culture system provides cells with the nutrients they require, as well as support to maintain homeostasis. If the conditions are not ideal, then the cells must adapt or they will die. Adaptation, though, is a stressor, and cellular stress has been associated with altered gene expression and/or regulation (e.g. imprinting). Therefore, to maximize the developmental potential of gametes and embryos, it is critical to provide suitable physico-chemical conditions, as far as current technology allows.

7.2.1 Temperature

Normal human body temperature is around 37°C. Although gametogenesis occurs at slightly lower temperatures, fertilization and embryo development occur at 37°C in vivo. Consequently, maintaining the cell cultures as close to 37°C as possible should be optimal, although this has not been established unequivocally [2]. Care should be taken to protect against exposure of gametes and embryos to temperatures significantly cooler or warmer than this, as that could adversely affect cellular metabolism and function. For example, there is some evidence that transient cooling of oocytes to room temperature causes disorganization of the meiotic spindle in some oocytes, with displaced chromosomes and a consequent risk of aneuploidy. Therefore, while it is possible for fertilization and embryo development to occur in oocytes that have been cooled to room temperature, this is not an optimal approach. For maintenance of the laboratory systems, and to support effective troubleshooting, temperature control is therefore an important aspect of the culture system.

Particular attention is required to maintain a stable temperature during follicular aspiration, transport of the aspirates to the "egg search" workstation, the egg search procedure, and subsequent handling of cumulus–oocyte complexes (COCs), as well as the resulting embryos.

7.2.2 pH

In addition to stable temperature control, gametes and embryos require the culture medium to be pH 7.2–7.4. At sea level, a culture environment containing ~6% CO_2 is required to maintain this pH range in a 25 mM bicarbonate solution (as is used in the majority of culture media). The concentration (or rather, the partial pressure) of CO_2 (pCO_2) required to maintain medium pH increases with altitude.

The approach of measuring the pH of cultures each morning, and then adjusting the amount of CO_2 in the incubator environment to meet a pH target, does not take into account fluctuations in atmospheric pressure that often occur throughout the day as the weather changes, which influence the pCO_2 required.

7.2.3 Oxygen

Oxygen levels in the reproductive tract are in the range of 2–8% [2], while ambient oxygen is ~20.9% at sea level. The earliest IVF labs cultured embryos under a gas phase of 5% CO_2/5% O_2/90% N_2 in special chambers placed inside incubators, but over time, the gas phase for culture changed to 5% CO_2-in-air. The reasons for this change were likely both economic and ergonomic, as special mix gas is more expensive, and not using it meant that the culture dishes could be placed directly onto the incubator shelves, rather than into special chambers. These "big-box" incubators, the standard type of incubators used in research laboratories, contain room air, to which CO_2 is added to reach the desired CO_2 concentration, using CO_2 controllers.

However, culture of human gametes and embryos under ambient pO_2 levels affects developmental potential, and has been reported to result in reduced cell number; reduced fetal development; disturbances of the epigenome, transcriptome, and proteome; and increased production of reactive oxygen species (ROS), which can cause DNA damage [2]. Therefore, it is now becoming the standard to culture gametes and embryos in a low-oxygen environment.

7.2.4 Osmolarity

Loss of water from the culture environment due to evaporation increases the osmolality of the culture medium: another stressor. Evaporative loss occurs during exposure to a dry environment in the laboratory and/or incubator. When preparing culture dishes for overnight equilibration, care must be taken to reduce the risk of evaporation from the microdroplets before the oil is added. However, there is evidence that even an oil overlay cannot provide long-term protection against evaporative loss: A strategy to manage cultures in a nonhumidified incubator is to replace the medium every 48 hours [2].

7.2.5 Culture Medium

Protection against significant changes in the culture medium is critical for optimal oocyte and embryo metabolism and homeostasis, but the chemical composition of the medium itself can also affect the outcome of ART. For example, even a five-minute exposure of fertilized mouse oocytes to a collection medium that did not contain amino acids resulted in fewer embryos reaching the blastocyst stage, with those that did reach the blastocyst stage having lower cell numbers [3].

Another important factor to consider is whether an IVF culture medium contains antioxidants. Antioxidants assist in reducing the incidence of ROS production, and in moderating its effects [4].

7.2.6 Contact Materials

Contact materials are all the consumables that come into direct contact with gametes and embryos. These include culture medium, dishes and other plasticware, pipettes, pipettor tips, other solutions, gases, and the laboratory environment.

Most clinical ART laboratories have an extremely limited ability to conduct embryo toxicity testing of the contact materials, and so several manufacturers have released cultureware in a certified "IVF range" that has been assayed by a 1-cell mouse embryo assay (MEA). In some jurisdictions, labs are required to use MEA-tested consumables, if they are available, regardless of the price.

Cost should never be the sole consideration when selecting consumables for use in the ART laboratory, particularly as it is often possible to negotiate pricing for good-quality items, based on ordering patterns and volume. The more important factors in choosing consumables are related to production quality, reproducibility, and performance in the culture system.

It is good practice to record for each treatment cycle the lot number of each of the contact materials used. In this way, should a recall be issued, it is relatively simple to identify and verify the affected patients/cycles.

7.2.7 Incubation System

In the more traditional IVF process, gametes are taken out of the incubator for insemination, and then daily for observations of fertilization and embryo development, with transfer into fresh culture medium on days 1 and 3 of culture. However, in many laboratories, particularly those using time-lapse systems, inseminated oocytes are left undisturbed for several days, or until the time of embryo transfer or cryopreservation.

When the gametes and embryos are outside the incubator, care must be taken to ensure that the observations and handling are conducted in either a temperature- and gas-controlled environment (such as an enclosed workstation) or are completed as quickly as possible, ideally within two minutes [5]. This is to reduce the risk of the gametes and embryos being exposed to ambient conditions, which will affect the temperature and pH of the culture medium.

Sufficient incubators should be available to minimize the number of times each incubator door is opened throughout the day [6]. This is because when the door of a big-box incubator is opened, its internal atmosphere is disturbed through exposure to room air and requires some time to reequilibrate, so repeated openings and closings expose all of the embryos in that incubator to these conditions.

7.2.8 Light

In nature, gametes and embryos are not exposed to light. Consequently, in many ART laboratories, room lighting is suppressed, but microscopy exposes gametes and embryos to light that is many times brighter [2]. The use of colored filters on the microscopes can reduce the exposure of oocytes and embryos to the more harmful blue end of the visible light spectrum.

The following sections consider the specific factors that should be taken into consideration when handling spermatozoa, oocytes, and embryos.

7.3 Spermatozoa

There is a common tendency in ART methodologies to overlook the relative importance of the male gamete, but the outcome of a cycle can certainly be influenced by how the semen sample is processed and the motile sperm preparation handled.

During their transit from the testes to the epididymides, spermatozoa undergo maturational changes that stabilize them for storage in the male reproductive tract. Therefore, before a spermatozoon can fertilize an oocyte, these changes must be reversed as part of the process of capacitation. Capacitation is a series of metabolic and physiological changes that occur during the transit of the spermatozoa through the female reproductive tract in vivo, or as part of the sperm preparation process for IVF, which leave the spermatozoa with the capacity to fertilize oocytes.

When capacitated spermatozoa reach the oocyte, they undergo the acrosome reaction, triggered by binding to the zona pellucida. The acrosome is a membrane-bound organelle covering the front of the sperm head, lying immediately under the plasma membrane. In the acrosome reaction, the outer acrosomal membrane and the overlying plasma membrane become more fluid, and the matrix inside the acrosome expands, causing localized contact, fusion, then loss of these membranes. The fertilizing spermatozoon then traverses the zona pellucida, binds to the oocyte plasma membrane via ligands in the equatorial segment exposed during the acrosome reaction, and the sperm and oocyte membranes fuse [7].

The fertilization process relies on the sperm membranes being sufficiently fluid to support fusion. It is therefore important to reduce their risk of exposure to ROS as this can cause reduced membrane fluidity, as well as DNA fragmentation. Since there is no active repair mechanism for nuclear DNA in the sperm head, DNA strand breaks can lead to failure of embryo development pre or postimplantation. The biggest contributors to ROS generation in semen are leucocytes and immature sperm cells, so it is critical to isolate the functional spermatozoa from the other cells in semen without pelleting all the cell types together, which is why whole semen should never be centrifuged.

Spermatozoa must also be carefully isolated from seminal plasma as it contains decapacitation factor(s) that reversibly inhibit capacitation and the acrosome reaction, and extended exposure to seminal plasma in vitro can inhibit sperm function [8]. It is for this reason that sperm washing and selection procedures must be started as soon as liquefaction has occurred, ideally within 30, but certainly no more than 60, minutes postejaculation. Apart from chain-of-custody questions, this is the main reason that semen samples are collected within the clinic – to remove travel time thereby minimizing exposure of the spermatozoa to seminal plasma.

7.3.1 Sperm Preparation Methods

There are many methods for preparing sperm suspensions for insemination, but those used most often are density gradient centrifugation, or direct swim-up from semen into culture medium [9, 10]. The common aim to is maximize the yield of functional spermatozoa while minimizing the risk of iatrogenic damage, such as physical separation of the head from the midpiece/tail or ROS generation [8]. Whichever method is selected, normozoospermic samples should yield a preparation with at least 90% motile spermatozoa [11].

7.3.2 Dealing with Unusual Sperm/Semen Samples

7.3.2.1 Extremely Low Sperm Concentration

For samples with relatively few motile spermatozoa, the semen can be layered over 1 ml of the upper layer suspension for a density gradient, and centrifuged (500 g; 20 min). This separates the spermatozoa from the seminal plasma, debris, and nonsperm cells, reducing the risk of iatrogenic ROS-generated damage.

7.3.2.2 Cryopreserved Semen

Frozen-thawed semen should first be diluted with a $5\times$ volume of sperm buffer added very slowly, and in stages, to protect the spermatozoa against osmotic shock during processing, as the freezing medium has a very high osmolarity. The diluted sample can then be processed as for fresh semen.

7.3.2.3 Extremely Low Motility

Because not all immotile spermatozoa are dead, there can be live spermatozoa in samples with 0% motile. In the HOS test, immotile spermatozoa are placed into a hypo-osmotic solution (~150, rather than 285, mOsm/kg), which causes the tail of live spermatozoa to swell and coil. These are collected and placed in standard culture media to reverse the membrane coiling, before being inseminated via intracytoplasmic sperm injection (ICSI).

7.3.2.4 Retrograde Ejaculation

This occurs when a man's semen passes back into the bladder at ejaculation. As sperm are sensitive to low pH, it is critical that the patient's urine be alkalinized before a sample is collected. The sample is centrifuged immediately, and the pellet(s) resuspended in sperm buffer before processing.

7.3.2.5 Surgically Retrieved Spermatozoa

Surgical sperm retrieval can be an option for patients with no spermatozoa in their semen. Percutaneous epididymal sperm aspiration (PESA) from the efferent ducts of either the cauda epididymis or vas deferens usually yields relatively clean samples with numerous motile spermatozoa, but there can be a high concentration of dead and senescent spermatozoa. The alternative is to retrieve spermatozoa directly from the testes, by testicular sperm aspiration, or by testicular sperm extraction where sections of seminiferous tubules are taken from the testes. While the absence of seminal plasma means that conventional sperm preparation methods are not required, ideally the motile spermatozoa are separated from the other cell types before selection for ICSI [12].

7.4 Oocytes

At the time of retrieval, "mature" oocytes are at the metaphase 2 stage of meiosis and remain at this stage until penetration by the fertilizing spermatozoon, when they undergo their final reduction division resulting in extrusion of the second polar body. It is the oocyte's mRNA that directs the first two rounds of cell division before activation of the embryonic genome. The success of the ART cycle, in terms of fertilization and embryo development, is heavily dependent upon the oocyte, which must undergo many physical and biochemical transformations.

Handling oocytes in vitro is therefore much more intricate than handling spermatozoa. Oocytes are very sensitive to changes in their environment, and this can affect their functional ability, so care must be taken to protect them from exposure to stressors. These stressors have already been discussed above, in Section 7.2, so the following are strategies to manage these exposures when handling oocytes.

7.4.1 Equilibration and Set-Up

An oocyte retrieval (or oocyte pick-up, OPU), requires prewarmed search dishes, into which the follicular fluid is transferred, as well as wash and culture dishes that contain medium. It takes several hours for culture medium to gas- and temperature-equilibrate, so any dishes and tubes containing medium must be prepared the day before and placed in an equilibration incubator overnight. Ideally, the tubes that will be used to collect the follicular fluid will also be prewarmed and labeled with the patient's name and other unique identifiers, as an extra check step when they are brought into the lab or workstation. All of the cultureware used should be from batches that have been QC-tested for IVF.

The workstation that is used for oocyte retrieval should maintain the temperature of the COCs close to 37°C, and certainly above 35°C, to reduce the risk of iatrogenic meiotic spindle depolymerization. To achieve this, the work surface might need to be kept slightly warmer than 37°C. To determine the best temperature for the work surface, it is best to do some "dummy runs" with the same volumes of medium (and oil, in the case of microdroplets of medium) that will be used and check the temperature inside the dish using a thermal probe. In addition, the work surface temperature to be used must be calibrated for every type of culture dish that will be used there [2].

7.4.2 Oocyte Retrieval

The timing of the OPU is a clinical decision, based on the kinetics of follicular growth and often on the amount of circulating estradiol. Once these criteria have been met, the ovulation process is triggered and the patient scheduled for OPU a few hours before ovulation is due to occur. By that stage, the mature COCs should be floating in the follicular fluid, rather than being attached to the follicle wall.

Before the OPU, a process of positive identification of the patient should be followed, where the patient tells the staff her name and other identifying details, rather than simply confirming that information. Ideally, the embryologist participates in this process to ensure that the correct patient's dishes are in the work area. This matters because sometimes the planned running order of cases is changed, and if the embryologist does not know whose oocytes are being collected, this greatly increases the risk of an inadvertent error in mixing patients' gametes. An alternative identification strategy is the use of electronic witnessing systems, where the patient's identity is confirmed via a system-generated ID card and must match the labeled dishes in the work area.

Once the patient has been prepared for the procedure, her ovaries are visualized via transvaginal ultrasonography, the follicles punctured, and the follicular fluid collected. Whether to flush the follicles is essentially a clinical decision. The flushing fluid, which should contain amino acids [3], must be at 37°C to reduce the risk of cooling the COCs, but it is virtually impossible to maintain this temperature in a syringe or down the thin length of a needle and tubing. The follicular (and flush) fluids are collected into sterile, prewarmed, labeled, culture tubes. The use of a tube-warmer is recommended at this stage, as simply holding the tubes by hand is not enough to maintain their temperature.

The contents of each tube are then transferred into search dishes and scanned under a dissecting microscope to identify any COCs. The search dishes have a diameter of 60 mm or more, so if the microscope is in a laminar flow hood, and the fan is left running, there is a risk of evaporative cooling, even if the dishes are on a warmed surface. An option to reduce this risk is to switch off the fan during the egg search procedure, or to use a warmed, humidified, and CO_2-controlled workstation.

There is also a significant risk of temperature loss when the COCs are held in a glass pipette or pipette tip – a temperature loss of 5°C per 5 s has been reported, irrespective of whether the pipette was prewarmed [2]. Therefore, as each COC is identified, it should be transferred immediately into the wash dish (37°C), and never held in the pipette while the rest of the search dish is checked. To modulate any effect of differences in the media compositions when moving oocytes and embryos between different culture media, a small volume of the medium into which they are being moved can be expelled around the oocyte or embryo before it is aspirated into the pipette.

Once the COCs have been retrieved and washed, they are placed in a fertilization medium and cultured until the time of insemination. Every time that gametes or embryos are moved from one dish or tube to another, an independent witness should verify that the correct patients' gametes or embryos are being processed, and that the labels on the old and new dishes are for the same patient. This can be done by having two people checking each other's work, or by the use of an electronic witnessing system. Whichever strategy is followed, it must be followed consistently, and done every time gametes or embryos are moved from one container to another, to minimize the risk of mix-up errors.

7.4.3 Insemination

Before performing the insemination, it is critical that the patient identity is checked and validated, as the insemination step is irreversible.

7.4.3.1 "Traditional" IVF

The COCs are left intact, and a suspension of washed, motile spermatozoa is added (in some labs, the COCs are moved into a microdroplet of the sperm suspension). It is best if the COCs are left intact, as this provides a matrix for the spermatozoa to enter, and the progesterone produced by the cumulus cells supports capacitation. Insemination must be done carefully, but sufficiently rapidly to not affect the temperature or pH of the preparations. Care must also be taken to ensure that there is no possibility of transfer of any spermatozoa onto or into the barrel of the pipettor, as this would represent a significant risk factor for cross-contamination of another sperm sample.

7.4.3.2 Insemination by ICSI

Because it is very difficult to access the oocyte through the cumulus and corona cells, oocytes for microinjection are denuded of their cumulus cells enzymatically and of their corona cells mechanically. The cumulus cells are in a hyaluronic acid matrix, so are dispersed by hyaluronidase treatment. Mechanical removal of the corona cells is managed using the flexible tips of a defined internal diameter (usually 175–200 μm, then 135–45 μm), to minimize the risk of oocyte damage.

Depending on whether the ICSI equipment is on the open bench or in a CO_2-controlled chamber, microinjection is performed in either HEPES- or MOPS-buffered media or bicarbonate-buffered medium, respectively.

After microinjection, the oocytes are washed, placed in fresh medium in equilibrated dishes, and returned to culture until the fertilization assessment on day 1. For time-lapse incubators, the injected oocytes are usually left in place until the day of embryo transfer or cryopreservation.

7.5 Embryos

Preimplantation embryos undergo significant physical transformation, developing over the course of four days from a single cell into a blastocyst with defined cell types. Although the biochemical requirements of the developing embryo differ from those of an oocyte, it shares the same requirements for physico-chemical control to support optimal development in vitro. Therefore, care must be taken to ensure that the cultures are maintained under stable conditions, with minimal exposure to ambient conditions. This can be managed by designating task-specific work areas in the laboratory, to give the shortest time between incubator and workstation.

As many of these requirements have already been outlined, this section presents additional considerations for embryo handling beyond those required for oocytes.

7.5.1 Fertilization Assessment

During the fertilization check 17 ± 1 hours postinsemination [11, 13], any remaining cumulus and corona cells that are interfering with a clear visualization of the oocyte are stripped away as quickly and gently as possible, usually using manufactured flexible plastic pipette tips. It is also important (especially in IVF cases, where this removal process can take some time) to only have as many oocytes per dish that can be stripped and graded within an acceptable time (i.e. within two minutes). Of course, if using a temperature- and gas-equilibrated enclosed workstation, then these timings become largely irrelevant, as pH and temperature can be maintained for a longer period. After the fertilization assessment, zygotes should be washed in the medium that they are about to be cultured in (to remove any of the fertilization medium, or any residual sperm etc.), placed into new dishes of preequilibrated medium, and returned to culture.

For ICSI-derived zygotes in a time-lapse incubator, the fertilization check is usually performed with the dishes in situ, so the medium is not changed at this step.

7.5.2 Embryo Culture to the Blastocyst Stage: Days 2–5

For laboratories that use a "single-step" medium, the embryos remain in the same type of medium throughout embryo development, although the medium might be refreshed partway through the culture period. For laboratories that use a sequential culture medium system, the embryos remain in "cleavage medium" from days 1–3, and if culture is to be continued beyond the cleavage stage, they are then transferred into a "blastocyst medium."

There is a question of whether to culture embryos individually or in groups. The argument for group culture is to capitalize on any coculture effects that might derive from beneficial substrates produced by the embryos; the argument against it is the possibility that embryos utilize substrates and leave depleted media and potential toxins as a product of cellular apoptosis, so individual culture protects an embryo against exposure to potential detrimental products from another embryo [14]. One approach that some labs take is to culture the higher- and lower-quality embryos in separate groups.

Key Messages

- Successful handling of gametes and embryos requires careful attention to all aspects of the laboratory systems and environment.
- These systems must respect the biology of the gametes and embryos, supporting their needs, rather than meeting lab scheduling constraints.
- Effective temperature control is required from the moment an oocyte is aspirated from its follicle until the embryo is transferred into the uterus.
- Medium pH and osmolarity must be maintained throughout the ART process.
- Fertilization and embryo culture should be in a low-oxygen environment.
- Effective risk management requires the use of at least two human-readable unique identifiers as well as witnessing of, at least, each step where gametes and embryos are moved from one container to another.

References

1. Mortimer D, Cohen J, Mortimer ST, Fawzy M, McCulloh DH, Morbeck DE, et al. Cairo consensus on the IVF laboratory environment and air quality: report of an expert meeting. *Reprod Biomed Online*. 2018;36:658–74.

2. Cairo 2018 Consensus Group. "There is only one thing that is truly important in an IVF lab: everything": Cairo consensus guidelines on IVF culture conditions. *Reprod Biomed Online*. 2020;40:33–60.

3. Gardner DK, Lane M. Alleviation of the '2-cell block' and development to the blastocyst of CFI mouse embryos: role of amino acids, EDTA and physical parameters. *Hum Reprod*. 1996;11:2703–12.

4. Morbeck DE, Paczkowski M, Fredrickson JR, Krisher RL, Hoff HS, Baumann NA, et al. Composition of protein supplements used for human embryo culture. *J Assist Reprod Genet*. 2014;31:1703–11.

5. Mortimer ST, Mortimer D. *Quality and risk management in the IVF laboratory*. 2nd ed. Cambridge, UK: Cambridge University Press; 2015.

6. ESHRE Guideline Group on Good Practice in IVF Labs, De los Santos MJ, Apter S, Coticchio G, Debrock S, Lundin K, et al. Revised guidelines for good practice in IVF laboratories (2015). *Hum Reprod*. 2016;31:685–6.

7. Mortimer D. The functional anatomy of the human spermatozoon: relating ultrastructure and function. *Mol Hum Reprod*. 2018;24:567–92.

8. Mortimer D. Sperm preparation methods. *J Androl*. 2000;21:357–66.

9. World Health Organization. *WHO laboratory manual for the examination and processing of human semen*. 5th ed. Geneva: World Health Organization; 2010.

10. Mortimer D, Mortimer ST. Density gradient separation of sperm for artificial insemination. In: DT Carrell, KI Aston, editors, *Spermatogenesis and spermiogenesis: methods and protocols*. Methods in Molecular Biology 927, New York: Springer (Humana Press); 2013. p. 217–26.

11. ESHRE Special Interest Group Embryology and Alpha Scientists in Reproductive Medicine. The Vienna consensus workshop on laboratory key performance indicators. *Hum Reprod Open*. 2017(2), doi.org/10.1093/hropen/hox011, and *Reprod Biomed Online* 2017;35:494–510 (simultaneous publication).

12. Björndahl L, Mortimer D, Barratt CLR, Castilla JA, Menkveld R, Kvist U, et al. *A practical guide to basic laboratory andrology*. Cambridge, UK: Cambridge University Press; 2010. p. 219–25.

13. Alpha Scientists in Reproductive Medicine and ESHRE Special Interest Group of Embryology. The Istanbul consensus workshop on embryo assessment: proceedings of an expert meeting. *Hum Reprod*. 2011;26:1270–83 and *Reprod Biomed Online* 2011;22:632–46 (simultaneous publication).

14. Wale PL, Gardner DK. The effects of chemical and physical factors on mammalian embryo culture and their importance for the practice of assisted human reproduction. *Hum Reprod Update*. 2016;22:2–22.

Noninvasive Morphological Selection of Oocytes

Giovanni Coticchio, Elena Borini, Catello Scarica, and Andrea Borini

8.1 Introduction

The mature human oocyte is the largest cell in the body; once fertilized by a sperm, it has also the capacity to direct preimplantation development and ultimately give rise to more than 200 cell types that constitute the fully formed individual. Such an astonishing characteristic and role in reproduction and the life cycle is not reflected in its shape and subcellular morphology. When released from the follicular environment and stripped of its companion cumulus cells in preparation for intracytoplasmic sperm injection (ICSI), the oocyte may be easily observed unstained at x200 magnification with a phase contrast microscope. Under such conditions, a typical oocyte, ideal according to the standards of IVF practice [1], appears as a spherical cell, enclosed by the glycoprotein shell of the zona pellucida (ZP) and displaying a cytoplasm with finely granulated, but rather inconspicuous and dull, texture (Figure 8.1). Many variations on this morphological theme, suspected to indicate a pathological condition on a cell scale, have been well-known to embryologists since the dawn of IVF. Indeed, if it were possible by simple morphological observation to discern and use selectively competent oocytes from those destined to developmental failure or associated with pathological clinical outcomes, IVF would gain significant benefit in terms of efficiency and safety. For such a reason, over more than three decades, numerous studies have been carried out seeking to establish possible associations between oocyte morphology and developmental competence. This quest, still ongoing, has been made difficult by several factors including (a) the need to preserve oocyte viability and therefore observe this cell noninvasively, (b) a general lack of understanding of possible relationships between oocyte phenotypes and cell function, (c) poor standardization of methods aimed at describing types and

magnitude of oocyte dysmorphisms, and (d) the static nature of the oocyte at the mature stage. Nevertheless, noninvasive oocyte selection based on morphology remains a central topic in clinical embryology and continues to evoke a passionate debate. This chapter describes the current knowledge on noninvasive assessment of oocyte morphology as an approach for gamete selection.

8.2 Stage of Maturation

The size of the mammalian oocyte in the primordial follicles is 20–30 mm, depending on the species. During follicular development, its volume increases 100-fold reaching its maximum in the early antral follicle. At this stage, the diameter of the human oocyte is 120 μm and will not increase over the subsequent phases of follicle development [2]. Oocytes collected in stimulated assisted reproduction technology (ART) cycles are fully grown in all cases. Generally, they are found at the metaphase II (MII) stage of meiosis (Figure 8.1) and ready for fertilization, but typically up to 20% appear meiotically immature, arrested at the prophase stage of meiosis or at intermediate stages between prophase and MII, presumably metaphase I (MI) [3]. Morphological observation allows these cases to be discerned: (a) prophase-arrested oocytes (Figure 8.2) displaying a large and visible nucleus, the germinal vesicle (GV); (b) MI oocytes not exhibiting the GV or the first polar body (1st PB) (Figure 8.3); and (c) MII oocytes devoid of the GV but showing the 1st PB, which appears extruded in the perivitelline space (PVS, the space between the oolemma and the ZP) but juxtaposed to the oocyte surface. According to such criteria, morphological assessment of oocyte maturity is straightforward. However, of note, if GV or MI oocytes are matured in vitro and extrude the 1st PB at a given time point, they will not reach the MII stage

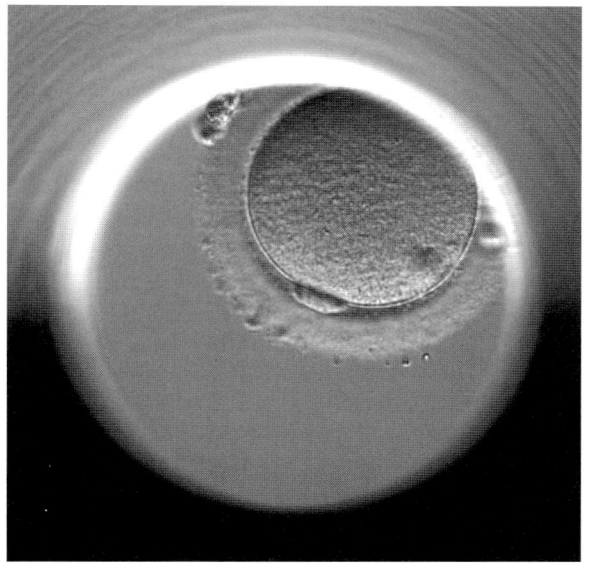

Figure 8.1 Mature oocyte enclosed into the glycoprotein shell of the ZP and displaying a cytoplasm with finely granulated, homogeneous texture

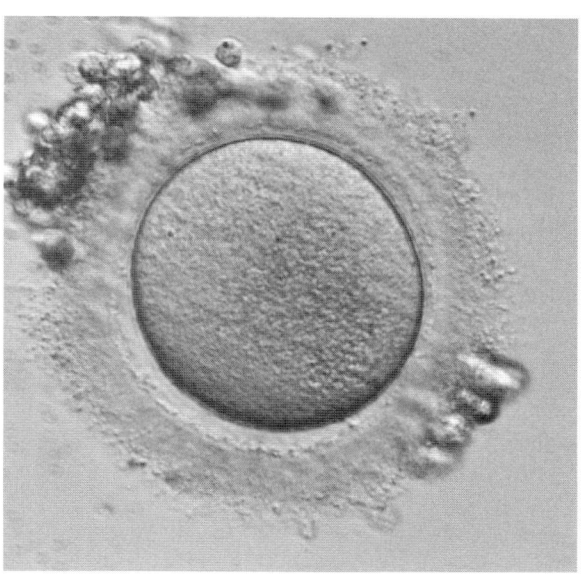

Figure 8.3 Immature oocyte at an intermediate stages between prophase and MII, presumably MI, and not showing the 1st PB

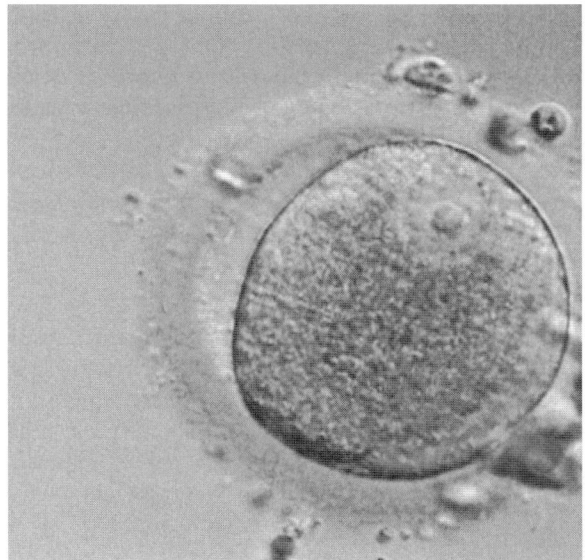

Figure 8.2 Immature prophase-arrested oocytes displaying a large and visible nucleus localised peripherally, the GV

before at least two hours of culture. In fact, the time of 1st PB extrusion is followed by a short period of a few hours during which oocytes progress through telophase I to finally reach MII [4].

8.3 Shape, Size, and Extracellular Correlates

8.3.1 Shape

The human oocyte, similar to those of other mammals, displays a regular spherical shape. A negligible flattening may occur at the site of the extrusion of the 1st PB. Occasionally, MII oocytes may present with a relatively elongated shape, characterized by two orthogonal axes of different length (Figure 8.4). This unusual profile Is likely to occur as a consequence of abnormal formation of the ZP and might therefore indicate significant alterations during folliculogenesis, with possible developmental implications. Isolated observations suggest that, following fertilization, an elongated shape of the oocyte can affect cell contacts between blastomeres. Under such conditions, at the 4-cell stage, blastomeres fail to develop the typical tetrahedral configuration, arranging themselves alternatively into a more planar organization. This morphology is associated with a delay in the times of compaction and blastocyst formation [5]. However, the evidence of an impact on embryo developmental competence and ultimately clinical outcome is lacking.

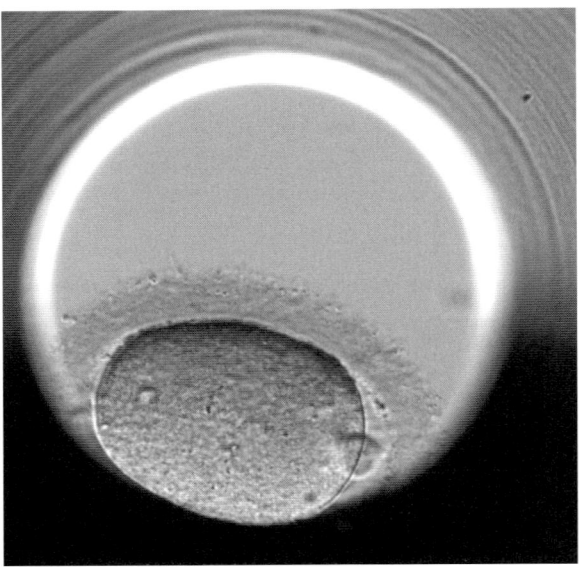

Figure 8.4 MII oocyte with elongated shape. The ZP is also elongated.

8.3.2 Size

By routine, nonquantitative observation, oocyte size is difficult to appraise comparatively. Oocytes of one or different cohorts may appear as the same size. On the other hand, by considering simple geometrical dimensions, small differences in diameter (almost imperceptible if not measured precisely) correspond to significant differences in volume. This might have importance for oocyte competence, because embryo development depends also on the amount of cytoplasm stored during oogenesis. Interestingly, recent data suggest that oocyte diameter (including the ZP) is negatively associated with female BMI, while oolemma diameter (excluding the ZP) is positively associated with fertilization and embryo utilization rates [6]. Therefore, oocyte diameter can represent a possible target for noninvasive assessment, especially because it is amenable to quantitative evaluation.

Oocytes of exceedingly large size, clearly discernible comparatively, are rare and represent a unique case. They are likely to derive from fusion of oogonia shortly before formation of the primordial follicle. They often display two polar bodies and two MII spindles, if analyzed by polarized light microscopy. They are therefore diploid and should not be used for treatment [7, 8].

8.3.3 Zona Pellucida

The ZP may display several morphological abnormalities, such as increased thickness, irregularities of the outer surface, or may appear unusually dark. Occasionally, limited parts of the ZP may show a gap (or "chamber") between internal and external layers. As mentioned before, ZP abnormalities might represent a downstream effect of perturbations of folliculogenesis and therefore indirectly reflect oocyte quality or have implications for sperm recognition and penetration during fertilization. However, oocyte morphology can only be assessed in ICSI cycles, where direct deposition of sperm into the oocyte cytoplasm bypasses the role of the ZP. ZP abnormalities have been less investigated compared to other dysmorphisms. Most studies do not indicate an association between abnormal ZP patterns and fertilization rates, embryo quality, or clinical outcomes [9]. Nevertheless, isolated reports suggest that ZP dysmorphisms may impact on implantation and pregnancy rates [10, 11]. Notably, electron microscopy analysis, although impossible to apply routinely and noninvasively, has allowed identification of specific ZP morphological abnormalities, described as numerous indentations and protuberances of the outer surface, extensive electron-light regions, and a thick inner surface. This phenotype, recurrent in isolated cases, was associated with low maturation rates, high cancellation rates, and reduced pregnancy rates [12].

8.3.4 Perivitelline Space

The PVS is the region delimited by the ZP and not occupied by the oocyte. Its volume has been assessed in relation to embryological and clinical outcome. Most studies ([13, 14, 15]) do not indicate significant relationships, except a few reports in which a large PVS was found to be associated with reduced embryo quality [16]. All such findings, however, are flawed by absence of quantitative criteria to define the size of the PVS, especially because this parameter depends on the relative size of the oocyte and the ZP.

Occasionally, cellular debris may be found in the PVS (Figure 8.5). A few reports suggest that such debris is associated with reduced fertilization rate and embryo quality or even the dose of gonadotropin used for ovarian stimulation [17], but their use in oocyte selection is marginal.

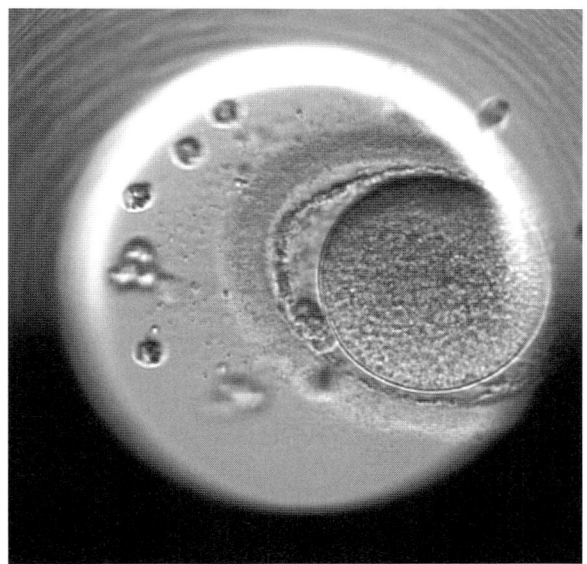

Figure 8.5 MII oocyte with cellular debris visible in the PVS

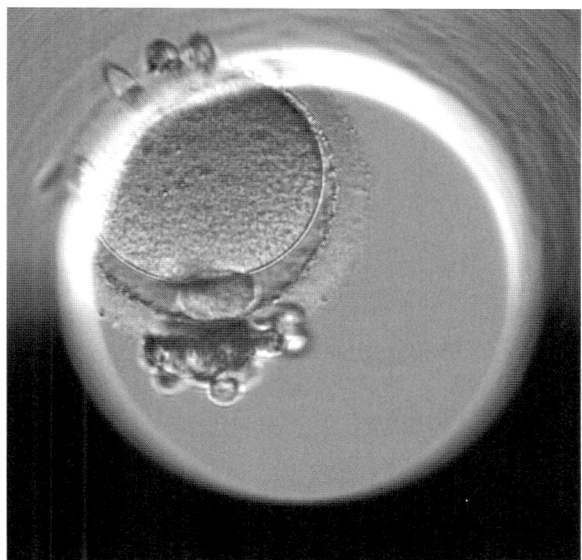

Figure 8.6 MII oocyte with large 1st PB

8.3.5 First Polar Body

The 1st PB is extruded to eliminate one of the two copies of each homologue chromosome at the first meiotic division. As a leftover material, it does not have a role in development, but could represent a biomarker of the function of the oocyte cytoskeleton at the cortical level. In fact, 1st PB extrusion requires coordinated action of an actomyosin structure, referred to as the Actomyosin cap [18]. Inadequate function of the cap caused by a variety of factors, for example in vitro maturation, may impact on the amount of cytoplasm eliminated with the 1st PB, with possible developmental implications [19].

The 1st PB can be assessed according to size, integrity, and smoothness of its surface. Most studies have failed to find an association between any of these characteristics and various parameters of development (fertilization, embryo quality) or clinical outcome ([15, 20, 21]). On the contrary, early studies on the 1st PB morphology reported strong negative associations between increased fragmentation, roughness, and size of the 1st PB and fertilization rates and embryo quality ([22, 23]). Collectively, evidence regarding the relationship between embryo quality and 1st PB morphology remains contradictory. However, although rare and occurring in only 2% of oocytes, an overtly large size (Figure 8.6) is the only 1st PB characteristic more convincingly associated with compromised embryo competence ([22, 23, 24]).

8.4 Intracellular Morphology

8.4.1 Vacuoles

Vacuoles may be found in oocytes at different maturation stages, in fertilized oocytes (Figure 8.7) and even blastomeres, inner cell mass, and trophectoderm. In mature oocytes (Figure 8.6), they are found only in a small proportion (3–4%) of specimens [25]. They may be found in different sizes and number. Analysis by transmission electron microscopy has shown a variety of ultrastructural features. Some vacuoles appear delimited by an uninterrupted membrane and simply filled with fluid. Other vacuoles display interruptions of the membranous envelope and various sorts of inclusions, such as fibrillar material and lipid droplets [26].

Assessment of a possible impact of vacuoles on development has been hindered by the fact that they may be found in different sizes and number, in addition to undergoing appearance, disappearance, and probably some degree of fusion during maturation, fertilization, and embryo cleavage. Regardless, adopting a quantitative approach of vacuole detection, Ebner and colleagues reported a negative association

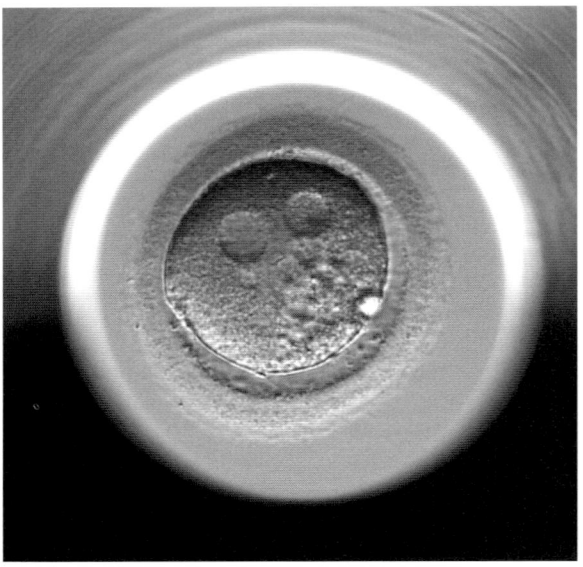

Figure 8.7 MII oocyte displaying multiple vacuoles with diameter ranging between 5 and 20 μm

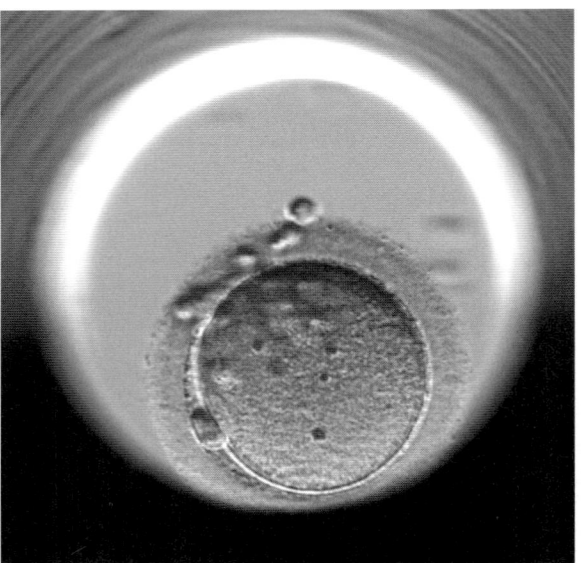

Figure 8.8 MII oocyte with multiple and partially clustered refractile bodies

between presence, size, and number of vacuoles and fertilization rate and blastocyst quality [27]. Rienzi et al. also reported lower fertilization rates in oocytes showing vacuoles [25]. Other studies did not confirm a relationship between oocyte vacuoles and fertilization or developmental rates ([14, 28]). This lack of consistency between different studies is not surprising because, in addition to size and number, possible vacuole impact might depend on position relative to crucial intracellular structures, such as the meiotic spindle. Also, at a practical level in the course of an ICSI procedure, care should be taken to avoid sperm deposition within a vacuole. In fact, it is possible that confinement of sperm within a closed environment delimited by a membrane may have implications for the release and action of the soluble sperm factor responsible for oocyte activation. In cases of oocytes with very large vacuoles, this might explain the observed reduced fertilization rates.

8.4.2 Refractile Bodies

Refractile bodies are abnormal morphological elements of different size (up to 8–10 μm in diameter) found in oocytes, usually isolated or present in small groups (Figure 8.8). They may represent the accumulation of lipofuscin, as suggested by positivity to lipofuscin-specific staining [29]. Depending on size, they display different ultrastructures. Smaller bodies (up to 1.5 μm) appear as an accumulation of matter with homogeneous electron density, delimited by an uninterrupted membrane and surrounded by many smaller lipid droplets. Larger refractile bodies appear to be formed by amorphous and irregular electron-dense material interspersed with lipid droplets partly enclosed by membranes [29]. Oddly enough, the incidence of oocytes displaying refractile bodies varies considerably (from 4.5% to 21.4%) between different studies [13, 25]. Such differences may be explained by the fact that refractile bodies may be alternatively classified as bull-eye inclusions [26] or simply overlooked because they are too small. Refractile bodies may represent relatively benign morphological abnormalities. In fact, while two reports indicated a negative association with fertilization and implantation rates ([30, 31]), the large majority of studies concluded that such morphological abnormalities are irrelevant to oocyte quality ([13, 25, 28]).

8.4.3 Smooth Endoplasmic Reticulum Clusters

The smooth endoplasmic reticulum (SER) is an essential organelle for cell function. In the oocyte, in

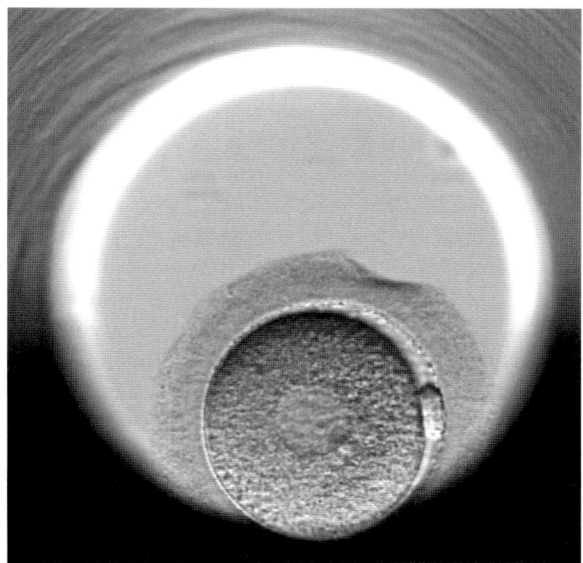

Figure 8.9 MII oocyte with large central SER

addition to its involvement in protein biosynthesis, it plays a crucial role in the generation of $Ca2^+$ cytoplasmic transients that trigger oocyte activation. However, this organelle is believed to give rise to a specific form of oocyte dysmorphism, referred to as SER clusters, believed to derive from coalescence or expansion of normal SER cisternae and tubules, as suggested by positivity to specific endoplasmic reticulum staining [32]. In mature oocytes, an average SER cluster element displays a circular shape on phase contrast observation, with a diameter of approximately 10 μm in diameter (Figure 8.9). However, the size may vary between 6–8 and 20 μm. In addition, SER clusters may be subject to size changes during maturation or prolonged incubation, since they are not usually noticed in GV oocytes, while medium-sized clusters observed in mature oocytes can expand over several hours of culture. The ultrastructure of SER clusters consists of a finely granulated matter delimited by a membrane and surrounded by mitochondria. SER clusters might be mistaken for vacuoles; however, "differential diagnosis" is based on the notion that the former are usually larger, translucent, and delimited by a thin margin, while the latter have the appearance of a cytoplasmic depression defined by a more marked outline [32].

SER clusters are relatively rare; they are found in 5–10% of all cycles and in 0.5–2.0% of all mature

oocytes. Similar to large vacuoles, care should be taken to prevent unintentional deposition of a micro-injected sperm into a SER element because this might hinder the action of the sperm factor responsible for oocyte activation and/or recruitment of free tubulin for the nucleation and growth of the sperm aster. The first major study on SER clusters immediately attracted the attention of IVF specialists. Although no impact was observed on fertilization rate in SER cluster-positive oocytes, development to blastocysts rate appeared somehow affected. More importantly, in one SER cluster-positive cycle, a baby was diagnosed with Beckwith-Wiedermann syndrome [32], a rare condition caused by epigenetic factors. Although isolated, this observation has led to numerous studies on a possible impact of oocyte SER clusters on ART outcome and safety. Collectively, these investigations failed to confirm obvious associations between SER clusters and rates of fertilization, cleavage, and development to blastocyst stage ([9, 25]). Nevertheless, cases of babies born with decreased weight and multiple malformations have raised significant concern [33], to an extent that the Alpha-ESHRE consensus on embryo assessment recommends that "oocytes with SER aggregates should not be inseminated" [1]. However, recent analyses carried out on a larger number of oocytes and babies born have ruled out that SER clusters are associated with reduced rates of fertilization and embryo development in vitro, or indeed short length of gestation, altered birthweight, or increased rates of malformation at birth ([34, 35, 36]). Therefore, there is no solid evidence supporting the exclusion of SER cluster-positive oocytes from use for treatment.

8.4.4 Granular Cytoplasm

In the majority of mature oocytes, the cytoplasm appears homogeneous, light, and finely granulated. However, a significant proportion (20–35%) of them displays a large cytoplasmic domain with a coarser darker granulation, usually positioned centrally (Figure 8.10). The cellular or ultrastructural nature of this morphological trait is unknown, but the magnitude and frequent occurrence of such a condition has prompted several investigations. The reported impact of the presence of granulated cytoplasm on embryo development or implantation is rare, while the majority of studies concluded that the

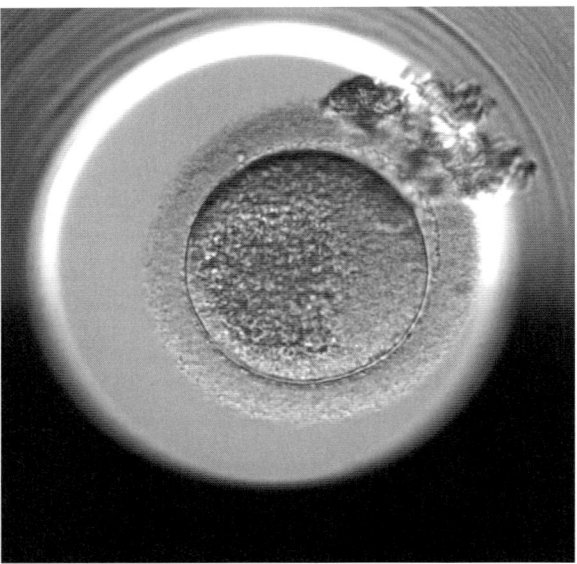

Figure 8.10 MII oocyte showing a very large partially eccentric domain of dark cytoplasm

developmental outcomes of oocytes showing this abnormality are not altered ([13, 14, 28]).

8.4.5 Combined Score

Oocytes may present with multiple morphological abnormalities, which might have an effect on oocyte quality, independently or cooperatively. Based on this concept, oocytes can be scored at the same time for multiple morphometric, intra- and extracellular abnormalities, and subsequently assessed for developmental ability. This approach to oocyte scoring and embryo morphological assessment performed on day 3 can be used together and additively to generate a stronger parameter to predict embryo implantation ability [37, 38]. Therefore, not only can information from different types of morphological abnormalities be expressed by a single value, but such parameters can be used in association with embryo score to predict implantation more successfully.

8.5 Conclusions

A multiplicity of morphological abnormalities, clearly visible with transmitted light microscopy, have been reported to be present in the majority of mature human oocytes collected in ART cycles. Such alterations indiscriminately involve the ZP, the 1st PB, and

the cytoplasm. Overall oocyte shape and size may also be affected. Collectively, attempts aimed at associating each of such dysmorphisms to a specific prognostic laboratory or clinical outcome have so far failed to provide unanimous answers. (See also Appendix Tables 8.1–8.3.) Among the reasons that have made these efforts fruitless is the fact that oocyte dysmorphisms are assessed subjectively and rarely quantified. While some dysmorphisms, such as ovoidal shape of the ZP, are considered relatively benign and usually do not represent a sufficient reason to exclude an affected oocyte from a cohort used for treatment, other abnormalities have repeatedly raised major concern. In particular, initial studies had indicated an epigenetic risk associated with SER clusters. However, more recent data seem to rule out the existence of specific health risks derived from the use of oocytes displaying such an alteration. Probably, the only two phenotypes more convincingly associated with developmental failure are oocytes of giant size, almost certainly derived from fusion of oogonia at premeiotic phases, or showing a very large 1st PB, presumably caused by perturbations of spindle positioning during meiotic maturation. Nevertheless, both types of oocytes are rare (each representing less than 2% of all mature oocytes) and their deselection is unlikely to impact on clinical outcome. Future studies aimed at establishing the possible relevance of oocyte dysmorphisms to embryo development and the health of the conceptus will require more rigorous methodology. This could be achieved with the adoption of enhanced image analysis technology and quantitative criteria, to increase reproducibility and sensitivity of oocyte morphological assessment.

Key Messages

- The scope of morphological oocyte selection is to improve ART treatment efficiency and safety, but not efficacy.
- Mature oocytes can be easily discriminated but can display multiple dysmorphisms.
- Oocyte dysmorphisms involve the ZP, oocyte size and shape, and oocyte cytoplasm.
- Attempts to associate specific dysmorphisms to different developmental fates have been hindered by:
  1. the need to preserve oocyte viability and therefore observe this cell noninvasively

2. a general lack of understanding of possible relationships between oocyte phenotypes and cell function
3. a poor standardization of methods aimed at describing types and magnitude of oocyte dysmorphisms
4. the morphologically static nature of the oocyte at the mature stage

- Some dysmorphisms, such as ovoidal shape of the ZP, are considered relatively benign.

- Initial studies indicated an epigenetic risk associated with SER clusters. However, more recent data seem to rule out the existence of specific health risks derived from the use of oocytes displaying such an alteration.
- Although rare, the only two phenotypes convincingly associated with developmental failure are oocytes of giant size, almost certainly derived from fusion of oogonia at premeiotic phases, or oocytes exhibiting a very large 1st PB.

References

1. ESHRE Special Interest Group Embryology and Alpha Scientists in Reproductive Medicine. The Istanbul consensus workshop on embryo assessment: proceedings of an expert meeting. *Hum Reprod*. 2011;26:1270–83.

2. Griffin J, Emery BR, Huang I, Peterson CM, Carrell DT. Comparative analysis of follicle morphology and oocyte diameter in four mammalian species (mouse, hamster, pig, and human). *J Exp Clin Assist Reprod*. 2006;3:2.

3. ESHRE Special Interest Group Embryology and Alpha Scientists in Reproductive Medicine. The Vienna consensus: report of an expert meeting on the development of ART laboratory performance indicators. *Reprod Biomed Online*. 2017;35:494–510.

4. Montag M, Köster M, van der Ven K, van der Ven H. Gamete competence assessment by polarizing optics in assisted reproduction. *Hum Reprod Update*. 2011;17:654–66.

5. Ebner T, Shebl O, Moser M, Sommergruber M, Tews G. Developmental fate of ovoid oocytes. *Hum Reprod*. 2008;23:62–6.

6. Weghofer A, Kushnir VA, Darmon SK, Jafri H, Lazzaroni-Tealdi E, Zhang L, et al. Age, body weight and ovarian function affect oocyte size and morphology in non-PCOS patients undergoing intracytoplasmic sperm injection (ICSI). *PLoS ONE*. 2019;14:e0222390.

7. Machtinger R, Politch JA, Hornstein MD, Ginsburg ES, Racowsky C. A giant oocyte in a cohort of retrieved oocytes: does it have any effect on the in vitro fertilization cycle outcome? *Fertil Steril*. 2011;95:573–6.

8. Rosenbusch B, Schneider M, Gläser B, Brucker C. Cytogenetic analysis of giant oocytes and zygotes to assess their relevance for the development of digynic triploidy. *Hum Reprod*. 2002;17:2388–93.

9. Rienzi L, Vajta G, Ubaldi F. Predictive value of oocyte morphology in human IVF: a systematic review of the literature. *Hum Reprod Update*. 2011;17:34–45.

10. Sauerbrun-Cutler MT, Vega M, Breborowicz A, Gonzales E, Stein D, Lederman M, Keltz M. Oocyte zona pellucida dysmorphology is associated with diminished in-vitro fertilization success. *J Ovarian Res*. 2015;8:5.

11. Shi W, Xu B, Wu LM, Jin RT, Luan HB, Luo LH, et al. Oocytes with a dark zona pellucida demonstrate lower fertilization, implantation and clinical pregnancy rates in IVF/ICSI cycles. *PLoS ONE*. 2014;9:e89409.

12. Sousa M, Teixeira da SJ, Silva J, Cunha M, Viana P, Oliveira E, et al. Embryological, clinical and ultrastructural study of human oocytes presenting indented zona pellucida. *Zygote*. 2015;23:145–57.

13. Balaban B, Urman B, Sertac A, Alatas C, Aksoy S, Mercan R. Oocyte morphology does not affect fertilization rate, embryo quality and implantation rate after intracytoplasmic sperm injection. *Hum Reprod*. 1998;13:3431–3.

14. Ten J, Mendiola J, Vioque J, de Juan J, Bernabeu R. Donor oocyte dysmorphisms and their influence on fertilization and embryo quality. *Reprod Biomed Online*. 2007;14:40–8.

15. Chamayou S, Ragolia C, Alecci C, Storaci G, Maglia E, Russo E, Guglielmino A. Meiotic spindle presence and oocyte morphology do not predict clinical ICSI outcomes: a study of 967 transferred embryos. *Reprod Biomed Online*. 2006;13:661–7.

16. Ferrarini Zanetti B, Paes de Almeida Ferreira Braga D, Souza Setti A, de Cássia Sávio Figueira R, Iaconelli A, Borges E. Is perivitelline space morphology of the oocyte associated with pregnancy outcome in intracytoplasmic sperm injection cycles? *Eur J Obstet Gynecol Reprod Biol*. 2018;231:225–9.

17. Hassan-Ali H, Hisham-Saleh A, El-Gezeiry D, Baghdady I, Ismaeil I, Mandelbaum J. Perivitelline space granularity: a sign of human menopausal gonadotrophin overdose in intracytoplasmic sperm injection. *Hum Reprod*. 1998;13:3425–30.

18. Jo YJ, Jang WI, Namgoong S, Kim NH. Actin-capping proteins play essential roles in the asymmetric division of maturing mouse oocytes. *J Cell Sci*. 2015;128:160–70.

19. Sanfins A, Plancha CE, Overstrom EW, Albertini DF. Meiotic spindle morphogenesis in in vivo and in vitro matured mouse oocytes: insights into the relationship between nuclear and cytoplasmic quality. *Hum Reprod*. 2004;19:2889–99.

20. Ciotti PM, Notarangelo L, Morselli-Labate AM, Felletti V, Porcu E, Venturoli S. First polar body morphology before ICSI is not related to embryo quality or pregnancy rate. *Hum Reprod*. 2004;19:2334–9.

21. Verlinsky Y, Lerner S, Illkevitch N, Kuznetsov V, Kuznetsov I, Cieslak J, Kuliev A. Is there any predictive value of first polar body morphology for embryo genotype or developmental potential?. *Reprod Biomed Online*. 2003;7:336–41.

22. Ebner T, Yaman C, Moser M, Sommergruber M, Feichtinger O, Tews G. Prognostic value of first polar body morphology on fertilization rate and embryo quality in intracytoplasmic sperm injection. *Hum Reprod*. 2000;15:427–30.

23. Ebner T, Moser M, Sommergruber M, Yaman C, Pfleger U, Tews G. First polar body morphology and blastocyst formation rate in ICSI patients. *Hum Reprod*. 2002;17:2415–18.

24. Ebner T, Moser M, Yaman C, Feichtinger O, Hartl J, Tews G. Elective transfer of embryos selected on the basis of first polar body morphology is associated with increased rates of implantation and pregnancy. *Fertil Steril*. 1999;72:599–603.

25. Rienzi L, Ubaldi FM, Iacobelli M, Minasi MG, Romano S, Ferrero S, et al. Significance of metaphase II human oocyte morphology on ICSI outcome. *Fertil Steril*. 2008;90:1692–1700.

26. Sousa M, Cunha M, Silva J, Oliveira E, Pinho MJ, Almeida C, et al. Ultrastructural and cytogenetic analyses of mature human oocyte dysmorphisms with respect to clinical outcomes. *J Assist Reprod Genet*. 2016;33:1041–57.

27. Ebner T, Moser M, Sommergruber M, Gaiswinkler U, Shebl O, Jesacher K, Tews G. Occurrence and developmental consequences of vacuoles throughout preimplantation development. *Fertil Steril*. 2005;83:1635–40.

28. De Sutter P, Dozortsev D, Qian C, Dhont M. Oocyte morphology does not correlate with fertilization rate and embryo quality after intracytoplasmic sperm injection. *Hum Reprod*. 1996;11:595–7.

29. Otsuki J, Nagai Y, Chiba K. Lipofuscin bodies in human oocytes as an indicator of oocyte quality. *J Assist Reprod Genet*. 2007;24:263–70.

30. Setti AS, Figueira RC, Braga DP, Colturato SS, Iaconelli AJ, Borges EJ. Relationship between oocyte abnormal morphology and intracytoplasmic sperm injection outcomes: a meta-analysis. *Eur J Obstet Gynecol Reprod Biol*. 2011;159:364–70.

31. Serhal PF, Ranieri DM, Kinis A, Marchant S, Davies M, Khadum IM. Oocyte morphology predicts outcome of intracytoplasmic sperm injection. *Hum Reprod*. 1997;12:1267–70.

32. Otsuki J, Okada A, Morimoto K, Nagai Y, Kubo H. The relationship between pregnancy outcome and smooth endoplasmic reticulum clusters in MII human oocytes. *Hum Reprod*. 2004;19:1591–7.

33. Akarsu C, Cağlar G, Vicdan K, Sözen E, Biberoğlu K. Smooth endoplasmic reticulum aggregations in all retrieved oocytes causing recurrent multiple anomalies: case report. *Fertil Steril*. 2009;92:1496.e1–e3.

34. Mateizel I, Van LL, Tournaye H, Verheyen G. Deliveries of normal healthy babies from embryos originating from oocytes showing the presence of smooth endoplasmic reticulum aggregates. *Hum Reprod*. 2013;28:2111–17.

35. Shaw-Jackson C. Implications on IVF patient care of discarding oocytes affected by smooth endoplasmic reticulum aggregates as recommended by the Alpha/ESHRE consensus. *J Assist Reprod Genet*. 2015;32:1705–6.

36. Shaw-Jackson C, Thomas AL, Van BN, Ameye L, Colin J, Bertrand E, et al. Oocytes affected by smooth endoplasmic reticulum aggregates: to discard or not to discard? *Arch Gynecol Obstet*. 2016;294:175–84.

37. Lazzaroni-Tealdi E, Barad DH, Albertini DF, Yu Y, Kushnir VA, Russell H, et al. Oocyte scoring enhances embryo-scoring in predicting pregnancy chances with IVF where it counts most. *PLoS ONE*. 2015;10:e0143632.

38. Bartolacci A, Intra G, Coticchio G, Aquila M dell', Patria G, Borini A. Does morphological assessment predict oocyte developmental competence? A systematic review and proposed score. *J Assist Reprod Gen*. 2022;39:3–17.

Appendix

Appendix Table 8.1. Studies reporting a negative impact of different oocyte dysmorphisms on fertilization rate

Dysmorphism	References							
	[28]	[13]	[22]	[32]	[5, 27]	[14]	[25]	[30]
Dark cytoplasm	—	—	—	n.a.	n.a.	—	—	—
Central granularity	—	—	—	n.a.	n.a.	—	—	—
SER clusters	n.a.	n.a.	n.a.	—	✓	n.a.	—	n.a.
Refractile bodies	—	—	—	n.a.	n.a.	n.a.	—	✓
Vacuoles	—	n.a.	n.a.	n.a.	✓	—	✓	✓
Abnormal oocyte shape	—	—	n.a.	n.a.	n.a.	—	—	n.a.
Abnormal zona	—	—	—	n.a.	n.a.	—	—	n.a.
Large PVS	n.a.	—	n.a.	n.a.	n.a.	—	—	✓
Large 1st PB	n.a.	n.a.	✓	n.a.	n.a.	n.a.	n.a.	✓

Legend: ✓ = detected; — = not detected; n.a. = not assessed

Appendix Table 8.2. Studies reporting a negative impact of different oocyte dysmorphisms on embryo development rate or quality

Dysmorphism	References							
	[28]	[31]	[13]	[22]	[5]	[14]	[25]	[37]
Dark cytoplasm	—	n.a.	—	—	n.a.	✓	—	n.a.
Central granularity	—	—	—	—	n.a.	—	✓	n.a.
SER clusters	n.a.	n.a.	n.a.	n.a.	✓	n.a.	—	n.a.
Refractile bodies	—	—	—	—	n.a.	n.a.	—	n.a.
Vacuoles	—	—	n.a.	n.a.	—	—	—	n.a.
Abnormal oocyte shape	—	n.a.	—	n.a.	n.a.	—	—	n.a.
Abnormal zona	—	n.a.	—	—	n.a.	—	—	n.a.
Large PVS	n.a.	n.a.	—	n.a.	n.a.	—	—	n.a.
Overall oocyte score	n.a.	n.a.	n.a.	n.a.	n.a.	n.a.	n.a.	✓

Legend: ✓ = detected; — = not detected; n.a. = not assessed

Appendix Table 8.3. Studies reporting a negative impact of different oocyte dysmorphisms on implantation rate

Dysmorphism	References							
	[31]	[13]	[32]	[5]	[15]	[10]	[25]	[37]
Dark cytoplasm	n.a.	—	n.a.	n.a.	—	n.a.	n.a.	n.a.
Central granularity	✓	—	n.a.	n.a.	—	n.a.	n.a.	n.a.
SER clusters	n.a.	n.a.	✓	—	n.a.	n.a.	n.a.	n.a.
Refractile bodies	✓	—	n.a.	n.a.	n.a.	n.a.	n.a.	n.a.
Vacuoles	✓	n.a.	n.a.	—	n.a.	n.a.	n.a.	n.a.
Abnormal oocyte shape	n.a.	—	n.a.	n.a.	n.a.	n.a.	n.a.	n.a.
Abnormal zona	n.a.	—	n.a.	n.a.	n.a.	✓	n.a.	n.a.
Large PVS	n.a.	—	n.a.	n.a.	—	n.a.	n.a.	n.a.
Overall oocyte score	n.a.	n.a.	n.a.	n.a.	n.a.	n.a.	✓	✓

Legend: ✓ = detected; — = not detected; n.a. = not assessedSummary

Prospects for Bioenergetics for Embryo Selection

Jonathan Van Blerkom

9.1 Introduction

The observer-based detection of seemingly abnormal cytoplasmic phenotypes ("dysmorphisms") in human metaphase II (MII) oocytes, and apparently aberrant patterns or ill-timing of developmentally essential stage-specific events during preimplantation embryogenesis (e.g. pronuclear membrane dissolution, uniform cytokinesis, morulation, and blastocyst formation), have formed the empirical basis of competence assessments. These observations have been used to guide oocyte and embryo selection in order to increase the likelihood of implantation and continued progression through gestation.

Such developmental selection criteria have been an integral part of clinical IVF since its inception over 40 years ago [1–8]. More recently, schemes to assess developmental competence using commercial time-lapse imaging systems allow continuous rather than static evaluation of the embryo during the preimplantation stages and are being used to complement or even replace embryologist-based assessments. Algorithms for embryo selection for transfer use similar, long-standing morphological characteristics but add an additional temporal and morphokinetic dimension from continuous monitoring that is not possible using snapshot static inspections even when these are timed to coincide with anticipated critical developmental landmarks [9]. Both static and dynamic imaging of development have supporters and detractors as to their actual power in assessing competence [10, 11, 12] and debate continues as to which specific characteristics are unambiguously associated with competence and outcome [13]. For the oocyte, however, time-lapse images offer little more than direct microscopic observations when used to select/deselect MII oocytes for insemination by intracytoplasmic sperm injection (ICSI). This is because the ooplasm appears largely static at MII and dysmorphisms and other cytoplasmic anomalies are already present if the oocyte has developed to this stage [1].

The developmental significance of empirical findings derived from outcome studies has provided some degree of validation for certain oocyte cytoplasmic phenotypes and temporal, morphological, and morphokinetic aspects of preimplantation embryogenesis employed to select for fertilization and embryo transfer. The recent application of deep DNA sequencing methods to preimplantation stage embryos that can detect aneuploidy and structural variants within the genome (e.g. duplications, deletions, inversions, and insertions) has become an important means of reducing "time to pregnancy" by allowing embryos to be ranked according to euploidy. While chromosomally abnormal embryos can self-identify through structural defects or arrested development prior to the morula stage, others can develop into apparently morphologically normal blastocysts capable of hatching within an expected time frame. However, the notion of selecting oocytes or embryos on the basis of markers of competence has been challenged by recent reports that embryos deemed likely to be compromised based on empirical criteria or DNA structural defects, including genetic mosaicism, have resulted in normal births [14]. It remains to be determined whether refinements in time-lapse imaging algorithms may offer more precise clues than currently exist for the detection of aneuploidy and other chromosomal defects that would negatively affect outcome in those embryos that outwardly appear to develop normally through the preimplantation stages.

Regardless of the method of competence assessment by observer-dependent or independent means, a fundamental question in understanding the biological basis of developmental competence is the extent to which the diverse cellular and chromosomal phenotypes observed for the human oocyte and embryo might have a common origin. It is in this context that the main theme of this chapter focuses on why "energy" has become such a key element in understanding how competence is established and maintained, and how this understanding has led to new methodologies in clinical IVF that can assess bioenergetic states associated with performance during the preimplantation stages and, more importantly, outcome.

9.2 Cellular Bioenergetics as the Driving Force in the Establishment of Developmental Competence

9.2.1 Historical Perspective on Cellular Bioenergetics and Developmental Competence

Cellular bioenergetics, which refers to the state of energy supply and demand at any specific stage during oogenesis or preimplantation embryogenesis, has long been suspected to be a primary driver of developmental competence in human IVF [15, 16] and has been proposed to offer the basis of a potential noninvasive biomarker of developmental competence [17]. Indeed, metabolic aspects of oogenesis that affect in vitro maturation and preimplantation embryogenesis have attracted growing interest as potential determinants of developmental success or failure and as possible causes of chromosomal abnormalities [18]. However, the availability of methods and instruments suitable for use in IVF programmes will be required if metabolic state analysis is to find a place. The following describes what cellular energy means in the context of developmental competence and why mitochondria have become the principal focus in this regard [19].

9.2.2 The Basis and Consequent Deficiencies of Bioenergetics

The biological basis for bioenergetics as a primary force in the establishment of developmental competence for the oocyte and the embryo from fertilization through gestation is that mitochondria are the primary source of high-energy nucleotide triphosphates such as ATP and GTP, whose production and utilization defines biogenetic state. This notion appears reasonable considering that energy deficiencies where cellular supply cannot meet demand are known to contribute directly or indirectly to a wide

variety of pathophysiologies such as neuropathies and myopathies, and diseases ranging from Alzheimer's to cancer [20–23]. Over a hundred defects in the oxidative phosphorylation process (OXPHOS diseases) that are known to impact the electron transport system result from pathogenic mitochondrial DNA (mtDNA) mutations that occur in the oocyte [24, 25]. These are transmitted to the offspring by virtue of the exclusive maternal inheritance of mitochondria. The degree to which normal bioenergetics are affected by such mtDNA mutations is highly variable owing to the so-called bottleneck that occurs during early oogenesis when the initial mitochondrial complement in the primordial germ cell undergoes significant numerical expansion.

The inheritance of a pathogenic mtDNA mutation is not necessarily uniform: oocytes with a single mtDNA genotype are said to be homoplastic while those with a wild and mutant genotype are termed heteroplasmic. The developmental and clinical consequences can be unpredictable, ranging from none to ultimately lethal, depending upon the magnitude of the mutant load, that is, the ratio of mutant to wild type genomes. Above certain mutation-specific thresholds these can be lethal during gestation or the cause of serious, if not life-threatening metabolic diseases (OXPHOS diseases) in affected individuals due to depressed bioenergetic capacity at critical high-energy-requiring developmental stages. The occurrence of bioenergetic deficiencies arising from OXPHOS diseases in young individuals and an age-related decline in overall cellular bioenergetic efficiency attributed to progressive mitochondrial dysfunction are the foundational biological principles of current research into determinants of developmental competence and normality from oocyte through early embryogenesis and subsequent gestation to birth.

9.3 What Is Cellular Energy in the Context of Developmental Competence in Clinical IVF?

While it is generally understood that a relationship exists between energy and outcome, there is perhaps less familiarity as to how energy is actually utilized at the subcellular level to support normal developmental competence. To better understand the basis of various methodologies designed to assess metabolism in individual oocytes and preimplantation stage for selective purposes, a brief discussion follows of the role of cellular bioenergetics as it applies to clinical IVF.

9.3.1 Cellular Bioenergetics and Its Role in Clinical IVF

While mitochondria are almost universally described as energy factories or the "powerhouses" of cells, a more apt analogy might view them as "mini-transformers" in the sense that they convert metabolites such as glucose, pyruvate, and certain fatty acids into high-energy nucleotides with ATP usually considered the primary currency of cellular energy. In this regard, it is also important to recognize that other nucleotide triphosphates such as GTP have specialized and critical roles in supporting normal cell functions that can impact developmental competence. A seemingly common misconception related to energetic issues that may affect oocytes and preimplantation embryos is that ATP can be considered a storage form of energy that is stable, long-lived, and therefore available as needed. However, under normal physiological conditions, the half-life of cytoplasmic ATP is measured in seconds, and is typically converted by

hydrolysis into a lower-energy form, ADP, in close proximity to its site of generation, the mitochondria. Where extracellular ATP exists, its half-life is measured in minutes with hydrolysis to ADP, AMP, and adenosine brought about by plasma membrane-bound ectonucleotidases.

The conversion of metabolic substrates (e.g. glucose) into high-energy nucleotides through a respiratory chain complex that resides in mitochondria involves discrete and well-defined steps in an electron transport process whose output is optimized by the availability of oxygen through an oxidative phosphorylation pathway (Figure 9.1). Because the attachment of a third phosphate group to a nucleotide (e.g. adenosine or guanine) is a higher-energy-requiring process than adding the first (AMP) or second (ADP) phosphate group, its removal during the hydrolysis of ATP to ADP, for example, frees the energy stored in this phosphor-anhydride bond, which is then transformed into biomechanical and biochemical work. The notion of energy in terms of a work function is essential in understanding causes of "systems failures" due to, for example, bioenergetic deficits that impact fertility at the gamete and embryonic levels.

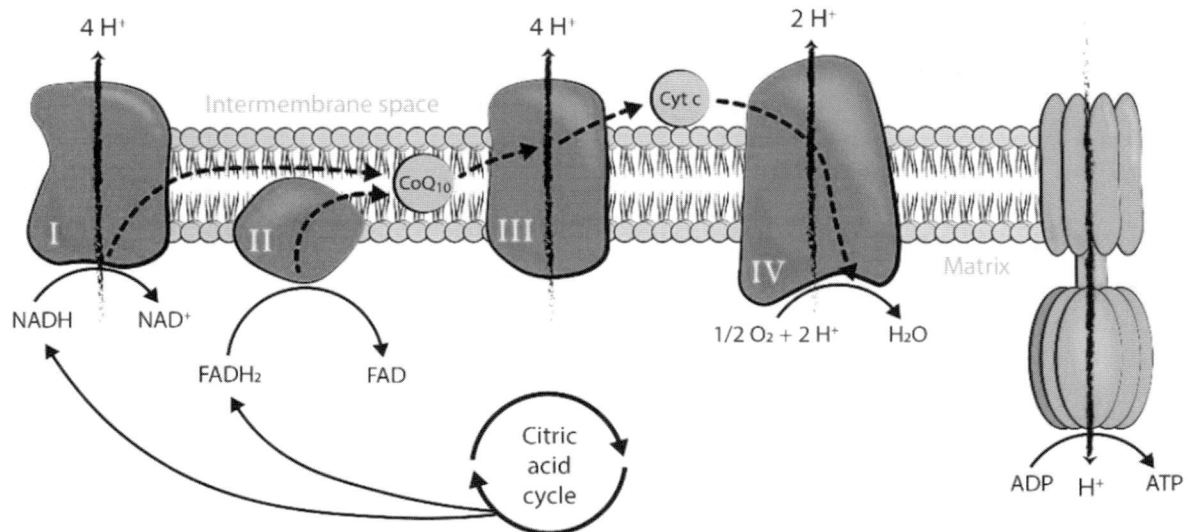

Figure 9.1 Production of adenosine triphosphate (ATP) by oxidative phosphorylation coupled to the mitochondrial electron transport chain

The four enzymatic complexes (I, II, III, and IV) and ATP synthase are represented in the inner mitochondrial membrane. ADP: adenosine diphosphate; Pi (inorganic phosphate); H^+: hydrogen ion (proton); NADH: nicotinamide adenine dinucleotide, reduced form; $FADH_2$: flavin adenine dinucleotide, oxidized form; O_2: oxygen; H_2O: water; Cyt c: cytochrome c; CoQ10: coenzyme Q10. In: Rodríguez-Varela C, Labarta E. Clinical application of antioxidants to improve human oocyte mitochondrial function: a review. *Antioxidants*. 2020;9(12):1197 (Fig. 1).

In cells, the hydrolysis of ATP (or GTP) is not spontaneous nor is this molecule as long-lived as it might be in an aqueous solution. Typically, its energy-relating hydrolysis to ADP is coupled with energy-dependent biological activities that can be generally considered to be "thermodynamically unfavorable," meaning that in the absence of an energy source, they fail to function, and cellular pathology or death can ensue. ATP-dependent "unfavorable" activities in the plasma membrane of cells that would also apply to oocytes and preimplantation embryos include the functional maintenance of (a) ion pumps, (e.g. Ca, K, Na), (b) water channels (aquaporins), (c) transporters (e.g. for glucose, amino acids, proteins), and (d) transmembrane receptors that involve cytosolic enzymatic reactions that activate signal transduction pathways or affect cytostructural stability and dynamics. For ATP-dependent processes, normal function requires the free energy released from the hydrolysis of ATP to be available at an ATP-binding domain with some classes of protein involved in essential cell processes containing an ATPase domain as well. Inorganic phosphate (Pi) liberated during hydrolysis is hydrated and used by molecules requiring phosphate, such as kinases, or recycled during the generation of new ATP molecules. Similar activities drive enzymatic reactions and non-G-protein signaling pathways within the cytoplasm.

Chemical energy is utilized to stabilize thermodynamically unstable reactions, which require such energy to promote and maintain their normal function (e.g. enzymes, cell membrane receptors, transporters, and proteins-involved signal transduction pathways). Mechanical energy is used to maintain cytoplasmic organization and cytoskeletal architecture and promote dynamic reorganizations that include normally occurring redistributions of subcellular components that include mitochondria, as well as pathways of vesicular traffic that are mediated by cytostructural elements such as actin microfilaments, microtubules, and associated motor proteins. The normal segregation of chromosomes during meiosis I and II in the oocyte and mitotic divisions in the preimplantation embryo is a primary example of mechanical energy utilization.

In the context of chemical- and mechanical-energy-requiring processes, ATP is widely held to be the fundamental currency of cellular bioenergetics arising primarily from mitochondria, with the highest levels generated by oxidative phosphorylation by

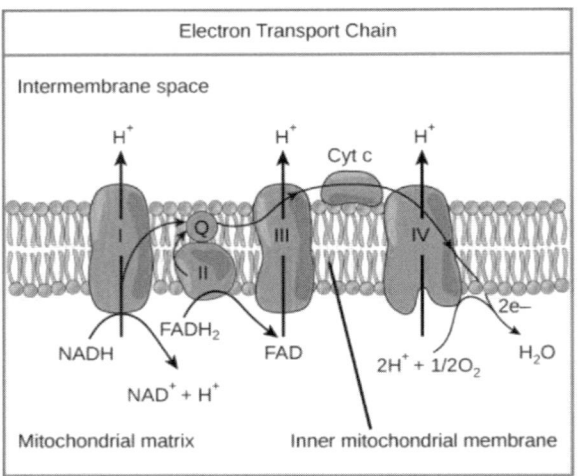

Figure 9.2 The electron transport chain is a series of electron transporters embedded in the inner mitochondrial membrane that shuttles electrons from NADH and FADH$_2$ to molecular oxygen. In the process, protons are pumped from the mitochondrial matrix to the intermembrane space, and oxygen is reduced to form water. In: https://openstax.org/books/biology/, Figure 7-10.

means of an electron transport chain located on the inner mitochondrial membrane (the cristae) (Figure 9.2). A secondary source derives from the citric acid cycle (also known as TCA or the Krebs cycle) in the mitochondrial matrix and occurs by means of the beta-oxidation of catabolized fatty acids. The flow of electrons from one protein to another in this membrane-bound transport chain complex promotes the pumping of protons across the inner mitochondrial membrane that establishes a chemiosmotic gradient whose magnitude, commonly denoted as $\Delta\Psi m$, is directly associated with the level of ATP production. The relative magnitude of this gradient can be approximated with mitochondria-specific fluorescent dyes such as JC1 to provide an indirect indication of the metabolic status of cytoplasm for oocytes and preimplantation stage embryos [18, 26–30] but its use clinically for selective purposes may be problematic owing to potential phototoxicity from UV excitation.

While ATP is the most abundant species supporting energy-requiring cell functions, other mitochondrially derived nucleotide triphosphates have critical bioenergetic and regulatory functions as well, such as GTP that is involved in the polymerization of spindle microtubules and the normal function of G-proteins. G-proteins represent a large family of GTP-dependent cell membrane receptors acting as "molecular switches" for signal transduction pathways by which extrinsic signals are transmitted internally from the plasma membrane to elicit a specific cytoplasmic or nuclear genomic response. CTP, TTP, and UTP have essential, albeit less, bioenergetic roles by serving as substrates for DNA and RNA biosynthesis. In addition, CTP is involved in posttranslational modifications such as glycosylation, and UTP is involved in glycogen synthesis and galactose metabolism, to mention a few of their functions.

9.4 Mitochondria as the Essential Energy Generator That Establishes Developmental Competence

Mitochondria are structurally complex organelles that likely originated as prokaryotes (α-proteobacteria) that entered primitive eukaryotic cells as an endosymbiotic organism some 1.45 billion years ago. Mitochondrial DNA (mtDNA) is a circular, double-stranded genome containing 16 569 base pairs encoding 37 genes: 2 RNAs, 22 tRNAs, and 13 proteins necessary for respiratory chain function. A 1 100 base pair region referred to as the D-loop (displacement loop) is a noncoding site that serves as the origin of mtDNA replication and the initiation of transcription for both heavy and light strands. In an evolutionary context and unlike its nuclear counterpart, mtDNA has remained largely unchanged with nearly all of the 1 300 proteins that comprise a human mitochondrion encoded by nuclear genes. In this sense, defects in mitochondrial function of nuclear origin could result from mutations that produce (a) functionally defective chaperones that normally vector proteins to mitochondria; (b) defects in the signal peptide that permits protein passage through the outer mitochondrial membrane, and for the preimplantation embryo; (c) structurally altered proteins that cannot promote transformational changes from the relatively low-activity "condensed" form that occurs in the oocyte and pre-blastocyst embryo to the more familiar (i.e. described in textbooks) elongated, structurally developed, and metabolically active "orthodox" form typical of somatic cells and the trophectoderm at the blastocyst stage [31, 32].

Since they represent the primary source of cellular energy, studies of stage-related changes in mitochondrial structure, function, and activity have become a nexus of interest with respect to the establishment and maintenance of developmental competence for the oocyte and preimplantation stage embryo.

9.4.1 Mitochondria Function and Dysfunction Relating to Development

Clinically, the relevant question is the extent to which putative bioenergetic deficits might be a proximal cause of infertility in women in general and, in particular, for those who require technological interventions by medically assisted conception. For the oocyte, early developmental defects and dysfunctions associated with a subthreshold numerical complement of organelles may compromise the normality of preovulatory oocyte meiotic maturation or development from fertilization through the pre- and early postimplantation stages. Because the number of mitochondria (as opposed to mtDNA copy number) is fixed in the MII oocyte, and significant replication (biogenesis) does not begin until well after implantation, a robust mechanism would seem to be required to allow approximately equivalent numerical distributions between daughter cells during the early cleavage stages when the structural organization and bioenergetic output of mitochondria is poorly developed (see Section 9.6). Unequal or disproportionate inheritance between blastomeres beginning at the first cleavage division may be a naturally occurring phenomenon in which blastomeres with inherited mitochondrial complements that fall below a threshold needed to provide sufficient levels of ATP and GTP are unable to progress as normal developmental processes are adversely affected.

Such disproportionate mitochondrial segregation between blastomeres has been identified in whole embryos and in isolated blastomeres of nascent human embryos by quantifying fluorescent intensities emitted by mitochondria-specific reporters followed by quantification of ATP levels in each corresponding cell [33]. These investigators reported that mitochondrial mass, estimated by quantification of fluorescent intensity, was directly related to cytoplasmic ATP content and differentially affected cytokinesis and blastomere fate. Early blastomeres with putative lower mitochondrial contents ceased dividing by the 4-cell stage, while others from the same embryo with higher intensities, presumed to reflect a relatively higher mitochondrial mass, continued to divide producing embryos with unequally sized blastomeres. The larger cells remained undivided or subsequently underwent lysis often resulting in a nonviable embryo.

Determining a blastomere-specific estimation of mitochondrial mass and associated bioenergetic status of individual cells may be useful for diagnostic purposes in instances of cleavage arrest or maturation or fertilization failure but not for selection for transfer or cryopreservation as mitochondria-specific fluorescent probes may not be suitable for clinical application in IVF. In addition, developmentally significant levels of disproportionate mitochondrial segregation between blastomeres would not be detectable by the noninvasive analytical methods discussed in Section 9.6 that use the intact, whole embryo to measure ATP levels, and detect oxygen depletion from culture medium or Raman spectroscopy to identify competence-related molecular by-products of metabolism. Van Blerkom et al. (2000) [33] reported that the net embryo mitochondrial fluorescent intensity and ATP concentrations of embryos showing disproportionate segregation at the blastomere level were largely similar to their counterparts showing uniform distributions; the difference for the former related solely to the dynamics of mitochondrial segregation.

9.4.2 Noninvasive Approaches to Assess Mitochondria Dispositions

Noninvasive methods currently used to estimate mitochondrial metabolism, organization, and function(s) in mammalian cells are currently under development for competence selection of human oocytes and preimplantation embryos in clinical IVF [34]. Some methods allow the detection of certain abnormal spatial organizations of mitochondria such as dense clustering or significant areas of reduced mitochondrial content, especially in the pericortical region, that may compromise meiotic maturation or the normality of development after fertilization. Their detection could have a central role in oocyte selection for fertilization when ICSI is used, or in the identification of subtle causes of fertilization failure, poor morphokinetic performance, or unexpected embryo arrest during in vitro culture.

9.5 mtDNA Copy Number and Developmental Competence

One early notion in clinical IVF was that developmental competence was directly related to mtDNA copy number in the oocyte [35] and preimplantation

stage embryo [36]. Here, it is important to emphasize that copy number is not equivalent to, or a proxy for, mitochondrial mass, that is, the actual number of organelles in the MII oocyte and cells of the preimplantation stage embryo. In this context, subnormal mtDNA content has been indicated as a cause of failed meiotic maturation, fertilization, or arrested cell divisions. Unusually high mtDNA copy numbers, especially at the blastocyst stage, may be developmentally toxic, presumably as a consequence of abnormally high levels of ATP generation when accompanied by corresponding levels of damaging reactive oxygen species that overwhelm any endogenous capacity for their neutralization (for review see [13, 27, 37]. However, whether mtDNA copy number is unambiguously related to outcome is currently a contentious issue given positive outcomes where mtDNA quantitation is indicated to be problematic in this regard.

With respect to normal developmental competence and mitochondria in general, and mtDNA content more specifically, levels are typically measured at the expanded blastocyst stage as an adjunct to preimplantation genetic testing for aneuploidy and structural defects (translocations, inversions, duplications, etc.) or known single-gene mutations. The utility of mtDNA quantitation in IVF for embryo selection to improve outcomes is unsettled as to its accuracy in predicting blastocyst developmental potential after transfer. Several large-scale studies indicate that mtDNA contents above a suggested threshold level have failed to confirm initially sanguine reports that this could be a definitive biomarker of competence [38, 39]. Because the methodology of mtDNA quantitation has often differed between reports that either support, or failed to confirm, copy number as a measure of competence at the blastocyst stage, and that outcome results based on mtDNA findings have been inconsistent, its value as a proxy for metabolism and developmental potential remains unclear. However, current indications suggest it may not be as robust a biomarker as previously thought for the peri-implantation stage human embryo [40, 41]. It is worth noting that the drive to improve outcome in human IVF in general has a history of promising methodologies that have failed to live up to their initial enthusiasm either because they are less than definitive for competence assessment, or not practical for most programmes given the considerable expense and complexity of instrumentation required.

The oocyte is the source of all mitochondria through the preimplantation and early postimplantation stages.

The mtDNA copy number and actual mitochondrial numbers in developmentally competent, fully grown, meiotically mature human oocytes has been confusing when a one-to-one correspondence has often been implied. Estimates have varied widely from 10 000 or less to over 100 000 actual organelles based on similar mtDNA values [37]. From transmission electron micrographs of MII human oocytes, including some of the earliest taken, it was obvious that such a correspondence was unlikely when genomic copy numbers in the hundreds of thousands or nearly one million were reported. However, a reasonable question to ask in the context of competence is whether there is a threshold mtDNA copy number for the human MII oocytes below which development is compromised? Some interesting findings in this regard that may be relevant for the human were reported by Wai et al. (2010) [42] for the mouse oocyte and embryo. They found that while as few as 4 000 mtDNA copies were consistent with fertilization and normal development through the preimplantation stages, 40 000–50 000 copies at MII was a "critical threshold" required for normal postimplantation embryogenesis. For the human, 100 000 copies at MII have been one critical threshold suggested for normal embryogenesis although higher levels have been indicated, such as described in the study by Santos et al. (2006) [43], where a mean copy number around 250 000 was considered consistent with fertilization and normal preimplantation embryogenesis. However, others have reported significantly lower levels in this regard [44]. Consequently, a distinction between mtDNA and mitochondrial numbers (i.e., mass) is often confused because early suggestions that each mitochondrion in a human MII oocyte contained a single genome are incorrect. However, what needs to be determined unambiguously, if findings from other species also apply to the human, is the minimal mtDNA copy and the minimal mitochondrial numbers compatible with meiotic maturation, fertilization, and pre-and early postimplantation embryogenesis.

9.5.1 Stage-Specific Spatial Reorganization of Mitochondria and Developmental Competence

Studies from this author's laboratory have indicated that spatial differences in cytoplasmic bioenergetics

likely occur in mouse oocytes, which are related to fertilizability [45, 46], and in which elevated levels of ATP generation are associated with mitochondria located directly below the oolemma, perhaps owing to proximity to the source of diffused oxygen. More recently, we revisited this notion by asking whether it may also manifest as corresponding higher temperatures in human oocytes that could be estimated using a permeable chemical intracellular thermometer ([47]: Cellular Thermoprobes, funakoshi.co.jp) whose fluorescent emission wavelength is a function of temperature calculated from 36.5° C (blue) to 37.5° C (red) by scanning laser confocal microscopic-derived color spectrum of temperature versus emission wavelength. The highest apparent temperature (red) was observed just beneath the oolemma (Figure 9.3: arrows, panels A, B) and at a somewhat lower level in dense mitochondrial clusters or aggregates (green/yellow: asterisks, panels A, B). The negative effect on competence associated with the presence of relatively large mitochondrial aggregates [29] may involve a change in local intracellular pH owing to higher levels of ATP hydrolysis, which can upregulate ATP production within the aggregate by virtue of increasing proton flow across the inner mitochondrial membrane [48]. Although speculative at present, it is an interesting possibility that the negative effects on competence described when such aggregates occur [29] could be associated with a change in local ambient redox potential that may perturb corresponding redox-sensitive signaling pathways [49].

The oocyte in panel A was cultured in an atmosphere of 6% CO_2, 5% O_2, and the balance N_2, while the one in panel B was cultured in room air. The higher oxygen concentration in room air was associated with "warmer" mitochondria occurring throughout the cytoplasm rather than being largely restricted to the subplasmalemmal cytoplasm. An oxygen concentration effect was a consistent finding suggesting that higher levels may more deeply diffuse into the ooplasm and upregulate respiratory activity in mitochondria that ordinarily would be less active.

Further supporting a physiological relationship between mitochondrial activity and cytoplasmic bioenergetics are findings that stage-specific ATP "bursts" occur during meiotic maturation of the mouse oocyte that are spatially localized and likely driven by corresponding, transient changes in local free calcium [50]. These bursts were stage and spatially related and developmentally significant with

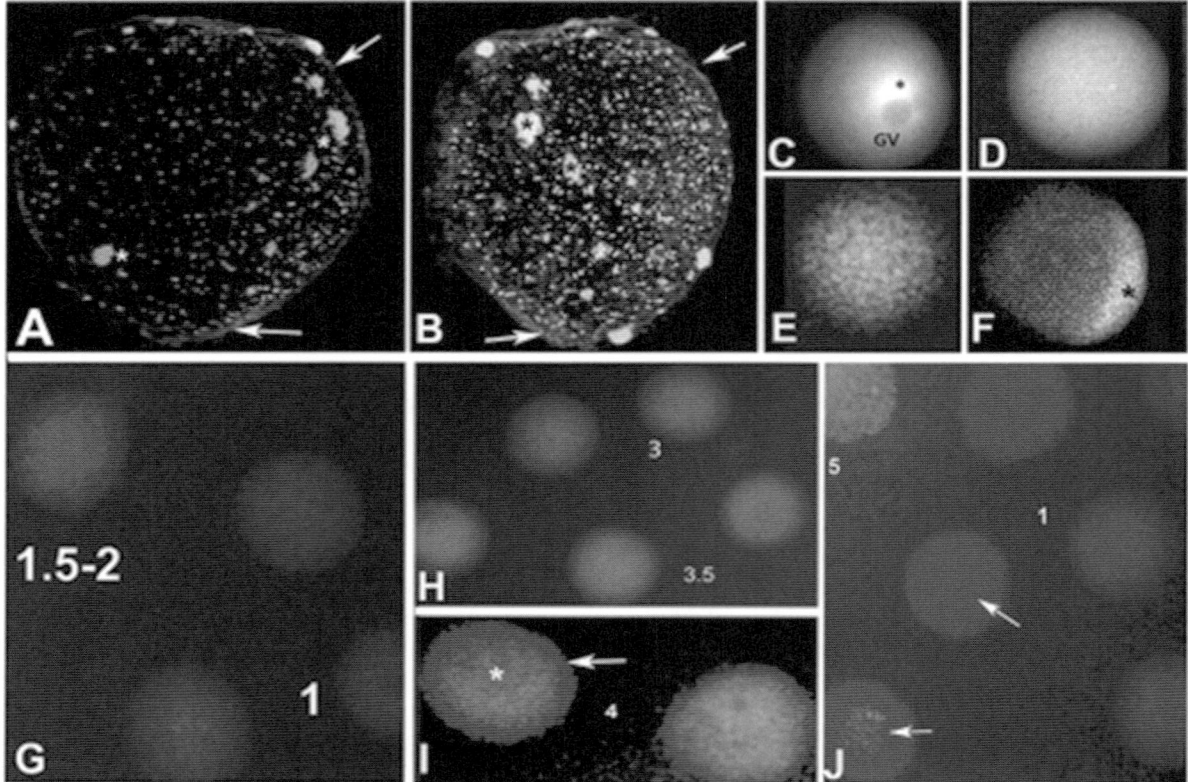

Figure 9.3 Panels A and B are images of a hemisphere of human MII oocytes showing differential intracellular temperatures revealed with a cell-permeable chemical intracellular thermometer whose fluorescent emission wavelength is a function of temperature. The temperature in the subplasmalemmal cytoplasm where a circumferential domain of high polarized mitochondria reside is slightly higher (arrows, red) than mitochondria in small clusters within the cytoplasm (green). The asterisks indicate larger mitochondrial aggregates that appear slightly warmer than those in smaller clusters. The oocyte in panel A was cultured in an atmosphere of 5% oxygen while the one in panel B was cultured in room air (~20% oxygen). The effect of the higher oxygen concentration is evident by the occurrence of red fluorescent mitochondria within the cytoplasm indicating that a higher intracellular availability of oxygen may upregulate mitochondrial respiratory activity and ATP production that would seem to be manifested by increases in temperature.
Panels C–J: Autofluorescent detection of NADH/NADPH in cohorts of human MII oocytes indicates differential intensities that can be related to ATP content and provide an indication of relative bioenergetic state. Panels C–D show typical autofluorescent phenotypes from a relatively uniform distribution (D) to one with numerous aggregates (E), or asymmetric localization (asterisk, F). The asterisk in panel C shows the typical pregerminal vesicle breakdown perinuclear accumulation of mitochondria.
Panels G–J indicate relative autofluorescent intensities in unfertilized human oocytes on a scale of 1 to 5 where 1 is the least intense and 5 the highest. These intensities were correlated with net ATP content and developmental performance in vitro after artificial (parthenogenetic) activation (see text for details). The arrows in panel J indicate small clusters/aggregates of mitochondria that can be detected by this autofluorescence method.

respect to competence as they occurred in mitochondrial clusters in which actin microfilaments were involved in their formation. For detection, the authors used the well-known bioluminescence produced by firefly luciferase, the same enzyme used to measure ATP in oocyte lysates in a luminometer using an ATP-driven luciferin-luciferase assays [51]. ATP bursts were imaged by the expression of luciferase after the injection at the GV stage of luciferase cRNA, a synthetic RNA molecule transcribed in vitro from a specific single-stranded DNA template. What these findings indicate is that the bioenergetic state of the ooplasm is not uniform and constant but rather dynamic with respect to stage and location; and that this state corresponds to important developmental events such as oocyte maturation and fertilization as supply and demand needs change during the cell cycle or as intercellular interactions/ communication develop.

The ability to detect and follow such changes at the single-cell level in living oocytes and early embryos on an ongoing basis during meiotic maturation, fertilization or cleavage has a high potential to (a) produce significant information and new insights into the physiological basis of energy-dependent intracellular processes that can better explain the biology of normal developmental competence ([37, 52] and (b) to reveal whether and what type of aberrations are downstream causes of developmental failure. Technologies that exist for this purpose have the potential to provide useful bioenergetic information for oocytes and embryos but may be too costly or difficult to incorporate in a routine practice. However, other methods for metabolic/bioenergetic assessments may be better suited in this regard, and can add a bioenergetic dimension to current selection criteria.

9.6 Oxygen Consumption Rates

Bioenergetic parameters associated with competence, such as net cytoplasmic ATP content, can be determined quantitatively for whole oocytes or embryos by direct measurements using ATP-dependent bio- or chemo-luminescence detected by a luminometer after destructive cell lysis. Obviously, this would be impossible in a clinical IVF setting for selection. However, similar measurements can be made noninvasively with using current metabolic analyzers that measure oxygen consumption rate (OCR) such as Agilent's Seahorse XF analyzers that are both highly sensitive and able to distinguish between glycolysis and mitochondrial respiration. The Seahorse instrument is widely used in research settings and measures fluxes in oxygen consumption and extracellular acidification rates (measure of proton efflux) to determine levels of ATP production. One drawback related to its use in a routine clinical IVF setting is cost and appropriate expertise that would generally be necessary, despite available analytical software. Nevertheless, in situ, noninvasive OCR measurements using sensitive oxygen microelectrodes is a well-recognized biomarker of metabolic activity for cultured cells, but for oocytes and preimplantation embryos, whether similar measurements can truly reflect developmental competence that improve outcome at a sufficiently high-confidence level to support its use remains to be determined. In this regard, it is encouraging that some early findings suggest an answer in the affirmative.

Muller et al. (2019) [53] used Seahorse technology to assess OCR in mammalian oocytes (bovine, mouse, and human) and embryos (bovine) and reported reproducible differences in respiration during meiotic maturation of the oocyte and preimplantation embryogenesis. These differences are likely directly related to overall mitochondrial bioenergetic activity and differential levels of ATP generation at specific stages for these two critical developmental phases. This is an important study because it demonstrates the sensitivity of this technology and shows that sequentially timed measurements can be made at certain landmark events such as germinal vesicle breakdown, polar body extrusion at MII for the oocyte and for the embryo, the morula-to-blastocyst transition, or at blastocyst "hatching." Furthermore, these authors noted (a) that oocyte bioenergetic levels could be assessed in both intact (cumulus enclosed) and denuded bovine oocytes and (b) the conditions used for OCR and ATP measurements were not toxic for fertilization and preimplantation development. That said, in clinical application for selective purposes, denuded oocytes would likely be candidates of choice because maturational status and the normality of cytoplasmic organization can be readily assessed and then, if necessary, further analysis by OCR methodology could be employed. Similar studies were reported for zebrafish embryos that showed no toxic effects of repeated OCR measurements during development with the Seahorse instrument [54].

Another promising, noninvasive method to assess oxidative phosphorylation rates in oocytes and preimplantation embryos that may have application in clinical IVF was described by Obeidat et al. (2018) [55]. Their design uses a novel "three electrode Clark sensor system" that was effective for assessing mitochondrial respiration in bovine and equine oocytes, and bovine embryos at the single oocyte/embryo level in microliter volumes. Based on animal studies, its construction and sensitivity clearly indicate a potential application in human IVF for oocyte and preimplantation embryo selection but, similar to other noninvasive methods for respiration-based competence assessment, threshold values will need to be determined with respect to outcome. Moreover, while efficacy has been shown, safety for human use will have to be demonstrated. However, an evaluation of the methodology and current findings suggest it may well have a place in IVF programs when standardized for setup, operation, and data analysis.

9.6.1 The Scanning Electrochemical Microscopic System for OCR Determination

Additional validation of OCR technology for competence determinations in clinical IVF comes from studies designed to establish the nature of a relationship between respiratory activity, mtDNA copy number, mitochondrial mass, and actual bioenergetic endpoints such as ATP content. To date, a few studies have made important contributions in this regard with another novel technology, the scanning electrochemical microscopic system (SECM) for single oocyte/embryo OCR determinations [56]. Yamanaka et al. (2011) [57] and Maezawa et al. (2014) [58] reported that differences in OCR in thawed vitrified human blastocysts related to the timing of the restoration of normal oxygen consumption could be used to identify those with the highest developmental potential. These investigators noted that inner cell mass (ICM)-containing blastocysts in the process of hatching, or which had fully hatched at specific times after thawing, had higher OCRs than those that remained zona intact. The success of hatching would likely be expected to be directly related to respiratory activity given that this morphodynamic process is energy requiring both to escape the confines of the zona pellucida and to maintain active fluid transport across the trophectoderm to keep the blastocyst cavity in an expanding state required for complete hatching and accomplishment of the alignment and adherence phases of implantation.

More recently, Morimoto et al. (2020) [59] reported that OCR rates measured by SECM were associated with a maternal-age-related decline in mitochondrial oxygen consumption that manifested morphologically as rate-limiting for the morula-to-blastocyst transition. A finding of particular relevance for competence assessments in this report was that mtDNA copy number and OCR were unrelated at any stage of preimplantation embryogenesis in their clinical IVF population from which measurements were obtained. This suggests that the well-known age-related decline in mitochondrial bioenergetic efficiency can affect embryonic stages and, as reported by Muller-Hocker et al. (1996) [60], may involve structural changes such as increased mitochondrial volume and reduced cristae numbers and size. Van Blerkom (2011) [37] proposed that if the magnitude of the polarity across the inner mitochondrial membrane ($\Delta\Psi$m) that maintains volume homeostasis does not transition to a higher state during a similar transition from a condensed to orthodox form at the end of the cleavage phase, mitochondrial swelling, internal structural disorganization, and significantly diminished ATP output would be a likely result.

Because the morphodynamic processes of the preimplantation embryo are energy-requiring and -driven processes, the simplest means of competence assessment at present for an IVF program may be observational, that is, whether embryos develop to an ICM-containing expanded blastocyst that can manifest signs of incipient hatching (e.g., the elaboration of focal transzonal cytoplasmic projections, termed zona breakers: Sathananthan et al., 2003 [61]) followed by complete, nonassisted emergence and maintenance of expansion after escape from the confines of the zona pellucida. The occurrence of focal transzonal trophectodermal projections that resemble "zona breakers" in form and kinetic activity observed in time-lapse studies of well-expanded human blastocysts reported by Van Blerkom (2019) [13] is consistent with the notion of zona breakers as a normal aspect of the hatching process in the peri-implantation human embryo. This is especially relevant where the zona may be unusually resistant to hatching for certain patients (e.g., maternal age related) or after thawing, where iatrogenic zona hardening may have occurred. In these instances, laser-assisted hatching can be beneficial but not all embryos will emerge, especially when the blastocoel has collapsed and not reformed during culture or after thawing, despite the presence of transzonal projections [13]. As noted above, Yamanaka et al. (2011) [57] and Maezawa et al. (2014) [58] used SECM methodology to show that a bioenergetic deficit existed in these situations and, even with mechanical hatching, a successful pregnancy was less likely to result, due most likely to an ATP deficiency.

The recent interest in mtDNA content in preimplantation-stage human embryos and developmental competence is controversial, but certain studies seem to shed some light on the nature of a possible relationship that is worth mentioning. The studies of Hashimoto et al. (2017) [62] were among the first to use OCR measurements based on the SECM system to correlate respiratory activity and mtDNA content during human preimplantation embryogenesis. Their findings indicate that while the mtDNA copy number during the preimplantation period could differ significantly between embryos, the mean copy number was largely stage related. A precipitous decline in mtDNA content occurred between MII and the 2-cell stage, followed by a relatively constant content at the whole embryo level up to the late morula, at which time a rise in copy number occurred in concert with blastocyst formation. This rise is temporally consistent with the similar structural development of mitochondria common during mammalian preimplantation embryogenesis as these organelles transition from a lower energetic condensed state to a higher energetic orthodox configuration. The hallmark of this transition is seen (a) structurally by their elongation and increased number of cristae that fully transverse a matrix of low electron density, and (b) by the expansion of the inner surface area of the inner mitochondrial membrane (the cristae) that is coincident with a higher $\Delta\Psi m$ state across the site of ATP generation [32, 37]. The rise in OCR begins around the morula stage before mtDNA copy numbers increase at the expanding blastocyst stage, which is consistent with the notion that it is the transition in mitochondrial structure and polarity to a higher level, rather than just more mtDNA copies alone, that contributes to the increased respiratory activity that is critically needed to support the process of blastocyst formation and associated energy-requiring morphodynamic processes.

In support of this notion are the findings of Morimoto et al. (2020) [59] that mtDNA copy number was unrelated to the maternal-age-related decline in mitochondrial oxygen consumption at any stage of preimplantation human embryogenesis. However, this would appear to conflict with the findings of Fragouli et al. (2015) [63] that mtDNA copy number increased significantly with advancing maternal age. In this regard, it may be worthwhile to examine whether mitochondrial mass and mtDNA content are related in the oocyte and preimplantation embryo with advancing maternal age if the latter is upregulated to compensate for a declining efficiency of mitochondria as suggested by Muller-Hocker et al. (1996) [60], which might include the ability to utilize ambient oxygen.

One caveat that needs to be emphasized with respect to bioenergetic assessments is that while OCR values have been shown to be a valuable biomarker of competence, if the only embryos available show subthreshold levels, in practice, their transfer would not be precluded because a normal outcome can occur based on current findings, although at a reduced probability.

9.7 Raman Spectroscopy as a Biomarker of Competence

While the results of Hashimoto et al. (2017) [62], Obeidat et al. (2018) [55], and others suggest that direct measurements of ATP production and the capacity to assess metabolic activity by OCR can be an important means for competence selection, it may not be practical in present iterations for most clinical IVF programs owing to cost, complexity, and expertise needed to assure high confidence. Raman spectroscopic analysis of spent culture media is an indirect means of metabolic profiling for competence assessment that uses unique spectral fingerprints of molecules identified from known databases. One limitation of this analytical method is associated with the physics of detection by laser-light excitation of the chemical bonds in molecules, which is reduced in low concentration because the Raman effect is induced by intense monochromatic laser light that changes in wavelength (usually in near infrared) if deflected by molecules in solution. This effect tends to be weakest for molecules at low concentration.

However, the demonstrable analytical power of Raman spectroscopy shown in other applications made it an appealing methodology for clinical IVF if it could detect molecules in spent culture media normally exported by preimplantation stage embryos during in vitro development, including those derived from metabolic processes that could be correlated with outcome alone [64, 65] or in conjunction with embryologist-based morphological observations [66]. As a potentially significant, biochemically based tool for selecting embryos within cohorts with the highest putative developmental competence, the importance of this capacity was twofold: (a) it was potentially operator-independent, that is, free of potential empirically associated (subjective) bias from observer-based morphological assessments and (b) that positive outcomes–based Raman-derived (metabolic) findings alone were largely independent of embryo performance in vitro, as characterized by the generally accepted performance morphological criteria for embryo grading [4].

Early favorable outcome results led to the introduction of a commercial instrument to generate a numerical Raman spectroscopic score using a proprietary algorithm derived from the detection of certain chemical bonds and associated molecules in spent culture media to assess the likelihood of a positive or negative outcome. Sadly, and despite initial encouraging outcome reports, the instrument that generated a numerical metabolic score that was independent of embryo development in vitro was found to be incapable of producing consistent and accurate information for competence assessment and was withdrawn from commercial sale.

From its infancy the clinical IVF field has not been immune from initial enthusiasm and excitement based on positive results for certain microscopic, biochemical, and analytical methods that were reported to significantly improve outcome, only later found to be less effective or ineffective as results from additional studies were reported. However, the biophysics of Raman spectroscopy are sound and well understood for cellular applications and, with the availability of comprehensive libraries of molecular fingerprints, offers the possibility that this method will be revisited, and its potential shown to have a role in improving outcome [66].

9.8 Noninvasive Autofluorescence as a Biomarker of Mitochondrial Bioenergetics in Clinical IVF

A potential approach to noninvasive competence selection relies on nontoxic, autofluorescence expressed by bioenergetic metabolites excited at specific wavelengths as a proxy for estimating metabolic activity that can enable the visualization of mitochondrial distributions such as those that may negatively impact on developmental competence.

One of the earliest demonstrations of the potential application of autofluorescence for continuous visualization of transient and stage-specific mitochondrial organization during the preimplantation stages was reported by Squirrell et al. (2003) [67] for rhesus monkey oocytes. They constructed a specially designed dual photon microscope at near infrared wavelength using a 1047-nm neodymium-doped, yttrium lithium fluoride-based ultrafast laser to detect mitochondrial autofluorescence. While this study was not focused on metabolic aspects of early development, it did demonstrate that mitochondria could be detected noninvasively and with no apparent toxicity to produce images very similar to those obtained in earlier studies with exposure to mitochondria-specific fluorescent stains such as rhodamine 123 ([68] Van Blerkom and Runner,

1984) or members of the MitoTracker family at specific stages of preimplantation development ([28, 33, 69]. Consistent with the report of Squirrel et al. are the findings of an intriguing study of preimplantation mouse development in vitro by Yokoo and Mori (2017) [70], who found that near-infrared laser irradiation significantly improved the quality of blastocysts and increased live birth rate with no apparent adverse effects on offspring. Whether near-infrared laser light enhancement of outcome for embryos exposed during the preimplantation stages involves a transient positive bioenergetic interaction with mitochondria is unknown, but is an interesting possibility worth investigating.

Similar to the Squirrel et al. (2003) [67] study, Sanchez et al. (2018) [71] used fluorescence lifetime imaging microscopy (FLIM) for metabolic imaging mitochondrial metabolism in mouse oocytes with normal and dysfunctional mitochondria. FLIM is a powerful quantitative technology used in cell biology for metabolic imaging of fluorophore-conjugated molecules and metabolism-associated molecules that autofluorescence at specific wavelengths [72] such as NAD (nicotinamide adenine dinucleotide), NADPH (nicotinamide adenine dinucleotide phosphate), and FAD (flavin adenine dinucleotide). Sanchez et al. (2018) [71] were able to quantify metabolic differences between wild type and mutant oocytes with dysfunctional mitochondria and detect reactive oxygen species generation at the blastocyst stage using a fluorescent ROS reporter, confirming what has been observed with cell cultures, namely, that FLIM was apparently developmentally benign for mouse embryos. As a research instrument, multiphoton microscopy using monochromatic laser light sources and bioinformatic algorithms for FLIM image analysis has clearly benefited basic cell biological studies [72]. However, issues of instrumentation cost and practicality will have to be resolved if general use in clinical IVF for competence assessment of individual oocytes and embryos is to be realized.

9.9 Application of Autofluorescence for Semiquantitative Estimations of Bioenergetic State at Relatively Low Cost for IVF Programs

We have investigated an alternative microscopic method for metabolism-associated "autofluorescence" based in part on the findings of Sikder et al. (2007) [73], who assessed mitochondrial distribution and bioenergetic activity noninvasively by live-cell imaging using conventional epifluorescence microscopy with excitation at 365 nm to visualize NADH and NADPH autofluorescence around 450 nm. They showed how this method could readily distinguish different cell types in culture solely on the basis of patterns of mitochondrial autofluorescence and changes in metabolism induced by altering culture conditions (atmosphere).

The following findings describe results to date from a pilot study to determine whether this type of imaging could be applied to human oocytes to detect (a) abnormalities in mitochondrial organization or distribution that have previously been reported to reduce developmental competence, (b) putative differences in fluorescent intensity that could be associated with bioenergetic activity, and (c) whether this method could be used in the IVF lab for selection purposes. Oocytes were chosen for the major portion of this preliminary work because they need to be denuded of cumulus and coronal cells to image the cytoplasm either for ICSI or after conventional insemination to confirm fertilization. It was also of interest to determine whether it could be a useful diagnostic of bioenergetic state in cases of failed fertilization and to assess similar metabolic activity in sibling, immature oocytes. After autofluorescent imaging, oocytes were prepared for net ATP content measurements by luciferin-luciferase chemiluminescence determinations [51].

Imaging studies were performed using the following microscopic platforms: (a) a Leica EVOS fluorescent microscope with an adjustable high-intensity LED light source with image processing and intensity quantitation using manufacturer supplied software, (b) an Olympus IX 82 widefield fluorescent microscope with imaging through a Hamamatsu OCRA R2 camera and image processing and fluorescent intensity quantification using Slidebook 6 software (3i, Denver, CO), and (c) empirical intensity estimates from a Nikon inverted microscope (Diaphot) with conventional epifluorescence and a 100-watt metal halide (mercury) lamp. While the first two microscopes are relatively costly and used primarily for research, similar intensities and mitochondrial distributions were obtained with the Nikon instrument, albeit at a somewhat lower overall intensity and resolution. For example, the images

shown in Figure 9.3 panels C–F were taken with a digital camera though a Nikon Diaphot microscope and shown unmanipulated in grayscale, which can improve resolution. For clinical IVF use, however, a high-intensity light source that is adjustable was found to be the most effective for imaging and quantifying autofluorescent intensities. Distinct differences in autofluorescence intensity were classified on a relative scale from 1 to 5 (RFI, relative fluorescent intensity) immediately prior to lysis for quantitation of net ATP content.

The RFI scale was determined across the entire oocyte at the same light level and exposure time on each microscopic platform to generate the values shown in panels G–J, with Type 1 being the lowest and Type 5 the highest. The most difficult to distinguish on each platform was Type 3 because some oocytes could be placed at the lower range of Type 4. In this instance, a value of 3.5 is assigned (panel H). Differences between Type 2 and 3 were occasionally difficult to clearly define and in these instances a 1.5 value was assigned (panel G). As discussed below, the slight differences for the 1.5 and 3.5 designations do not appear to be too relevant for competence determinations. However, with experience, intensity designations can become a routine exercise. Oocytes could be further classified by their pattern of autofluorescence as follows: (a) largely uniform intensity across the ooplasm (panel D); (b) nonuniform distributions with higher fluorescent intensity asymmetrically localized (asterisk, panel F); (c) clustered fluorescence and a low-intensity signal in the pericortical cytoplasm as indicated by an asterisk and arrow in panel I, respectively; (d) a puncta-like distribution within the cytoplasm that corresponds to mitochondria occurring in aggregates (asterisk, panel I) and less typically, panel E. These types of aggregation patterns have been described in human oocytes using mitochondria-specific fluorescent reporters [28, 29] and by transmission electron microscopy [74]. Additional support for a mitochondrial association with autofluorescence patterns is indicated by an asterisk in the GV-stage oocyte in panel C, where a pronounced perinuclear mitochondrial accumulation normally occurs prior to its breakdown [68, 75]. Of particular interest for this pilot study with respect to selection for fertilization at the oocyte stage were those exhibiting a uniform pattern of autofluorescence and based on the following bioenergetic and in vitro performance findings: Types 3–4 would be most likely to be developmentally competent in comparison to those showing heterogenous patterns of mitochondrial clustering or significant aggregation (see above in this section).

Whether NADH/NADPH autofluorescence alone could be a reasonable approximation of bioenergetic state for competence assessment was further tested by measuring ATP contents in oocytes with each numerical grade. To date, the average net ATP content (pmol/oocyte) for 139 MII oocytes showing no grossly evident cytoplasmic dysmorphisms or abnormalities that failed to fertilize after conventional IVF were as follows: (a) Types 1 and 2: 0.79–1.04, (b) Types 3 and 4: 1.24–1.63, (iii) Type 5: 2.33–2.75. These values are within the range previously measured by Van Blerkom et al. (1995) [51] for human oocytes selected only based on meiotic maturity. Types 3 and 4 were grouped together for this initial analysis. Very similar ATP values were measured in 53 immature oocytes between the GVB and MI stages that were identified at the first check for fertilization, 12–14 hours postinsemination.

Whether the excitation and emission wavelengths used in this study could be developmentally toxic could not be tested by intentionally inseminating exposed oocytes solely for experimental purposes. However, according to protocol, oocytes that were immature at follicular aspiration, but which spontaneously matured to MII could be used for such purposes under the provision that they are not inseminated. In this regard, after exposure to visualize and measure autofluorescence, oocytes were "activated" in the presence of either a calcium ionophore (A23187) or $SrCl_2$ followed by in vitro culture for up to five days. The ability to progress through the preimplantation stages in a timely manner similar to their normally fertilized counterparts was indicative of an early level of developmental competence. To date, 73% (53/64) activated with 31% (16/53) developing to an expanded blastocyst stage; all showed Type 3/4 intensity prior to activation. None classified as Type 1 or 2 progressed beyond the 6- to 10-cell stage and cell divisions were often irregular (i.e., nonuniform blastomeres). Type 5 oocytes were relatively infrequent as were Type 1, although for the latter they mostly occurred as a major portion of a patient-specific cohort where large numbers of oocytes (≥ 15) were retrieved and/or in patients with women with polycystic ovarian syndrome. In both instances, after parthenogenetic activation, none progressed

beyond the 4-cell stage. A preliminary conclusion from these findings is that bioenergetic levels below and above certain thresholds, that may be detectable by this method, are developmentally toxic.

Collectively, the findings from this pilot study suggest a developmentally relevant association may exist between the intensity of autofluorescence and ATP content and, consequently, serve as a useful proxy of bioenergetic state. One caveat that needs to be noted concerns the meiotic status of the oocytes used in this preliminary study, namely, that they were immature at follicular aspiration but had spontaneously completed maturation to MII in vitro. Studies of MII oocytes at aspiration will be necessary to confirm these findings and provide threshold intensity levels assessed by improved empirical grading methods or by instrument-based measurements that can be related to bioenergetic state. However, findings discussed above strongly indicate that this approach is developmentally benign and suitable for oocyte and embryo selection in a clinical setting. Additional studies will likely determine whether (a) an autofluorescence intensity relationship exists between mitochondrial mass and mtDNA content in the oocyte and (b) the extent to which bioenergetic state at the blastomere level is a function of the uniformity of the inherited mitochondrial complement. If demonstrated, potential negative downstream effects already associated with early disproportionate mitochondrial segregation [33] may be used to deselect those embryos showing this phenotype.

Of particular interest regarding competence is whether a subthreshold mitochondrial mass/mtDNA copy number can occur that is able to support meiotic maturation and fertilization-associated events including pronuclear formation and early cleavage divisions, but that is insufficient to permit the persistence of normal preimplantation embryogenesis to the hatched blastocyst stage. The rationale for this notion is that mitochondrial mass may be a critical factor in establishing developmental competence because, with each cell division beginning at fertilization, the number of mitochondria is theoretically halved as they segregate into daughter cells with no additional organelles arising until well after implantation. A subnormal threshold in the oocyte inherited by the embryo may be insufficient to support higher energy levels required by cells as development progresses through the preimplantation stages despite the structural transition from condensed to orthodox states. Transmission electron microscopic images of human GV-stage oocytes that failed to reinitiate meiosis in vivo after controlled ovarian stimulation and ovulation induction indicate a mitochondrial density that is often substantially lower than in normally maturing siblings [74], providing tentative support for the notion that the size of the mitochondrial complement in an MII oocyte is likely to be a primary determinant of bioenergetic capacity and therefore developmental competence.

9.10 Concluding Remarks

In its simplest iteration, developmental competence is the ability of an MII oocyte to be fertilized and by upregulating free calcium levels after sperm penetration, to "activate" the process of embryogenesis by (a) promoting the endpoint of meiosis, the emission of a half set of sister chromatids in the second polar body at telophase II, (b) initiating cortical granule exocytosis to prevent polyspermy penetration, (c) establishing intracellular conditions for the formation of a normal first mitotic spindle, and (d) generating free calcium oscillations that establish the temporal pattern for the first and subsequent cell divisions. The normal occurrence of these early physiological events is energy dependent with appropriate levels of ATP and GTP generation necessary for progression to the blastocyst stage, followed by hatching, implantation, and continued gestation to birth.

In this context, several basic themes have been embedded in current notions of how developmental competence is established. One is that it is largely established in the oocyte prior to fertilization and a second and related theme is that cellular energy is a principal driver of competence from the preovulatory resumption of arrested meiosis at the GV stage through gestation. It is for this reason that considerable efforts have been undertaken to determine, noninvasively, the bioenergetic state of the oocyte and preimplantation embryo such that as a biomarker of competence, it could be included in clinical IVF programs to select the oocyte and embryo "most likely to succeed." Consequently, the present focus of this chapter has been on the oocyte rather than the embryo for the very reason that mitochondria and the normality of their maternal inheritance can be directly tied to competence. Analytical tools that measure bioenergetic state exist and, if they can be effectively applied in clinical IVF, they will have an important role in selection so as to bias the IVF procedure toward a positive outcome.

Each of the methods described above – from mtDNA quantification, OCR measurements, Raman spectroscopic assessments of metabolism, to FLIM – requires highly sensitive and often costly instrumentation. Each has the potential to detect and quantify metabolic levels by nondestructive and nontoxic means that can provide developmentally useful information. The findings from the pilot study for NADH/NADPH autofluorescence present a potentially less costly opportunity that may be better suited for most IVF programs if confirmed as a viable means of competence assessment that improves outcome. Application of such a lower-cost analytical platform may be of particular utility where accessibility, availability, and affordability are major barriers to advanced fertility treatments [76]. We have also found that RFI determinations have utility as a diagnostic tool for failed fertilizations and instances where cytokinesis unexpectedly ceased or was asymmetric during cleavage.

Given the central role of bioenergetics in human gametogenesis and embryogenesis, the essential question that was not answered in this chapter is which current or commercially available method(s) for detection or quantification might be worthwhile for consideration in IVF programs. If cost and expertise are not prohibitive, it would appear that commercially available OCR methodologies such as Agilent Seahorse analysers have been proven to be reliable and valuable for relating metabolism to developmental viability in both animal and human studies. Raman spectroscopy of spent culture medium remains an intriguing possibility based on its sensitivity and the broad range of molecules that can be identified when they occur at detectable levels, but it remains to be determined whether an effective commercially viable Raman-based instrument dedicated to IVF can be produced. FLIM is also an effective means to detect differential bioenergetics and mitochondrial distributions that are competence-related, but cost and current complexity can be significant factors for routine clinical use. The NADH/NADPH autofluorescent method has promise but will need additional studies, with actual outcome results, in order for its effectiveness in evaluating developmental potential to be validated. Until these methodologies can transition from basic research to the clinic, perhaps evaluations from experienced embryologists (the "observers") will remain a central element in competence assessments. However, in the present era of computer-based image analysis for assessing the normality of morphodynamic aspects of early embryogenesis, and the biochemical identification of micro-and macromolecules in culture medium that may be released by a developmentally competent or incompetent embryo, it is possible to envisage a time that in one form or another, accurate assessments of bioenergetic state alone, or in combination with other assessment methods, will generate observer-independent algorithms that can facilitate gamete and embryo selection. It is also likely that metrics that address the issue of chromosomal normality can be included based on the most recent findings that DNA present in blastocoelic fluid [77] and in spent embryo culture medium can be used for determination of ploidy [78, 79] (see Chapter 15), which adds an important component to a bioenergetic-focused selection paradigm. However, until selection becomes automated and multifaceted with each metric independently validated, measures of bioenergetics need to be considered because energy states at important developmental landmarks or transitions underlie competence.

However, perhaps the simplest measure of competence in the near term and in the absence of IVF-appropriate instrumentation for accurate metabolic assessments, may be what the embryo demonstrates by its performance in vitro from fertilization onward. Oocytes with inherited mitochondrial mass deficiencies and mutations that negatively affect OXPHOS, or where an idiopathic inability to supply sufficient levels of nucleotide triphosphates becomes functionally compromising, will likely self-select by failing to achieve MII or, if fertilized, will fail to support appropriately aligned and juxtaposed pronuclei after sperm penetration, or normal development during the pre-implantation stage. The current role of an observer in competence assessment should not be overlooked as it has yet to be clearly shown whether cost-effective OCR or autofluorescence methodologies appropriate for general use in clinical IVF can effectively distinguish between a blastocyst with a normally formed ICM from one in which it is absent, scant, or poorly organized. Until such a time when noninvasive competence selection can truly become operator-independent, the recognized morphological and morphokinetic signs of developmental distress or dysfunction that would diminish the likelihood of a positive outcome will remain a central element in oocyte and embryo selection. However, these currently applied approaches may well be significantly refined in the future by the addition of noninvasive methods including perhaps the simplest, the autofluorescent signatures of mitochondrial bioenergetic substrates and coenzymes such as NADH and FAD.

Key Messages

- Bioenergetic state and capacity are related to developmental competence and outcome in clinical IVF.
- Measurements of bioenergetic state at different stages of preimplantation embryogenesis can assist oocyte and embryo selection for fertilization and transfer, respectively.
- Semiquantitative assessments of bioenergetic states can be performed at low cost with existing expertise present in a typical IVF unit.

References

1. Van Blerkom, J. Occurrence and developmental consequences of aberrant cellular organization in meiotically mature human oocytes after exogenous ovarian hyperstimulation. *J Electron Microsc Tech*. 1990;16: 324–46.

2. Van Blerkom J, Henry G. Oocyte dysmorphism and aneuploidy in meiotically mature human oocytes after ovarian stimulation. *Hum Reprod*. 1992;7:379–90.

3. Meriano J, Alexis J, Visram-Zaver S, Cruz M, Casper R. Tracking of oocyte dysmorphisms for ICSI patients may prove relevant to the outcome in subsequent patient cycles. *Hum Reprod*. 2001;16:2118–23.

4. Alpha Scientists in Reproductive Medicine and ESHRE Special Interest Group of Embryology. The Istanbul consensus workshop on embryo assessment: proceedings of an expert meeting. *Hum Reprod*. 2011;26:1270–83.

5. Braga D, Setti A, Figueira R, Machado R, Iaconelli A, Borges E. Influence of oocyte dysmorphisms on blastocyst formation and quality. *Fertil Steril*. 2013;100:748–54.

6. Rienzi L, Ubaldi F, Iacobelli M, Minasi M, Romano S, Ferraro S, et al. Significance of metaphase II human oocyte morphology on ICSI outcome. *Fertil Steril*. 2008;90:1692–700.

7. Rienzi L, Vajta G, Ubaldi F. Predictive value of oocyte

morphology in human IVF: a systematic review of the literature. *Hum Reprod Update.* 2011;17:34–45.

8. Dal Canto M, Guglielmo M, Renzini M, Fadini R, Moutier C, Merola M, et al. Dysmorphic patterns are associated with cytoskeletal alterations in human oocytes. *Hum Reprod.* 2017;32:750–7.

9. Dolinko A, Racowsky C. Time-lapse microscopy for embryo culture and selection. In: Nagy Z, Varghese A, Agarwal A, editors. *In vitro fertilization*, Cham: Springer; 2019, p. 227–45.

10. Rienzi L, Capalbo A, Stoppa M, Romano S, Maggiulli R, Albricci L, et al. No evidence of association between blastocyst aneuploidy and morphokinetic assessment in selected population of poor-prognosis patients: a longitudinal cohort study. *Reprod BioMed Online.* 2015;30:57–66.

11. Wu Y, Lazzaroni-Tealdi E, Wang Q, Zang L, Barad DH, Kushnir VA, et al. Different effectiveness of closed embryo culture system with time-lapse imaging (EmbryoScope™) in comparison to standard manual embryology in good and poor prognosis patients: a prospectively randomized pilot study. *Reprod Biol Endocrinol.* 2016;14:49–57.

12. Fishel S, Campbell A, Montgomery W, Smith R, Nice L, Duffy S, et al. Live births after embryo selection using morphokinetics versus conventional morphology: a retrospective analysis. *Reprod BioMed Online.* 2017;35:407–16.

13. Van Blerkom, J. The role of mitochondria in the establishment of developmental competence in early human development. In: Nagy Z, Varghese A, Agarwal A, editors. *In vitro fertilization*. London: Springer; 2019. p. 897–915.

14. Patrizio P, Shoham G, Shoham Z, Leong M, Barad DH, Gleicher N. Worldwide live births following the transfer of chromosomally "abnormal" embryos after PGT/A: results of a worldwide web-based survey. *J Assist Reprod Genet.* 2019;36:1599–607.

15. Martin K, Hardy K, Winston, R, Leese H. Activity of enzymes of energy metabolism in single human preimplantation embryos. *J Reprod Fertil.* 1993;99:259–66.

16. Leese H. Metabolism of the preimplantation embryo: 40 years on. *Reproduction* 2012;143:417–27.

17. Leese H, Conaghan J, Martin K, Hardy K. Early human embryo metabolism. *BioEssays.* 1993;15:259–64.

18. Wilding M, De Placido G, De Matteo L, Marino M, Alviggi C, Dale B. Chaotic mosaicism in human preimplantation embryos is correlated with a low mitochondrial membrane potential. *Fertil Steril.* 2003;79:340–6.

19. Kim J, Seli E. Mitochondria as a biomarker of IVF outcome. *Reproduction.* 2019;157:235–42.

20. Breuer M, Koopman W, Koene, M, Noetteboom, M, Rodenburg RJ, Willems PH, Smeitink JAM. The role of mitochondrial OXPHOS dysfunction in the development of neurologic diseases. *Neurobiol Dis.* 2012;51:27–34.

21. Shoffner J. Oxidative phosphorylation defects and Alzheimer's disease. *Neurogenetics.* 1997;1:13–19.

22. Chandra D, Singh K. Genetic insights into OXPHOS defect and its role in cancer. *Biochim Biophys Acta.* 2011;1807:620–5.

23. Ashton T, Gilles McKenna W, Kunz-Schughart LA, Higgins GS. Oxidative phosphorylation as an emerging target in cancer therapy. *Clin Cancer Res.* 2018;24:2482–90.

24. Tuppen E, Blakely L, Turnbull D, Taylor R. Mitochondrial DNA mutations and human disease. *Biochim Biophys Acta.* 2010;1797:113–28.

25. de Laat P, Rodenburg R, Smeitink J. Mitochondrial oxidative phosphorylation disorders. In: Blau N, Duran M, Gibson K, Dionisi Vici C, editors. *Physician's guide to the diagnosis, treatment, and follow-up of inherited metabolic diseases.* Berlin, Heidelberg: Springer; 2014. p. 337–59.

26. Van Blerkom J. Mitochondria in human oogenesis and preimplantation embryogenesis: engines of metabolism, ionic regulation and developmental competence. *Reproduction.* 2004;128:269–80.

27. Van Blerkom J. Mitochondria as regulatory forces in oocytes, preimplantation embryos and stem cells. *Reprod. BioMed Online.* 2008;16:553–69.

28. Van Blerkom J, Davis P, Mathwig V, Alexander S. Domains of high-polarized and low-polarized mitochondria may occur in mouse and human oocytes and early embryos. *Hum Reprod.* 2002;17:393–406.

29. Wilding M, Dale B, Marino M, di Matteo L, Alviggi C, Pisaturo ML, et al. Mitochondrial aggregation patterns and activity in human oocytes and preimplantation embryos. *Hum Reprod.* 2001;16:909–17.

30. Wilding M, Fiorentino A, De Simone M, Infante V, De Matteo L, Marino M, Dale B. Energy substrates, mitochondrial membrane potential and human preimplantation embryo division. *Reprod BioMed Online.* 2002;5:39–42.

31. Stern S, Biggers J, Anderson A. Mitochondria and early development of the mouse. *J Exp Zool.* 1971;176:179–92.

32. Van Blerkom, J, Manes C, Daniel J. Development of preimplantation rabbit embryos in vivo and in vitro. I. An ultrastructural comparison. *Devel Biol.* 1973;35:262–82.

33. Van Blerkom J, Davis P, Alexander S. Differential mitochondrial inheritance between blastomeres in cleavage stage human embryos: determination at the pronuclear stage and relationship to microtubular organization, ATP content and developmental competence. *Hum Reprod.* 2000;15:2621–33.

34. Sanchez, T, Seidler M, Gardner D. Needleman D, Sakkas D. Will noninvasive methods surpass invasive for assessing gametes and embryos? *Fertil Steril.* 2017;108:730–7.

35. May-Panloup P, Chretien MF, Malthiery Y, Reynier P. Mitochondrial DNA in the oocyte and the developing embryo. *Cur Top Dev Biol.* 2007;77:51–83.

36. Wells D. Mitochondrial DNA quantity as a biomarker of blastocyst implantation potential. *Fertil Steril.* 2017;108:742–7.

37. Van Blerkom J. Mitochondrial function in the human oocyte and embryo and their role in developmental competence. *Mitochondrion.* 2011;11:797–813.

38. Fragouli E, Sapth K, Alfarawati S, Wells D. Quantification of mitochondrial DNA predicts the implantation potential of chromosomally normal embryos. *Fertil Steril.* 2013;100: Supplement S1.

39. Murakoshi Y, Sueoka K, Takahashi K, Sato S, Sakurai T, Tajima H, Yoshimura Y. Embryo developmental capability and pregnancy outcome are related to the mitochondrial DNA copy number and ooplasmic volume. *J Assist Reprod Genet.* 2013;30:1367–75.

40. Victor A, Brake A, Tyndall J, Griffin D, Zouves CG, Barnes FL, Viotti M. Accurate quantitation of mitochondrial DNA reveals uniform levels in human blastocysts irrespective of ploidy, age, or implantation potential. *Fertil Steril.* 2017;107:34–42.

41. Victor A, Griffin D, Gardner D, Brake A, Zouves CG, Barnes FL, Viotti M. Births from embryos with highly elevated levels of mitochondrial DNA. *Reprod BioMed Online.* 2019;39:403–12.

42. Wai T, Ao A, Xiaoyun Zhang X, Cyr D, Dufort D, Shoubridge EA. The role of mitochondrial DNA copy number in mammalian fertility. *Biol Reprod.* 2010;83:52–62.

43. Santos T, El-Shourbagy S, St John J. Mitochondrial content reflects oocyte variability and fertilization outcome. *Fertil Steril.* 2006;85:584–92.

44. Shoubridge E, Wai T. Mitochondrial DNA and the mammalian oocyte. *Curr Top Dev Biol.* 2007;77:87–111.

45. Van Blerkom J, Davis P. Mitochondrial signaling and fertilization. *Mol Hum Reprod.* 2007;13:59–770.

46. Van Blerkom J, Zimmerman S. Role of ganglioside GM1 and associated membrane proteins in the development of a functionally polarized oolemma at fertilization. *Reprod BioMed Online.* 2016;33:458–75.

47. Hayashi T, Fukuda N, Uchiyama S, Inada N. A cell-permeable fluorescent polymeric thermometer for intracellular temperature mapping in mammalian cells. *PLoS ONE.* 2015;10(2):e0117677.

48. Aw T-Y. Intracellular compartmentalization of organelles and gradients of low molecular weight species. *Int Rev Cytol.* 2000;192:223–53.

49. Krishtalik L. pH-dependent redox potential: how to use it correctly in the activation energy analysis. *Biochim Biophys Acta.* 2003;1604:13–21.

50. Yu Y, Dumollard R, Rossbach A, Lai A, Swann K. Redistribution of mitochondria leads to bursts of ATP production during spontaneous mouse oocyte maturation. *J Cell Physiol.* 2010;224:672–80.

51. Van Blerkom J, Davis, P, Lee, J. ATP content of human oocytes and developmental potential and outcome after in-vitro fertilization and embryo transfer. *Hum Reprod.* 1995;10:415–24.

52. Van Blerkom J. The mitochondria in early development. *Semin Cell Dev Biol.* 2009;20:191–200.

53. Muller B, Lewis N, Tope A, Leese HJ, Brison DR, Sturmey RG. Application of extracellular flux analysis for determining mitochondrial function in mammalian oocytes and early embryos. *Sci Reports.* 2019;9:16778.

54. Bond S, McEwen K, Yoganantharajah P, Gibert Y. Live metabolic profile analysis of zebrafish embryos using a seahorse XF 24 extracellular flux analyzer. In: Félix L, editor. *Teratogenicity testing.* Methods in Molecular Biology 1797, New York: Humana Press; 2018. p. 393–401.

55. Obeidat Y, Evans A, Tedjo, W, Chiccob AJ, Carnevale E, Chena TW. Monitoring oocyte/embryo respiration using electrochemical-based oxygen sensors. *Sens Activators B Chem.* 2018;276:72–81.

56. Utsunomiya T, Goto K, Nasu M, Kumasako Y, Araki Y, Yokoo M, et al. Evaluating the quality of human embryos with a measurement of oxygen consumption by scanning electrochemical microscopy. *J Mammal Ova Res.* 2008;25:2–7.

57. Yamanaka M, Hashimoto S, Amo A, Ito-Sasaki T, Abe H, Morimoto Y. Developmental assessment of human vitrified warmed blastocysts based on oxygen consumption. *Hum Reprod.* 2011;26:3366–71.

58. Maezawa T, Yamanaka M, Hashimoto S, Amo A, Ohgaki A, Nakaoka Y, et al. Possible selection of viable human blastocysts by monitoring morphological changes. *J Assist Reprod Genet.* 2014;31:1066–104.

59. Morimoto N, Hashimoto S, Yamanaka, N, Nakano T, Satoh M, Nakaoka Y, et al. Mitochondrial oxygen consumption of human embryos declines with maternal age. *J Assist Reprod Genet.* 2020;37:1815–21.

60. Muller-Hocker J, Schafer S, Weis S, Munscher C, Strowitzki T. Morphological-cytochemical and molecular genetic analyses of mitochondria in isolated human oocytes in the reproductive age. *Mol Hum Reprod.* 1996;2:951–8.

61. Sathananthan H, Gunasheela S, Menezes J. Mechanics of human blastocyst hatching in vitro. *Reprod BioMed Online.* 2003;7:228–34.

62. Hashimoto S, Morimoto N, Yamanaka M, Matsumoto H, Yamochi T, Goto H, et al. Quantitative and qualitative changes of mitochondria in human preimplantation embryos. *J Assist Reprod Genet.* 2017;34:573–80.

63. Fragouli E, Spath K, Alfarawati S, Kaper F, Craig A, Michel CE, et al. Altered levels of mitochondrial DNA are associated with female age, aneuploidy, and provide an independent measure of embryonic implantation potential. *PLoS Genet.* 2015;11:e1005241.

64. Seli E, Sakkas D, Scott R, Kwok SC, Rosendahl SM, Burns DH. Noninvasive metabolomic profiling of embryo culture media using Raman and near-infrared spectroscopy correlates with reproductive potential of embryos in women undergoing in vitro fertilization. *Fertil Steril.* 2007;88:1350–7.

65. Scott, R, Seli E, Miller, K, Sakkas D, Scott K, Burns DH. Noninvasive metabolomic profiling of human embryo culture media using Raman spectroscopy predicts embryonic reproductive potential: a prospective blinded pilot study. *Fertil Steril.* 2008;90:77–83.

66. Zhao Q, Yin, T, Peng J, Zou Y, Yang J, Shen A, Hu J. Noninvasive metabolomic profiling of human embryo culture media using a simple spectroscopy adjunct to morphology for embryo assessment in in vitro fertilization (IVF). *Int J Mol Sci.* 2013;14:6556–70.

67. Squirrell J, Schramm R, Paprocki A, Wokosin D, Bavister B. Imaging mitochondrial organization in living primate oocytes and embryos using multiphoton microscopy. *Microsc Microanal.* 2003;9:190–201.

68. Van Blerkom J, Runner M. Mitochondrial reorganization during resumption of arrested meiosis in the mouse oocyte. *Amer J Anat.* 1984;171:335–55.

69. Sun Q, Wu G, Lai L, Park K, Cabot R, Cheong HT, et al. Translocation of active mitochondria during pig oocyte maturation, fertilization and early embryo development in vitro. *Reproduction.* 2001;122:155–63.

70. Yokoo M, Mori M. Near-infrared laser irradiation improves the development of mouse pre-implantation embryos. *Biochem Biophys Res Com.* 2017;487:415e418.

71. Sanchez T, Wang T, Pedro M, Zhang M, Esencan E, Sakkas D, et al. Metabolic imaging with the use of fluorescence lifetime imaging microscopy (FLIM) accurately detects mitochondrial dysfunction in mouse oocytes. *Fertil Steril.* 2018;110:1387–97.

72. Leng-Chun, C, Lloyd W, Chang, C-W, Sud D, Mycek MA. Fluorescence lifetime imaging microscopy for quantitative biological imaging. *Method Cell Biol.* 2013;114:457–88.

73. Sikder S, Reyes J, Moon C, Suwan-apichon O, Elisseeff JH, Chuck RS. Noninvasive mitochondrial imaging in live cell culture. *Photochem Photobiol.* 2007;81:1569–71.

74. Makabe S, Van Blerkom, J. *Atlas of Human female reproduction.* London: Taylor & Francis; 2006.

75. Van Blerkom J. Microtubule mediation of cytoplasmic and nuclear maturation during the early stages of resumed meiosis in cultured mouse oocytes. *PNAS.* 1991;88:5031–5.

76. Van Blerkom J, Hennigan C, Ombelet W. Design and development of simplified, low-cost technologies for clinical IVF: applications in high- and low-resource settings. In: Nagy Z, Varghese A, Agarwal A, editors. *In vitro fertilization.* Cham: Springer; 2019. p. 193–206.

77. Magli MC, Albanese C, Crippa A, Tabanelli C, Ferrarretti AP, Gianaroli L. Deoxyribonucleic acid detection in blastocoelic fluid: a new predictor of embryo ploidy and viable pregnancy. *Fertil Steril.* 2019;111:77–85.

78. Ben-Nagi J, Odia R, Vinals Gonzalez X, Heath C, Babariya D, SenGupta S, et al. The first ongoing pregnancy following comprehensive aneuploidy assessment using a combined blastocenetesis, cell free DNA and trophectoderm biopsy strategy. *J Reprod Infertil.* 2019;20:57–62.

79. Huang L, Bofale B, Tang Y, Lu S, Sunney Xie X, Racowsky C. Noninvasive preimplantation genetic testing for aneuploidy in spent medium may be more reliable than trophectoderm biopsy. *PNAS.* 2019;116:14105–12.

Static Morphological Assessment for Embryo Selection

Thomas Ebner

10.1 Introduction

Since fertilization is the result of the fusion of two gametes, it is obvious that not only the corresponding zygote but also the corresponding embryo are highly dependent on the initial quality of spermatozoon and oocyte. At virtually every developmental stage, static assessment of morphology on one or more days is still the practice most commonly used for preimplantation embryo selection, although it has to be emphasized that time-lapse video cinematography has gained ground. An international expert group aimed to standardize morphological evaluation among clinics and suggested a rough timing (relative to the time of insemination or sperm injection on day 0) when daily observations should be performed, and the respective stage of development assessed [1]. These timings agreed by the consensus participants closely corroborate those published by the esteemed Sir Robert Edwards in 1981 [2]. As observed by Sir Edwards, the preimplantation human embryo follows a specific timeline (Figure 10.1). The question at hand is which of these stages, and what morphological features should be assessed, when undertaking static evaluations in the clinical embryology laboratory.

10.2 Zygote Stage

Regardless of whether gametes are brought together using conventional IVF or by intracytoplasmic sperm injection (ICSI) the chronological order of oocyte activation and fertilization is the same with several differences, namely that in ICSI the essential steps of cumulus penetration, zona pellucida binding, and membrane fusion are bypassed. However, once the sperm is in the ooplasm its head will decondense to form the male pronucleus. More or less simultaneously, a female counterpart appears in the cortical spindle region next to the polar bodies. The latter is then drawn toward the center of the oocyte by

microtubules originating from the male pronucleus until both pronuclei appose. Within each pronucleus several nucleoli mark the active sites of rRNA synthesis. As development proceeds, these nucleoli tend to fuse and polarize until pronuclear membrane breakdown occurs.

Considering the said dynamics, the arising characteristic pattern of zygote or pronuclear stage can be nothing but a snapshot. Nevertheless, over the years characteristics of the pronuclear stage have been widely used as predictive parameters of blastocyst formation, implantation, and pregnancy [3, 4, 5].

Around the beginning of the new millennium, it became clear that asynchrony in the formation and polarization of nucleoli may impair further development of the embryo [5]. It should be noted that regular fertilization requires the presence of two polar bodies and two pronuclei. Three-pronuclear zygotes from polyspermy or nondisjunction as well as parthenogenetically activated oocytes must not be used for in vitro culture and transfer; and zygotes with one pronucleus should only be used when none with two pronuclei (binucleate) are available. So when speaking of pronuclear score in Section 10.2.1, this always refers to the binucleate zygote.

10.2.1 Pronuclear Pattern

The basis of most day 1 grading systems is a combination of both nucleoli size/number and distribution [3, 4]. The positioning of the nucleoli is preferably polarized at the pronuclear junction and nucleoli scattered all over the karyoplasm will be associated with a negative prognosis [3]. Later on, a refined simplified grading system was described allowing for an accurate prediction of embryo quality by a single-observation scoring [4]. Fewer parameters for consideration and so less time required for evaluation in a single static observation, and so less stress to the zygote, are the main advantages of the Tesarik versus

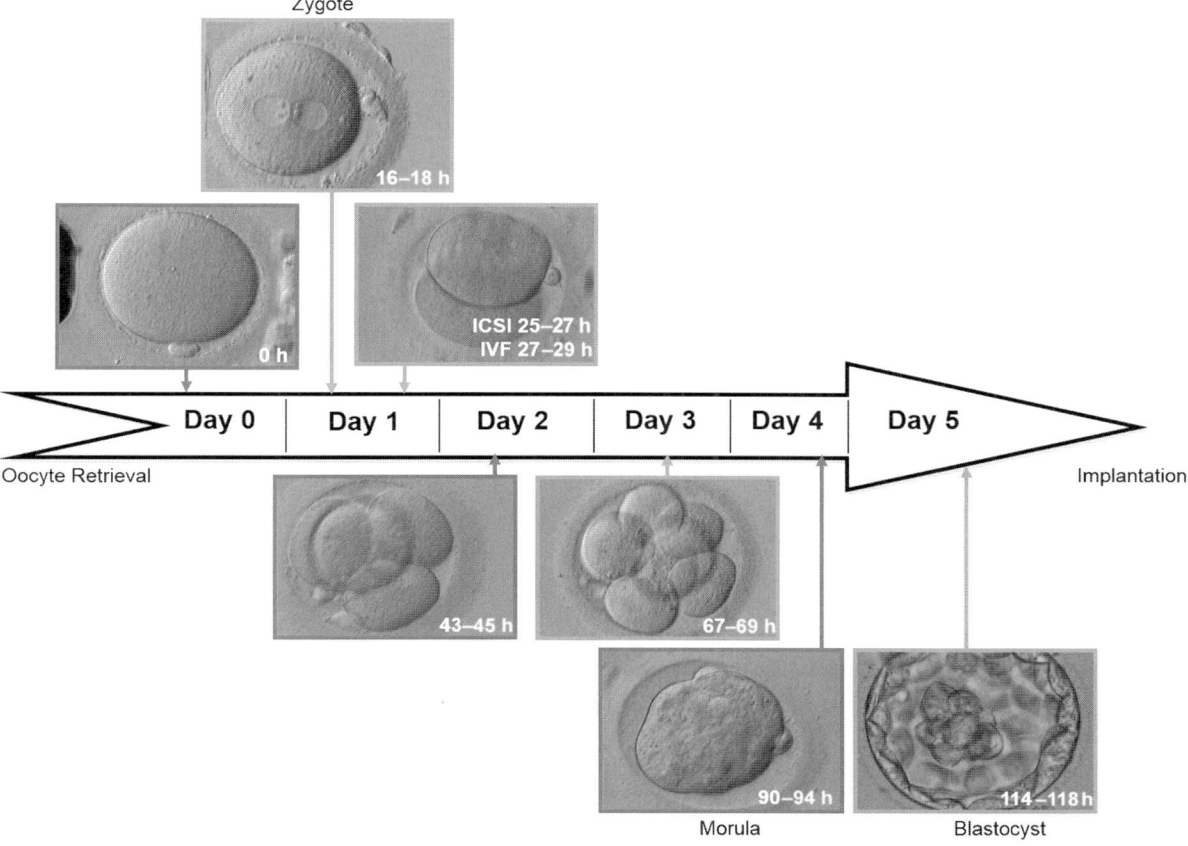

Figure 10.1 Suggested timeline of preimplantation development

the Scott scoring system [3, 4]. In fact, for the ease of the analysis, pronuclear symmetry, for example the equality of nuclei within each pronucleus, is the most striking predictive parameter at zygote stage. This is also reflected in the commonly used Z-score of Scott et al. (2000) [5] who observed a decline in blastocyst formation with ascending scores (Figure 10.2).

There are only a few scenarios in which even the best pronuclear pattern would have a bad developmental prognosis [5], these being a peripheral location or nonabuttal of the pronuclei as well as unequal size of the same (difference >10 μm). These abnormal pronuclear arrangements would reflect sperm- (nonabuttal, unequal size) or oocyte-borne problems. Zygotes showing all these dysmorphisms have the tendency to arrest in development and so it is recommended that they are not selected for transfer when there are potential alternatives, whether at the cleavage stage or after extended culture.

10.2.2 Cytoplasmic Halo

Additional prognostic power is attributed to the cytoplasmic appearance of the zygote [5, 6]. In detail, a microtubule-mediated withdrawal of mitochondria and other cytoplasmic components to the perinuclear region leaves a subplasmalemmal zone of translucent cytoplasm, the so-called halo. The physiological role of this redistribution of cell organelles in human zygotes is unclear but it is speculated that the observed central clustering may be involved in maturation of mitochondria, reactive oxygen species avoidance, and/or appropriation of ATP.

Contrary to popular belief, a large prospective study showed that there is no reason to exclude zygotes with extreme halos (e.g., >20 μm) from culture and it was proven that any kind of halo effect is beneficial [6]. The only problem with the halo effect as a selection tool is that $>80\%$ of zygotes do express

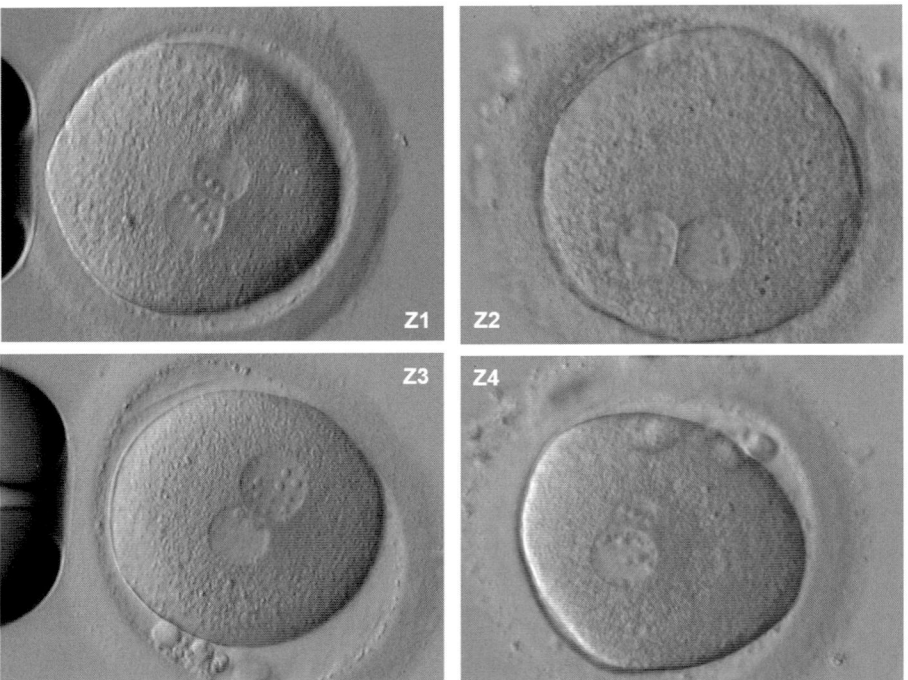

Figure 10.2 Zygote score according to Scott et al. (2000) [5]. Z1: aligned nucleoli, equal; Z2: aligning nucleoli, equal nucleolar size and number; Z3: unequal alignment of nucleoli, differences in nucleolar number and size; Z4: unequal sized pronuclei.

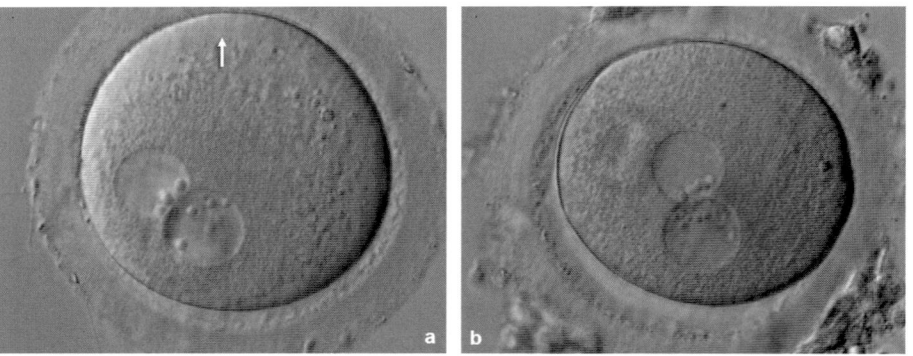

Figure 10.3 Zygotes showing presence (a) or absence (b) of a cytoplasmic halo (indicated by the arrow)

this typical cytoplasmic appearance (Figure 10.3) so that the halo most often is used together with other prognostic parameters at the zygote stage including distance and location of pronuclei and number and polarity of nucleoli to name but a few [7]. This cumulative pronuclear score [7] revealed that nucleolar pattern and cytoplasmic halo appeared as the most important factors predictive of implantation for fresh

and cryopreserved zygotes, while pronuclei position was specifically relevant for frozen-thawed zygotes.

The final phase of the zygote stage is marked by pronuclear membrane breakdown (also referred to as pronuclear fading). From this event onward it takes 3–4 hours before the M-phase of the first cell cycle ends and the zygote subsequently cleaves. In the absence of a time-lapse system, pronuclear membrane breakdown and early cleavage are useful predictive tools.

Recommendations

- Zygote scoring should always be done at the light microscopical level (at least x200 magnification) since a binocular microscope (usually below x20 magnification) will not allow accurate identification of pronucleus number and nucleoli disposition.

- For the same reason, individual culture of zygotes is recommended since the scoring of grouped zygotes would be impractical and complicate tracking of the respective zygote score once the zygote enters first mitosis.

- If zygote scoring is part of the routine evaluation, pronuclear pattern should be prioritized over halo formation.

- In the absence of a time-lapse system, undocumented zygotes (e.g. cleavage without proper identification of 2PN) should be seen as lower-priority candidates for transfer.

- Those zygotes of poorest prognosis (score Z4) show peripheral location or nonabuttal of the pronuclei as well as unequal size of the same and are associated with poor outcome.

10.3 Cleavage Stage

Cleavage stage is the period after fertilization when the zygote starts to develop into a multicellular organism. Practically, it spans the period between first mitosis on day 1 and late on day 3 when tight junctions begin to form between the cell membranes, compaction ensues, and the morula forms (day 4).

10.3.1 Timing for Static Assessments

Alpha Scientists in Reproductive Medicine and the ESHRE Special Interest Group of Embryology (2011) highlighted that standardized timing of observations from hours postinsemination is critical for comparing results between different laboratories [1]. Moreover, these experts presented expected stages of development at each of their nominated time points postinsemination. For static assessment of cleavage stage, the time points agreed on were 2-cell: 26 ± 1 h for ICSI (plus 2 h for IVF), 4-cell: 44 ± 1 h (IVF and ICSI), and 8-cell: 68 ± 1 h (IVF and ICSI) (Figure 10.1). Based on this timeline, the authors also postulated that, on average, embryos that cleave more slowly or more quickly than expected are likely to be abnormal and have a reduced implantation potential. Indeed, the delay of mitotic cleavages and subsequent rearrangements of the individual blastomeres seems to be associated with viability of embryos considering that prolonged cell cycles reflect DNA repair processes and cellular rearrangement prior to cleavage. For increased mitotic activity, however, the situation is less clear [8, 9] since the extent to which culture conditions (e.g. culture media) may influence mitotic rate and compaction behavior is unpredictable [1].

10.3.2 Cell Number and Stage-Appropriateness

During cleavage, the cytoplasmic volume remains essentially the same as that of the zygote, being simply allocated to numerous smaller nucleated cells, the blastomeres. For normal development, the number of blastomeres doubles with every cell cycle that, by definition, is "an orderly sequence of events in which a cell duplicates its contents and then divides into two" [10], p. 2653). As a consequence, the volume of the daughter cells will be approximately half of the volume of the original blastomere that divided. While the first cell cycle ends with the beginning of the first mitosis, the second embryonic cell cycle begins with two blastomeres that subsequently divide forming a 4-cell embryo showing four more or less identically shaped cells. A resulting day 2 embryo of regular morphological appearance would show a crosswise arrangement of four blastomeres with three cells lying side by side, thus forming a tetrahedron. Any change in cleavage plane orientation may result in a planar 4-cell embryo showing a consistent contact area between blastomeres. It has been hypothesized that in such scenarios cell division has probably not been fully completed due to a defect in the male centrosome that is responsible for the first mitosis [11].

Logically, during the third cell cycle, four blastomeres cleave one after the other until the 8-cell stage is reached. It should be noted that in humans, compaction usually starts around the fourth cell cycle so that 14–16 individual cells without signs of compaction are seen rather rarely.

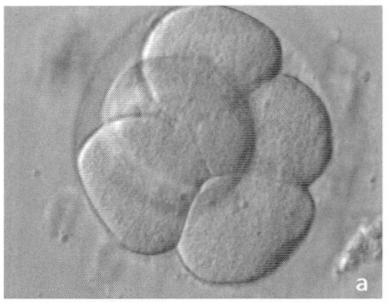
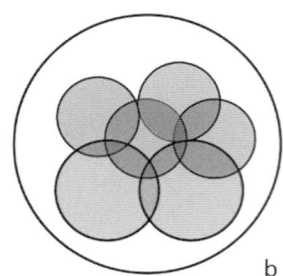
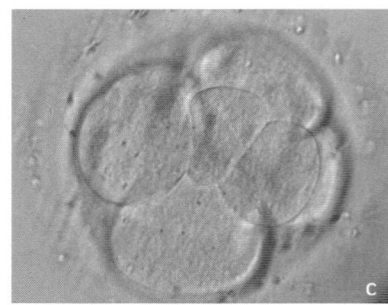

Figure 10.4 Differences in stage-appropriateness at 6-cell stage. Schematic drawing (b) illustrates correct formation of blastomeres. Deviations either derive from trichotomous mitosis (a) or incorrect order of cleavages (c).

10.3.3 Blastomere Symmetry

From this ideal physiological model described above it is evident that within a cleaving embryo identical cell sizes are only possible at the 2-, 4-, 8-, and 16-cell stage. To put it differently, a 6-cell embryo with six identically shaped cells (Figure 10.4a) can never be normal and most probably is the result of a trichotomous mitosis at the zygote stage. This scenario would involve two mitotic spindles in the zygote causing three (instead of two) identical daughter cells. If this irregular cleavage is then followed by three regular blastomeric cleavages an embryo would end up with six blastomeres of identical size.

For any other cell stage not representing the beginning or end of an embryonic cell cycle – for example the 3-, and 5- to 7-cell stages – only two different cell sizes are possible (e.g. the size of the mother cell and that of the daughter cell generation). To continue the logic of the 6-cell embryo example above, the only stage-appropriate formation of blastomeres would be achieved if two cells of a 4-cell embryo have already cleaved (with two more to go) ending up in two larger and four smaller cells (Figure 10.4b). Therefore, the embryo shown in Figure 10.4c cannot be considered stage-appropriate since it shows four large and two small cells.

In principle, embryo development can be classified into three categories: slow-, normal-, and fast-cleaving embryos. This classification is based on cell number on day 3 and has identified 7–9 cells as the normal range [12]. Consistent with this, others [8] reported a 65% aneuploidy rate in blastocysts derived from day 3 embryos with ≥10 cells. However, improvements in culture media and other conditions, including low O_2 tension, might result in euploid embryos with >9 cells on day 3; Pons et al. (2019) showed that embryos with >11 blastomeres on day 3 had the same likelihood of forming a euploid blastocyst and resulting in a healthy live birth as 8-cell embryos [13]. Of note, there is growing evidence that embryos with a higher mitotic rate can be normal [9].

10.3.4 Fragmentation

Assessment of cell number, stage-appropriateness, and blastomere symmetry should be relatively easy parameters to assess, at least in an ideal model as indicated in Section 10.3.2. In reality, however, the presence of cytoplasmic fragmentation can interfere with regular cleavage and, depending on its extent, may hinder accurate scoring of embryo morphology. Nevertheless, apart from blastomere number, fragmentation is the major criterion for scoring and selecting cleavage-stage embryos for transfer.

In principle, any membrane-bound extracellular cytoplasmic volume that shows no nucleus (e.g. has no DNA content) and thus is not able to sustain itself should be considered a fragment. Fragmentation is nonhomogenous, particularly with regards to size, which makes it difficult to distinguish larger fragments from smaller blastomeres. It has been suggested, however, that entities <45 μm in day 2 embryos and <40 μm in embryos on day 3 should be classified as fragments and those larger than these cutoffs classified as blastomeres [14]. The fact that the formation of fragments is highly dynamic and that they can form and be reabsorbed [15] at virtually any developmental stage further complicates scoring of embryo morphology during cleavage stages.

The challenges presented to accurate assessment of fragmentation may have been the major driving force for the development of computer-controlled, morphometric analysis tools of blastomere size that allow for the accurate calculation of the actual amount of fragmentation in human embryos [16]. However, since such sophisticated techniques are not available to most clinical embryologists, fragmentation must be estimated with less objective approaches, typically by visual assessment of this dysmorphism. Usually, the degree of fragmentation is expressed as a percentage and defined as the volume of the perivitelline space and/or cleavage cavity occupied by anucleate cytoplasmic fragments [17]. An international expert group defined the relative degrees of fragmentation as mild (<10%), moderate (10–25%), and severe (>25%). However, these percent values are "based on the cell equivalents," so for a 4-cell embryo, 25% fragmentation would equate to one blastomere in volume [1].

Alikani et al. (1999) stressed that apart from the extent of fragmentation, the spatial distribution of fragments is also of relevance [17]. These authors defined five patterns of fragmentation (Figure 10.5). According to this grading scheme fragmentation type I is minimal in volume and mostly associated with one single blastomere. Localized fragments accumulating in the perivitelline space comprise type II, whereas more blastomeres are involved in the formation of scattered fragmentation of type III. Pattern IV includes the presence of larger fragments that is also the case for pattern V, but in this worst grade, fragments appear apoptotic/necrotic with a characteristic granularity and cytoplasmic contraction.

Of note, microsurgical removal of fragments results in changes in blastomere organization and has been associated with an overall 4% increase in implantation rate [17]. Two hypotheses may explain this effect. Either the removal of anucleate fragments may prevent the embryo from secondary degeneration or it could restore the spatial relationship of blastomeres within the embryo that would then facilitate normal cell-cell contact. Regardless of whether fragmentation is assessed based on volume or pattern, it is evident that the effect on treatment outcome will worsen with the number of fragments present [17, 18]. There is evidence that a wide range of chromosomal abnormalities [19] and apoptotic phenomena are found in fragmented embryos. Heavily

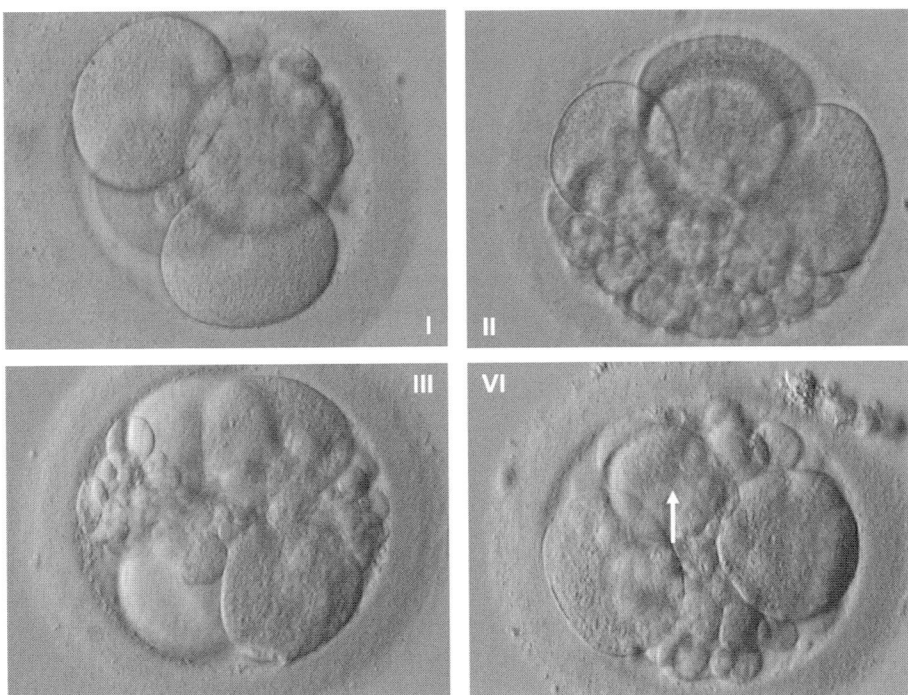

Figure 10.5 Day 2 fragmented embryos showing different fragmentation patterns according to Alikani et al. (1999) [17]. Type I: minimal in volume; type II: localized fragments; type III: scattered fragments potentially occupying cleavage cavities; type IV: large fragments (arrow) included resembling blastomeres. It should be noted that type 5 fragmentation, characterized by apoptotic appearance, is not depicted.

fragmented embryos (e.g. >50%; type IV and V pattern), in particular, are associated with a significantly higher rate of malformations [18] and a lower live birth rate [17].

10.3.5 Uneven Cleavage and Multinucleation

Any type of fragmentation will have a profound influence on cell size and uniformity. It is logical that a blastomere that loses cytoplasm due to fragmentation will automatically be of reduced size, which may result in unevenly sized blastomeres that are not stage-appropriate. Hardarson et al. (2001) [15] compared day 2 transfers of 4-cell embryos with and without evenly sized blastomeres and found that both implantation and pregnancy were negatively affected by uneven cleavage. According to these authors, this impact was the result of a higher rate of aneuploidy (29.4% vs. 8.5%).

Uneven cleavage is often accompanied by multinucleation [15], which basically involves all nuclear phenotypes (binucleation, ≥3 nuclei or micronuclei) that differ from the normal blastomere constitution represented by the presence of one nucleus at interphase of its blastomeric cell cycle. The assumed correlation between uneven cell size and genetic structure is supported by the finding that binucleated blastomeres are noticeably larger than mononucleated ones.

Multinucleation at the 2-cell stage is more frequent than at the 4- or 8-cell stage [20], but it is unclear whether the increased number of cells (in combination with the presence of fragments) hinders accurate detection. This is supported by time-lapse video sequences that indicate that multinucleation is underestimated in human embryos. To make things even more complicated, a certain capacity for self-correction during early cleavage divisions has been hypothesized [21]. Coexistence of different multinucleation phenotypes, coupled with the possibility of missed detection, may explain the conflicting conclusions regarding the potential negative impact of multinucleated cells on outcome.

There is evidence that multinucleation not only affects blastulation [22] but also compromises ongoing implantation [15, 20]. However, embryos with multinucleated cells can develop into euploid blastocysts resulting in healthy babies [21]. Not least because of the reported correlation between multinucleation and controlled ovarian hyperstimulation [20]. This dysmorphism, together with stage-specific cell size and fragmentation, should be one of the pillars of all morphological scoring systems in use [1] since all three of them have independent prognostic power to predict live birth [23].

Recommendation

- On day 2, tetrahedral blastomere configuration is considered to represent the normal status; planar embryos, however, represent a poor prognosis subgroup of embryos.
- Embryo scoring after expression of the embryonic genome is considered to be more predictive than done before this event. In other words, day 3 could be prioritized over day 2 morphology.
- Fragmentation of embryos is a dynamic process so it should be clear that static scoring of fragmentation has its limitations.
- The more blastomeres that are involved in the process of fragmentation the more severe is the impact on further fate.
- Morphokinetic data have shown that considerably more embryos have multinucleated cells than previously estimated on the basis of static observation. As such, multinucleation may only play a secondary role in embryo evaluation in the future.
- Stage-appropriateness is the most underestimated parameter in embryo scoring.
- At any mitotic stage, signs of compaction between blastomeres is a positive predictor.

10.4 Compaction/Morula

While embryos at earlier cleavage stages (e.g. before activation of the embryonic genome around the 8-cell stage) resemble an accumulation of solitary blastomeres with a rather low level of biosynthesis, the compaction phase is characterized by increased biosynthetic rates and the capacity to metabolize glucose more efficiently. In addition, the compacting embryo is capable of actively regulating ionic gradients, thus controlling its internal environment.

Compaction and formation of the morula are dynamic processes that are pivotal for blastocyst formation and establishment of the two cell lineages, the inner cell mass (ICM) and trophectoderm (TE). This crucial function is reflected by metabolic, molecular, and cellular changes, which are spatially and temporally regulated. In parallel, stage-specific modulations of gene expression are indicative of such changes [24].

As soon as any two cells within a multicellular embryo start to fuse, compaction is considered to have got underway [10]. It is important to stress that compaction is species-specific and for human embryos there is no fixed time point of the beginning of this event; however, normal compaction usually does not happen before day 3. Using static morphological assessment, the precise timing of this initial step of compaction is almost impossible to observe. Even with time-lapse technology its annotation has a high intra- and interobserver variability due to the increased number of cells and the type of compaction.

Two extreme timings of compaction have been discussed. Precocious compacting at the 2- to 4-cell stage, on the one hand, can result in formation of trophoblastic vesicles missing predecessor cells of the ICM. On the other hand, 14- to 16-cell embryos without evidence of compaction were thought to be of reduced capacity to blastulate [25]. However, this concept has been refuted by [26] who differentiated noncompacting embryos on day 5 from compacting (some areas of compaction) and fully compacted embryos. In this study, 14-cell embryos without signs of compaction showed excellent blastulation rates. However, compaction beginning on day 4 was a positive predictor of blastocyst formation, for example an 8- or 10-cell embryo without any sign of compaction had a worse outcome compared to a compacting 8- or 10-cell embryo [26]. Moreover, the more blastomeres involved in the compacting mass, the more likely a good-quality blastocyst will form [25, 26]. Any loss of cytoplasm due to fragmentation or excluded cells will severely impair day 5 development and implantation potential [26].

Recommendation

- The proportion of blastomeres undergoing compaction is indicative of further development to blastocyst stage.
- The more cytoplasm is lost from the compacting morula due to fragmentation or exclusion of blastomeres, the worse is the prognosis.

10.5 Blastocyst

On around day 4, the outer cells of the morula acquire their typical epithelial phenotype and form a selective barrier that is crucial for inward transport of water (by means of $Na^{[2]+}$ pumps) and subsequent expansion of the embryo due to passive influx of water [24]. Once intracellular fluid accumulation leads to the formation of a visible blastocoel, initiation of the blastocyst stage is set [10]. Again, the exact time of the beginning of blastulation is almost never detectable by means of static morphological assessment. Although good pregnancy results are achievable with day 4 transfers there is a strong tendency toward transfers at blastocyst stage on days 5, 6, or even 7. Apart from a better synchronization between the endometrium and the developmental stage of the embryo, blastocyst transfer allows for grading of the ICM and TE lineages as selection criteria. Together with the grade of expansion, the ICM and TE are part of every blastocyst scoring scheme worldwide [27].

10.5.1 Expansion

Evaluation of embryos on day 5, the typical day of blastocyst scoring, may include embryos developing more slowly and so at the morula stage to those fully expanded or even hatching blastocysts. These discrepancies in rate of development reflect variabilities in cell numbers. In this context, a high mitotic activity (reflecting the grade of expansion) is a reliable indicator of blastocyst viability and developmental capacity [27]. Thus, the size of the blastocyst available for transfer is of major importance.

Gardner et al. (2000) [27] specified six subclasses of blastocysts according to the size of the blastocoel and the grade of expansion. In detail, grades 1 and 2 are referred to as early blastocysts dependent on whether the blastocoel reaches half the volume of the blastocyst or not. At the full blastocyst stage (grade 3), two distinct cell lineages, the ICM and TE, are recognisable. Once the zona pellucida starts to thin due to intracellular pressure and the blastocyst increases in size, it is referred to as an expanded blastocyst (grade 4). Grades 5 and 6, finally, comprise hatching and completely hatched blastocysts. Regarding cell numbers, early blastocysts usually have no more than 30 cells, full blastocysts approximately consist of 60, and expanded blastocysts have >100 cells [28].

10.5.2 Inner Cell Mass

Hardy and colleagues (1989) were some of the first to identify differences in the growth rate of the TE and ICM. In general, the mitotic rate of the latter is approximately 1.5 times lower than that of the TE; however, the overall proportion of the ICM is relatively high, for example 34% of all cells on day 5, 51% on day 6, and 37% on day 7 [29]. Consequently, Gardner et al. (2000) [27] used cell number and cohesiveness of the embryoblast to subdivide the ICM into grades A–C according to whether it appeared tightly packed, loosely grouped. or composed of few cells only. Others [30] tried to quantitatively evaluate the ICM. These authors emphasized the importance of size and shape of the cell mass. It turned out that ICM was the only parameter that was significantly related to implantation with smaller ICMs (e.g. less than 3 800 μm[2]) showing lowest implantation rates. The problem with these data, however, is that the size of the embryoblast is closely related to the degree of expansion. In other words, the ICM gets smaller due to an increased cohesion of ICM cells as the blastocyst expands. Richter et al. (2001) [30] pooled grades 3–5 blastocysts and thus introduced a certain bias that might explain the fact that their results could not be confirmed by others [31].

Evaluation of ICM shape applying a Roundness Index (length of the ICM divided by width) is a rather imprecise approach [31, 32], so the suggested better implantation [30] of blastocysts with slightly elongated ICMs (compared to round or more ovoid ICMs) is disputable. One way to avoid such inconsistencies in ICM scoring would be to implement (semi) automatic quantification systems, so as to precisely measure the ICM size [32].

10.5.3 Trophectoderm

Historically, TE morphology was considered to be of lesser relevance than ICM quality when considering each of these parameters as predictive of implantation. This dogma changed when Swedish scientists [33] published the predictive strength of TE grade over ICM for selecting the best fresh or vitrified-warmed blastocyst for transfer. Since that date, evidence has accumulated indicating that accurate assessment of TE morphology is the most relevant parameter in prediction of live birth [31. 34]. This indeed makes sense since TE cells drive invasion and represent progenitor cells of the placenta.

As with ICM, TE grading is done focusing on the number and cohesion of (sickle-cell-shaped) cells. According to this grading system [27], quality A would refer to a cohesive epithelium, whereas a grade B TE would be characterized by a reduced cell count showing one or more gaps within the cell lineage. The worst case, grade C, would be a trophectoderm consisting of very few larger cells potentially having less physiological impact due to a lower number of tight junctions.

Figure 10.6 illustrates one of the major problems associated with static morphological assessment at the blastocyst stage. Routinely, only one cross-sectional circumference of the blastocyst is evaluated and what can be compensated in the case of the ICM (due to the fact that this is a three-dimensional cell mass) may cause a deviation in TE grading depending on the angle of view.

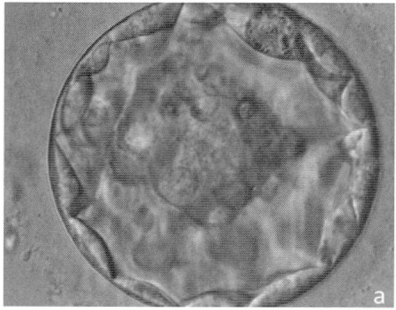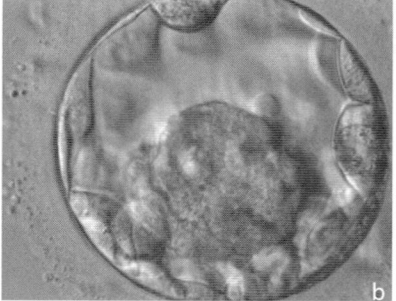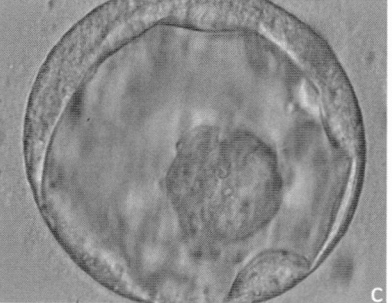

Figure 10.6 Different images of one and the same blastocyst. Depending on the angle of view of the trophectoderm, the quality varies from A to C. It should be noted that image c was taken three hours after a and b, respectively.

It seems that morphological evaluation of TE is a rather subjective interpretation of cell number and cohesion. Again, more automatic approaches would allow for optimal quantification of TE thickness, cell number, and, particularly, TE regularity ([32] and see Chapter 11).

Recommendations

- It should be noted that blastocyst culture does not eliminate genetically abnormal embryos.
- Day 4 blastocysts have a good prognosis and can be considered for transfer.
- There is a correlation between size of the blastocoel and blastocyst cell number.
- In terms of live birth prediction, quality of the trophectoderm should be given priority over quality of the inner cell mass.
- The size of the inner cell mass is dependent on the degree of cohesion of the same. As a consequence, assessment of inner cell mass size and shape is of less use in blastocyst scoring.
- Fragmentation and/or exclusion of blastomeres from the blastocyst has a distinct effect on cell number and should be taken into consideration when scoring blastocysts.

10.6 Cumulative Morphological Scoring

It can be justifiably claimed that static morphological assessment throughout the first six days of preimplantation development is the most regularly used method for noninvasively selecting the best embryo candidate for transfer. As with all biomarkers, limitations in predicting healthy live birth are evident since aneuploidy markers (e.g. giant oocytes) are rare.

In order to optimize prediction of preimplantation development and implantation behavior embryologists tended to switch from single static observations to multiday scoring. The more predictive biomarkers that were identified, the higher was the chance for a given embryo to form a blastocyst and to result in a pregnancy [35, 36].

The question arises as to which developmental stage(s) should be prioritized since static morphological assessment always requires incubator openings that, in turn, will stress the embryos and potentially harm their development depending on the time out of

the incubator. With respect to this, a predictive model for selection of day 3 embryos [37] was set up and led to the findings that day 1 evaluation had the poorest predictive value and that day 2 or day 3 evaluations alone were sufficient for morphological selection of cleavage stage embryos. Indeed, the superiority of cleavage stage morphology over pronuclear score has been confirmed [38]. Moreover, numerous studies indicate that the stage of development on day 5 provides the highest predictive value for embryo viability, with limited to no predictive value attributable to embryo morphology on day 3 (reviewed by [39]).

However, not even the most optimized scoring scheme can guarantee the identification of a cleavage-stage embryo or blastocyst that will result in the birth of a heathy baby. The inadequacy to select euploid embryos using limited noninvasive techniques such as static assessment of embryo growth may in part account for this scenario. Another related problem is the fact that scoring zygotes and embryos is linked to regular working hours of the lab. This is a default since time-lapse imaging has shown that various crucial cleavage events occur during hours after insemination that coincide with nighttime and are consequently missed or cannot be used as a selection criterion.

More dynamic methods are desirable, and advantages of time-lapse incubators cannot be ignored. However, embryo assessment, even with the most precise time-lapse morphokinetic annotations combined with machine learning and artificial intelligence, will undoubtedly continue to benefit from static morphological assessment.

Key Messages

Day 1

- Zygote scoring should always be done at the light microscopical level (at least x200 magnification) since a binocular microscope (usually below x20 magnification) will not allow accurate identification of pronucleus number and nucleoli disposition.
- If zygote scoring is part of the routine evaluation, pronuclear pattern should be prioritized over halo formation.
- Those zygotes of poorest prognosis show peripheral location or nonabuttal of the pronuclei as well as unequal size of the same.

Days 2 and 3

- On day 2, tetrahedral blastomere configuration is considered to represent the normal status; planar embryos represent a poor prognosis subgroup of embryos.
- Embryo scoring after expression of the embryonic genome is considered to be more predictive than when done before this event. In other words, day 3 should be prioritized over day 2 morphology.
- Fragmentation of embryos is a dynamic process, so it should be clear that static scoring of fragmentation has its limitations. However, the more blastomeres that are involved in the process of fragmentation, the more severe is the impact on further fate. It is not recommended to artificially remove fragments, particularly in the case of minor or localized fragmentation.
- Morphokinetic data have shown that considerably more embryos have multinucleated cells than previously estimated on the basis of static observation. As such, multinucleation may only play a secondary role in embryo evaluation in the future.

Day 4

- As with any other mitotic stage, signs of compaction between blastomeres on day 4 is a positive predictor.

- At the morula stage, the proportion of blastomeres undergoing compaction is indicative of further development to blastocyst stage. The more cytoplasm lost from the compacting morula due to fragmentation or exclusion of blastomeres, the worse is the prognosis.
- Day 4 blastocysts have a good prognosis and can be considered for transfer.

Day 5

- Blastocyst culture does not eliminate genetically abnormal embryos.
- In terms of live birth prediction, quality of the trophectoderm should be given priority over quality of the inner cell mass. Although a correlation between size of the blastocoel and blastocyst cell number is expected, blastocyst expansion is the least important selection criterion.
- The size of the inner cell mass is dependent on the degree of cohesion of the same. As a consequence, assessment of inner cell mass size and shape should be given low priority in blastocyst scoring.
- Fragmentation and/or exclusion of blastomeres from the blastocyst has a distinct effect on cell number and should be taken into consideration when scoring blastocysts.

References

1. Alpha Scientists in Reproductive Medicine and ESHRE Special Interest Group of Embryology. The Istanbul consensus workshop on embryo assessment: proceedings of an expert meeting. *Hum Reprod.* 2011;26:1270–83.

2. Edwards RG, Purdy JM, Steptoe PC, Walters DE. The growth of human preimplantation embryos in vitro. *Am J Obstet Gynecol.* 1981;141:408–16.

3. Scott LA, Smith S. The successful use of pronuclear embryo transfers the day following oocyte retrieval. *Hum Reprod.* 1998;13:1003–13.

4. Tesarik J, Greco E. The probability of abnormal preimplantation development can be predicted by a single static observation on pronuclear stage morphology. *Hum Reprod.* 1999;14:1318–23.

5. Scott LA, Alvero R, Leondires M. The morphology of human pronuclear embryos is positively related to blastocyst development and implantation. *Hum Reprod.* 2000;15:2394–403.

6. Ebner T, Moser M, Sommergruber M, Gaiswinkler U, Wiesinger R, Puchner M, Tews G. Presence, but not type or degree of extension, of a cytoplasmic halo has a significant influence on preimplantation development and implantation behaviour. *Hum Reprod.* 2003;18:2406–12.

7. Senn A, Urner F, Chanson A, Primi MP, Wirthner D, Germond M. Morphological scoring of human pronuclear zygotes for prediction of pregnancy outcome. *Hum Reprod.* 2006;21:234–9.

8. Luna M, Copperman AB, Duke M, Ezcurra D, Sandler B, Barritt J. Human blastocyst morphological quality is significantly improved in embryos classified as fast on day 3 ($\geq$10 cells), bringing into question current embryological dogma. *Fertil Steril.* 2008;89:358–63.

9. Shebl O, Haslinger C, Kresic S, Enengl S, Reiter E, Oppelt P, Ebner T. The hare and the tortoise: extreme mitotic rates and how these affect live birth. *Reprod Biomed Online.* 2021;42:332–9.

10. Ciray HN, Campbell A, Agerholm IE, Aguilar J, Chamayou S, Esbert M, Sayed S. Proposed guidelines on the nomenclature and annotation of dynamic human embryo monitoring by a time-lapse user group. *Human Reprod.* 2014;29:2650–60.

11. Ebner T, Maurer M, Shebl O, Moser M, Mayer RB, Duba HC, Tews G. Planar embryos have poor prognosis in terms of blastocyst formation and implantation. *Reprod Biomed Online.* 2012;25:267–72.

12. Munné S. Chromosome abnormalities and their relationship to morphology and development of human embryos. *Reprod Biomed Online.* 2006;12:234–53.

13. Pons MC, Carrasco B, Parriego M, Boada M, González-Foruria I, Garcia S, et al. Deconstructing the myth of poor prognosis for fast-cleaving embryos on day 3. Is it time to change the consensus? *J Assist Reprod Genet.* 2019;36:2299–305.

14. Johannson M, Hardarson T, Lundin K. There is a cutoff limit in diameter between a blastomere and a small anucleate fragment. *J Assist Reprod Genet.* 2003;20:309–13.

15. Hardarson T, Hanson C, Sjögren A, Lundin K. Human embryos with unevenly sized blastomeres have lower pregnancy and implantation rates: indications for aneuploidy and multinucleation. *Hum Reprod.* 2001;16:313–18.

16. Hnida C, Engenheiro E, Ziebe S. Computer-controlled, multilevel, morphometric analysis of blastomere size as biomarker of fragmentation and multinuclearity in human embryos. *Hum Reprod.* 2004;19:288–93.

17. Alikani M, Cohen J, Tomkin G, Garrisi GJ, Mack C, Scott RT. Human embryo fragmentation in vitro and its implications for pregnancy and implantation. *Fertil Steril.* 1999;71:836–42.

18. Ebner T, Yaman C, Moser M, Sommergruber M, Pölz W, Tews G. Embryo fragmentation in vitro and its impact on treatment and pregnancy outcome. *Fertil Steril.* 2001;76:281–5.

19. Munné S, Alikani M, Tomkin G, Grifo J, Cohen J. Embryo morphology, developmental rates, and maternal age are correlated with chromosome abnormalities. *Fertil Steril.* 1995;64:382–91.

20. Van Royen E, Mangelschots K, Vercruyssen M, De Neubourg D, Valkenburg M, Ryckaert G, Gerris J. Multinucleation in cleavage stage embryos. *Hum Reprod.* 2003;18:1062–9.

21. Balakier H, Sojecki A, Motamedi G, Librach C. Impact of multinucleated blastomeres on embryo developmental competence, morphokinetics, and aneuploidy. *Fertil Steril.* 2016;106:608–614.e2.

22. Alikani M, Calderon G, Tomkin G, Garrisi J, Kokot M, Cohen J. Cleavage anomalies in early human embryos and survival after prolonged culture in-vitro. *Hum Reprod.* 2000;15:2634–43.

23. Rhenman A, Berglund L, Brodin T, Olovsson M, Milton K, Hadziosmanovic N, Holte J. Which set of embryo variables is most predictive for live birth? A prospective study in 6252 single embryo transfers to construct an embryo score for the ranking and selection of embryos. *Hum Reprod.* 2015;30:28–36.

24. Coticchio G, Lagalla C, Sturmey R, Pennetta F, Borini A. The enigmatic morula: mechanisms of development, cell fate determination, self-correction and implications for ART. *Hum Reprod Update.* 2019;25:422–38.

25. Tao J, Tamis R, Fink K, Williams B, Nelson-White T, Craig R. The neglected morula/compact stage embryo transfer. *Hum Reprod.* 2002;17:1513–18.

26. Ebner T, Moser M, Shebl O, Sommergruber M, Gaiswinkler U, Tews G. Morphological analysis at compacting stage is a valuable prognostic tool for ICSI patients. *Reprod Biomed Online.* 2009;18:61–6.

27. Gardner DK, Lane M, Stevens J, Schlenker T, Schoolcraft WB. Blastocyst score affects implantation and pregnancy outcome: towards a single blastocyst transfer. *Fertil Steril.* 2000;73:1155–8.

28. Dumoulin JCM, Derhaag JG, Bras M, Van Montfoort APA, Kester ADM, Evers JLH, et al. Growth rate of human preimplantation embryos is sex dependant after ICSI but not after IVF. *Hum Reprod.* 2005;20:484–91.

29. Hardy K, Handyside AH, Winston RM. The human blastocyst: cell number, death, and allocation during late preimplantation development in vitro. *Development.* 1989;107:597–604.

30. Richter KS, Harris DC, Daneshmand ST, Shapiro BS. Quantitative grading of human blastocyst: optimal inner cell mass size and shape. *Fertil Steril.* 2001;76:1157–67.

31. Ebner T, Tritscher K, Mayer RB, Oppelt P, Duba HC, Maurer M, et al. Quantitative and qualitative trophectoderm grading allows for prediction of live birth and gender. *J Assist Reprod Genet.* 2016;33:49–57.

32. Santos Filho E, Noble JA, Poli M, Griffiths T, Emerson G, Wells D. A method for semi-automatic grading of human blastocyst microscope images. *Hum Reprod.* 2012;27:2641–8.

33. Ahlström A, Westin C, Reismer E, Wikland M, Hardarson T. Trophectoderm morphology: an important parameter for

predicting live birth after single blastocyst transfer. *Hum Reprod.* 2011;26:3289–96.

34. Bakkensen JB, Brady P, Carusi D, Romanski P, Thomas AM, Racowsky C. Association between blastocyst morphology and pregnancy and perinatal outcomes following fresh and cryopreserved embryo transfer. *J Assist Reprod Genet.* 2019;36:2315–24.

35. Balaban B, Urman B, Isiklar A, Alatas C, Aksoy S, Mercan R, et al. The effect of pronuclear morphology on embryo quality parameters and blastocyst transfer outcome. *Hum Reprod.* 2001;16:2357–61.

36. Lan KC, Huang FJ, Lin YC, Kung FT, Hsieh CH, Huang HW, et al. The predictive value of using a combined Z-score and day 3 embryo morphology score in the assessment of embryo survival on day 5. *Hum Reprod.* 2003;18:1299–1306.

37. Racowsky C, Ohno-Machado L, Kim J, Biggers JD. Is there an advantage in scoring early embryos on more than one day? *Hum Reprod.* 2009;24:2104–13.

38. Berger DS, Zapantis A, Merhi Z, Younger J, Polotsky AJ, Jindal SK. Embryo quality but not pronuclear score is associated with clinical pregnancy following IVF. *J Assist Reprod Genetics.* 2014;31:279–83.

39. Racowsky C, Combelles CMH, Nureddin A, Pan Y, Finn A, Miles L, et al. Day 3 and day 5 morphological predictors of embryo viability. *Reprod Biomed Online.* 2003;6:323–31.

Dynamic Morphological Assessment for Embryo Selection

Alison Campbell

11.1 Historical Perspective and Background

Until quite recently, it had not been possible, within the IVF laboratory, to continuously assess or monitor preimplantation human embryos in vitro. Assessments of fertilization status, for example, and of subsequent cell cleavage and embryo development, were limited to once daily at most, so as to minimize the potential damaging exposure to the less controlled environment outside of the incubator. It remained this way, with reasonable success, for several decades. However, over the last 10 years, the development of time-lapse imaging incubation devices, and their implementation into clinical IVF laboratories, has been increasingly utilized and now offers an alternative for embryo assessment. Time-lapse imaging brings a dynamic, as opposed to the traditional static, approach to monitoring the developmental events of the early human embryos in vitro, enabling photographs to be automatically collected at regular intervals throughout the laboratory-based life of the embryo. This avoids the need to remove the embryos from the protective and optimized incubation conditions so the embryologist can microscopically assess them. Along with this comes the facility to precisely and automatically time stamp each cell division or developmental event, be it anomalous or typical. The combination of morphological and dynamic, or kinetic, assessment has been termed morphokinetics.

Static, visual inspection of embryo morphology was discussed in Chapter 10 by Thomas Ebner. In brief, very commonly in IVF the "best" available embryo, in terms of its morphology alone, is chosen from a cohort of embryos, between two and six days following insemination, to be transferred to the uterus. This crucial decision is made on the series of static observations but is often heavily weighted to the

appearance of the embryos on the day of scheduled embryo transfer.

Failure to select a viable embryo for transfer will inevitably remove the chance of a positive outcome in an IVF treatment cycle, and failure to preferentially select a viable embryo from a cohort of embryos will delay time to pregnancy and birth. With highly successful cryopreservation programs available in most fertility clinics, it is likely that transferring a patient's embryos consecutively (following vitrification and warming) will have the same end result (or the same cumulative pregnancy rate), as selection to prioritize the embryos according to their expected potential to implant. However, to minimize the emotional (and sometimes the financial) burden on patients, identification and selection of the most viable embryo should be a priority. With advancing maternal age being the most negatively impactful factor on fertility, time is of the essence and delays should be avoided when at all possible.

Sequential observations of the developing embryos in vitro, whether they are static and daily, or several times hourly using time-lapse imaging, assists in building up an informative log of the embryo's in vitro developmental history. This detail has been linked to the quality or viability potential of the embryo and sheds light on its timeline through and after fertilization. We know that several of the developing embryo's morphological features are most accurately assessed in relation to time, and evidence and guidelines suggest that the assessment of these should ideally be performed within designated, evidence-based, and specified time windows [1].

The observation of morphology over time (morphokinetics) as an indicator of embryonic competency is not new but has become more sophisticated and clinically utilizable due to technological advancements and the introduction of time-lapse imaging devices in the IVF laboratory.

11.2 Considerations When Implementing Time-Lapse Imaging in the IVF Laboratory

There are several time-lapse imaging devices available. Before making a selection for use, capabilities, specification, and user requirements should be considered carefully. As with any new laboratory equipment, a clear rationale is required, and a cost-benefit and evidence assessment should be conducted in order to assist in selecting the most appropriate device for the particular setting. Other important considerations include supplier reliability and responsiveness, device capacity, culture conditions (dry/humid), alarm system compatibility, software and algorithm availability, consumable cost, and other requirements such as plastic-ware and gases, service contract arrangements, space requirement, user-friendliness, monitoring arrangements, training availability, support, and operating procedures/ laboratory protocols for use.

Time-lapse devices differ widely in their specification in terms of the type of microscopy used, light exposure, frequency and quality of image collection, software, and the number of focal planes. It is always advisable to speak to specialist colleagues about their own experiences and to attend a workshop, or obtain a demonstration device, to give first-hand experience of using the device prior to making a choice. A comprehensive change control plan, service-level agreement, and validation plan are recommended once the selection has been made. As most time-lapse devices currently rely on manual, or semiautomatic annotation of the time-lapse images, staff training in annotation and a quality assurance schedule is critical and should be specified from the outset [2]. A basic example of a user requirement specification for a time-lapse device is provided to enable comparison of specifications and capabilities in Table 11.1.

Table 11.1. Example of equipment specification template for a time-lapse imaging system

Equipment	Time-lapse device					
Model reference						
Manufacturer						
Scope and application	A time-lapse incubator for CO_2/reduced O_2 incubation and morphokinetic assessment facilitated by annotation of inseminated human oocytes and embryos in an IVF laboratory.					
Date						
Completed by						
	Basic requirements					
Ref	Priority	Description		Function provided	Verified	Date
	Hi M Lo			Y N ?		
1		O_2/CO_2 mix utilizing N_2 from a generator				
2		Integrated data logging				
3		External independent monitoring facility				
4		Maximum external dimensions = n x n x n				
5		Software/API for data merging				
6		Budget				
7		Running cost/consumables				
8		Capacity				
9		Quality standards met				

Table 11.1. *(cont.)*

Equipment	Time-lapse device			
Model reference				
Manufacturer				
Scope and application	A time-lapse incubator for CO_2/reduced O_2 incubation and morphokinetic assessment facilitated by annotation of inseminated human oocytes and embryos in an IVF laboratory.			
Date				
Completed by				

Basic requirements

Additional requirements

Ref	Priority	Description	Function provided	Verified	Date
	H M L		Y N ?		
9		Alarm connectivity compatibility			
10		Easy to clean			
11		Servicing frequency			
12		Number of focal planes = n			
13		Minimum image quality			
14		Software – ease of use, flexible, adaptable			
15		Annotation (manual/auto)			
16		Remote support			

Key performance indicators (KPI) from manufacturers data

Ref	Priority	Description	Meets KPI	Verified	Date
	H M L		Y N ?		
1		e.g. maximum temperature change after door opening = n			
2		Temperature recovery time after door opening = <n seconds			
3		Maximum CO_2 dip after door opening= n%			
4		CO_2 recovery time after door opening= <n seconds/ minutes			

Maintenance /servicing and warranty

Ref	Priority	Description	Meets requirements	Verified	Date
	H M L		Y N ?		
1		Serviceable by current service contractors			
2		Reliable historical service from manufacturer/ distributor			
3		Serviceable by distributor			
4		Warranty from installation date			
5		Lead time for callout			

Table 11.1. (*cont.*)

Equipment	Time-lapse device				
Model reference					
Manufacturer					
Scope and application	A time-lapse incubator for CO_2/reduced O_2 incubation and morphokinetic assessment facilitated by annotation of inseminated human oocytes and embryos in an IVF laboratory.				
Date					
Completed by					
	Basic requirements				
	Total costs				
Ref	Provider	Item description	Cost	Verified	Comment	Date
1		Device				
2		Delivery				
3		Alarm				
4		Installation				
5		Gases				
6		IT				

11.3 Uses of Time-Lapse Imaging and Assessment

There are several approaches to using time-lapse devices in fertility laboratories. They can be used simply as an undisturbed incubator, whereby the embryologist or technician can view the developing embryos using the acquired photographic images, at the time points already proposed by consensus guidelines. Such data can provide useful information, allow a more complex and analytical approach to be taken, or can be applied somewhere in between. This will be covered in Section 11.5.4 in more detail.

Due to the high magnification and image quality provided by most time-lapse imaging, such devices provide a useful platform for training and teaching. The facility to pause, rewind, and study the images enables the student to learn and evaluate clinical material without rushing or imposing risk on the embryos caused by environmental stress, outside of the protected culture environment. The time-lapse device can also be used to enable increased flexibility in working patterns within the IVF laboratory. With the capabilities to "turn back the clock," and rewind the time-lapse videos, embryologists can make their assessments conveniently within their working day.

For example, an insemination could take place at 11 am, and fertilization assessment can be conducted optimally using the time-lapse images of 16–18 hours later. Without time lapse, insemination at this time of day would require intervention for assessment of fertilization between 3 am and 5 am.

A new level of second opinion is now possible – particularly useful within a small team – such that a colleague can later look at the same image, or series of them, that were originally assessed. Finally, there are also multiple opportunities for the study of embryo morphokinetics, anomalies of development, and to make novel observations that would not be possible without this tool.

11.4 Morphokinetics and Annotation: What Can and What Should Be Recorded?

On review of time-lapse images, generally viewed as a video, the embryologist or technician can manually (or automatically) annotate the images using the device software, in order to obtain a detailed log of the embryo's morphokinetic profile, along with any other observable variables required. There are many different approaches to this practice, from limited

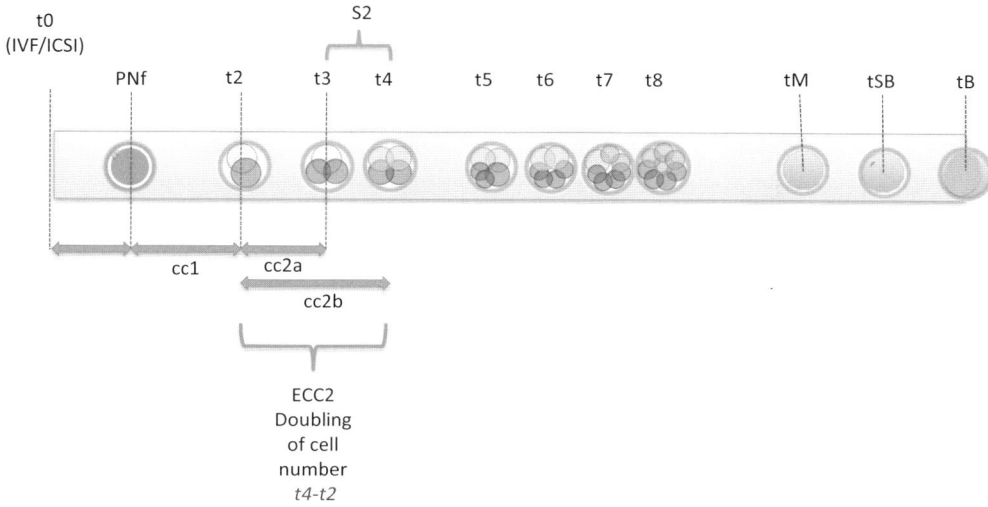

Figure 11.1 Schematic of time-lapse nomenclature. Adapted from Campbell A, Fishel S, editors. *Atlas of time lapse embryology*. Boca Raton, FL: CRC Press; 2015.

annotation (of pronuclear number and cell number) to very detailed annotation that may incorporate novel observations, sometimes clustered over several consecutive image frames. The approach adopted will likely depend on the output required. The laboratory operating procedure may dictate that the time-lapse device is simply used as a regular incubator, but that the embryos are viewed on the device monitor rather than removing them from the culture environment. On the other hand, great details may be collected for each embryo with the intention of applying or devising algorithms for embryo selection.

Annotation practice and nomenclature are based on the times (t) from IVF or intracytoplasmic sperm injection to pronuclear appearance (tPNa) and fading (tPNf) and through each cell division – generally to eight cells (t2 to t8), and from morula formation (tM), start of blastulation (tSB), the full blastocyst (tB), and expanded blastocyst (tExB). Using common time-lapse nomenclature, cell cycles for each blastomere are coded "cc" such that cc2, for example, describes the second cell cycle, calculated as t3–t2 (Figure 11.1).

Conventional, static, light microscopical observations, unlike time-lapse imaging, do not facilitate the detailed assessment of timings of mitoses, or enable the observation of anomalous cleavage events of the in vitro preimplantation embryo. Furthermore, without time-lapse, transient characteristics such as number of pronuclei, multinucleation, or cell merging can easily be missed when embryos are limited to a single observation. Time-lapse imaging and analysis ensure that such phenomena can be observed and recorded, which allows them to be considered when embryo selection takes place. Approaches to using time-lapse imaging in the IVF lab range from simple to complex (Table 11.2).

Since the introduction of time-lapse imaging within clinical IVF, novel variables have been described and their associations with viability are being studied. Examples include the appearance, number, and dynamics of blastocoelic threads, or strings; the angle between the polar bodies; filopodia-like structures at the cleavage furrow; and episodes of blastocyst expansion and collapse. Even without vast morphokinetic data and analyses, it is logical that if an embryo cleaves irregularly or erroneously, deviating from what we understand of cell biology and mitosis, that it may be less viable, at least, than an embryo which develops typically and according to our biology textbooks. Time lapse offers this insight and huge opportunity for research studies (Video 11.1).

11.5 Practical Tips for Working with Time Lapse

Four areas that may require particular consideration, attention, and skill for those introducing time-lapse imaging are dish or slide preparation, annotation standards and consistency, information for patients, and data handling.

117

Table 11.2. Examples of simple, moderate, and complex approaches to the use of time-lapse imaging in the IVF lab

Simple	Used primarily as an uninterrupted incubation system. Limited assessment of images (with or without annotation). For example, assessment of number of pronuclei, early divisions, and/or blastocyst development.
Moderate	Assessment, with annotation, of the process of development from fertilization to blastocyst development (e.g. annotation of fertilization and t2–tB); with attention given to erroneous development or behavior. For example, trichotomous division of one blastomere, "direct cleavage," which has been reported to be associated with poor viability. The use of commercially available, or published, algorithms may sit in this category.
Complex	Assessment and recording of the variables above, with additional focus given to the annotation of further novel variables such as blastocoel collapse, vacuolation, cell merging, polar body dynamics, etc. for within-house algorithm development and validation. This approach is most conducive to research studies.

11.5.1 Dish or Slide Preparation

Embryologists are already familiar in working with aseptic technique and understand the need to work swiftly to minimize evaporation of culture medium during dish preparation. The same principles apply when preparing dishes, or "slides," for time-lapse incubators but with additional practical challenges to consider. Time-lapse incubation, being undisturbed, sits well with the use of single-step culture medium; rather than sequential media so the dishes are often prepared and then used for five, six, or even seven days continuously. We know that over this period, evaporation can occur, potentially causing shifts in osmolality that can harm or stress oocytes, zygotes, or embryos. Being mindful of the need for evaporation minimization is vital, so working swiftly and using cold medium and oil on a nonheated workbench is recommended, prior to equilibration. One dish should be prepared at a time, for the same reason. Another dish preparation tip, particularly important when working with time-lapse, is to remove any bubbles within the dish after its preparation and before use that may obscure the oocyte or embryo and impact the quality of the time-lapse image collected. The use of a stereo microscope to perform dish preparation and bubble identification and removal is advisable.

11.5.2 Annotation Standards

Although automated, or semiautomated, time-lapse video analysis and interpretation is likely to be increasingly used in the future, so far, data generated from these devices have primarily come from manual image assessment and recordings of the events observed (that is, by "annotation"), on human review of the time-lapse images viewed as videos. Due to the manual nature of data collection, to minimize subjectivity and maximize data quality, rigorous training of practitioners and quality assurance is required to assure the output and value of a clinical time-lapse offering. The use of intraclass correlation coefficients, for example, enables assessment of different practitioners and the reproducibility of annotations of the morphokinetic variables. Where there are multiple practitioners involved in time-lapse data collection, the risk of subjectivity and inconsistency is enhanced, and intrapractitioner annotation variation may also exist. Minimization of this subjectivity can be achieved by clear definition of key variables, and with strict annotation practice, set out within the standard operating procedure. Guidelines for nomenclature and annotation are available to encourage international consistency and to allow compilation of large data in the future [3].

11.5.3 Information for Patients

When introducing time-lapse imaging in the IVF lab, the level of information provided to patients will likely relate to the approach taken by the embryology laboratory and clinic to its application. For example, if the time-lapse device functionality is not used to assess the developing embryos in a more detailed manner than standard methodologies, there may be no additional information available for the patient, who may not even have awareness of the type of incubator or monitoring method used. However, if the clinic is actively utilizing the time-lapse images to provide information about the developing embryos, and perhaps also for preferential selection, these details can be shared with the patients to inform, support, and advise them. Furthermore, some clinics make the time-lapse videos available to patients through a portal, or use them as an aide for consultation such that the additional information gleaned may enhance patient acceptance of their treatment and their subfertility, and help them plan their next steps. The impact for the IVF patient, of incorporating time-lapse monitoring of embryo development, therefore appears to go beyond clinical outcome.

11.5.4 Time-Lapse Data Handling and Analysis

The quantity of data obtained from time-lapse imaging increases in scale rapidly. This is expected as around 10 focal plane images are collected every 5–10 minutes for each embryo from insemination through to embryo transfer (so over 120 hours or more), along with patient demographic, clinical, and outcome data. To be able to link the time-lapse data export with clinical databases, a unique identifier should be used to log each patient onto the time-lapse device (Figure 11.2). Completion and accuracy of annotation and outcome data are crucial to maximize the outputs, particularly if algorithms are planned.

The morphokinetic data of a specific, transferred embryo where the outcome is known has been commonly referred to as being of "known implantation data" or "KID." This outcome may be a pregnancy test result (positive or negative), gestational sac, fetal heart, miscarriage, embryo ploidy, or a live birth.

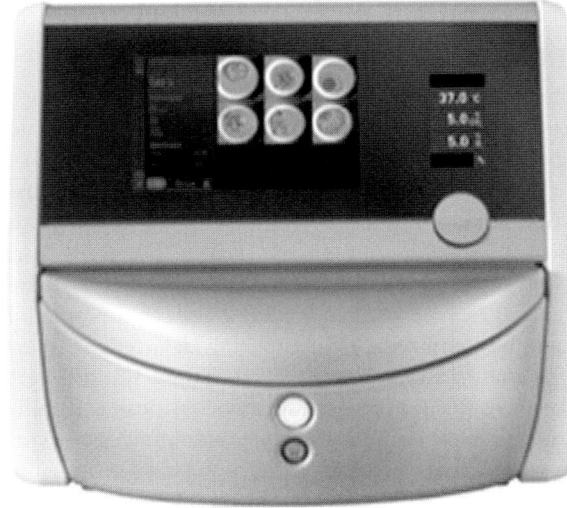

Figure 11.2 Example of a time-lapse imaging device. EmbryoScope Flex (image provided by Vitrolife, Sweden).

Morphokinetic data can be compared between embryos giving positive or negative implantation data (KID+ or KID−) in order to identify significant variables, or to build selection algorithms. All data can be utilized following a single embryo transfer, or a double embryo transfer with a negative outcome (as the fate of all of these individual embryos is known). Using data following multiple embryo transfer resulting in the same number of fetal hearts/babies born is best avoided as it can be problematic without the use of genetic fingerprinting to ascertain the chorionicity or zygoticity.

Annotation data, consisting of timings, morphologies, anomalies, irregularities, novel phenomena, and durations of embryo developmental events, have been retrospectively analyzed against such outcome measures and these data can also be used to derive predictive selection algorithms, or to identify simple preferential selection (or deselection) criteria, for prospective use in the IVF laboratory.

11.6 Time-Lapse Algorithms for Embryo Selection

Early adopters of clinical time-lapse imaging in IVF used a hierarchical approach to time-lapse algorithm development whereby embryos were classified based on them reaching developmental milestones, along with the relative timings associated with them. Significant differences were reported between implanted and not implanted embryos for six early morphokinetic variables [4]. Since then, many time-lapse algorithms have been published that differ in the significant variables identified, outcome measures used, and the timings of specified developmental events. There have been several reports of unsuccessful transfer of algorithms between clinical settings but also of the value of generic algorithms, which are now commercially available through device manufacturers [5, 6, 7]. Best practice should always be to validate any time-lapse algorithms, retrospectively and in-house, on large data prior to clinical application, and to assess the performance of the algorithm regularly.

11.7 Does Time-Lapse Imaging Bring Clinical Benefits?

Morphokinetic analysis is considered by many time-lapse users to provide more informed embryo selection compared with traditional, static morphology. Using this morphokinetic information, selection algorithms have been developed, published, and independently evaluated, although evidence of their performance, compared with traditional morphological selection, and their transferability between clinical settings, is inconsistent. This may in part be due to the lack of standardization and the heterogeneity in the application of time-lapse imaging.

Perhaps confounded by the varied approaches to the implementation of time-lapse imaging in IVF laboratories, and the associated heterogeneity of studies and algorithms reported within the literature, a definitive uplift in clinical outcomes with the use of time-lapse imaging has not been firmly proven. A Cochrane review of 2019, including nine randomized controlled trials, concluded that there was insufficient evidence of improved outcomes (live birth rate, miscarriage rate, and clinical pregnancy rate) when time-lapse was compared with conventional methods [8]. Despite this finding, it is generally accepted that time-lapse imaging is safe and that the undisturbed culture and continuous monitoring that time lapse offers should provide the most stable environment for development, and more critical embryo assessment and selection. A number of large retrospective studies have reported enhanced outcomes, but more studies are required [6].

Artificial intelligence (AI) is being introduced in many areas of medicine, including reproductive medicine. A recent multicenter large retrospective analysis of information gleaned from time-lapse imaging utilized a deep learning trained model to predict clinical pregnancy with higher accuracy than time-lapse algorithms have, to date, reported. Prospective studies are now required to assess the potential clinical impact of AI approaches, which sit well with time-lapse technology [9].

11.8 Human Embryo Morphokinetics and Chromosomal Anomalies

Aneuploidy is believed to be the largest cause of embryo implantation failure and miscarriage. Aneuploidy is prevalent in human oocytes and embryos, with incidence increasing with maternal age. Preimplantation genetic testing for aneuploidy (PGT-A) is aimed at identifying aneuploidy to enable the preferential selection of euploidy.

Identification of the most viable embryo for transfer has become increasingly important to maximize success following fertility treatment and to reduce the number of multiple pregnancies and births. Whether PGT-A improves outcomes has been continuously debated and large randomized controlled trials are few, and often outdated by the time of completion and technology progresses. Despite PGT-A being generally considered effective at identifying embryo ploidy, and enhancing outcomes in some studies, there are limitations and challenges to this approach. The removal of several trophectoderm cells for testing requires technical expertise and training and specific equipment. The procedure, and especially the genetic testing, can be expensive and time-consuming. Furthermore, the approach and invasive nature of this test has resulted in concerns being raised regarding its ethics and reliability.

Prior to the introduction of time-lapse imaging, there had been a few reports in the scientific literature of associations between blastocyst morphology and aneuploidy, and of delayed development of aneuploidy embryos, around the time of blastulation. With the introduction of time-lapse imaging in IVF laboratories offering PGT-A came the opportunity to study the morphokinetics of euploid and aneuploid embryos, and to assess whether differences existed that could be associated with the copy number of chromosomes within the cells of the developing embryos.

11.8.1 Is There an Association between Embryo Ploidy and Morphokinetics?

Since 2012, there have been several time-lapse-based reports of associations between early human embryo development and ploidy. In particular, the timing of early cleavage events was reported to be tightly clustered in euploid human embryos, compared with their aneuploid counterparts [10]. This study was followed by others that also considered whether there was a difference in the morphokinetics of euploid and aneuploid embryos, by comparing data from blastocysts that had undergone PGT-A. Some, but not all – like the early nontime-lapse reports – found significant periblastulation delays in aneuploid embryos. However, there is heterogeneity between time-lapse studies considering and comparing the morphokinetics of euploid and aneuploid embryos, and most have not reported an association between early morphokinetics and ploidy, suggesting that euploid and aneuploid embryos may develop similarly until around the maternal to zygotic genomic transition.

A systematic review of 2018 covered 13 time-lapse publications that considered morphokinetics and ploidy. It highlighted the heterogeneity of these studies, which varied in the stage of embryo biopsy, the clinical indications for PGT-A, incubation conditions, outcome measure, and statistical methodology and concluded that the intervals between cleavage events appeared to have more relevance than the specific timings, when considering the potential selection of euploid embryos. In addition, the review concluded that most of the studies, which involved extended culture to the blastocyst stage, reported significant differences between periblastulation morphokinetics of aneuploid and euploid [11]. More studies are needed to elucidate fully the possible association between morphokinetics and embryo ploidy. Early time-lapse markers are arguably simpler and more objectively annotated, but it appears that they may not be as reliably representative of embryo viability as the later morphokinetic variables.

This area of clinical research is particularly challenging, in part due to the heterogeneity of patient factors and clinical practices, but also because embryo ploidy is not truly binary, as ploidy mosaicism exists within the human embryo. Furthermore, there is evidence to suggest that laboratory factors, such as culture media, humidity, or oxygen tension, could impact embryo aneuploidy [12].

11.8.2 Are There Practical Synergies between Time-Lapse Imaging and PGT-A?

Time-lapse imaging in the IVF laboratory may complement PGT-A in several ways. Frequent acquisition of time-lapse images avoids the need to remove the embryo culture dish from the optimized conditions in order to assess the developing embryos. This has advantages for PGT-A practice as the embryologist can perform numerous assessments of the embryos in order to optimize the timing of facilitative laser breaching (if performed) and of the biopsy procedure. This information could also be helpful to inform patients and to set their expectations about the number and the quality of blastocysts available. This morphokinetic detail could also be utilized to prioritize blastocysts for biopsy, especially if the number of blastocysts to be biopsied was restricted due to

capacity or cost. If proven to offer superior selection, time lapse could also provide the potential for ranking euploid embryos for transfer when patients are fortunate enough to have more than one.

Time-lapse imaging in the field of IVF is a vibrant and continuously emerging field that could benefit patients and help further our understanding of human preimplantation development [13].

Key Messages

- Human embryos in vitro are not all equal in their capacity to make a viable pregnancy. How we assess and select between them is of great importance. Time-lapse is providing embryologists with more detailed information that may improve knowledge and selection accuracy, compared with standard approaches.
- Time-lapse imaging is a useful tool in the IVF laboratory offering several benefits:
  1. information and advanced embryo assessment and selection
  2. a teaching, training, and supervising tool
  3. ease of obtaining a second opinion
  4. increased flexibility in workflow
  5. research and development opportunities
- Time-lapse algorithms for embryo selection can be adopted from the published literature, developed in-house, or obtained commercially from device manufacturers. Validation of algorithms should always be performed prior to prospective use.
- Implementing time-lapse imaging requires careful planning. Important considerations include choice of device, annotation policy, the use of algorithms, and data handling. Collaboration with expert users and utilizing published guidelines for use and nomenclature is recommended.
- There are potential synergies between time-lapse imaging and PGT-A:
  1. Real-time images can be utilized to optimize the timing of laser breaching (to facilitate herniation) and biopsy, for PGT-A, without removing the embryos from the incubator until necessary.
  2. Time-lapse algorithms may be useful in selecting between euploid embryos.
  3. Where PGT-A is not available or permitted, time lapse may provide more information than standard selection and a more precise, noninvasive selection tool.

References

1. Alpha Scientists in Reproductive Medicine and ESHRE Special Interest Group of Embryology. The Istanbul consensus workshop on embryo assessment: proceedings of an expert meeting. *Hum Reprod.* 2011;26:1270–83.

   Alpha Scientists in Reproductive Medicine and ESHRE Special Interest Group of Embryology. The Istanbul consensus workshop on embryo assessment: proceedings of an expert meeting. *Reprod Biomed Online.* 2011;22:632–6.

2. Campbell A, Fishel S, editors. *Atlas of time lapse embryology.* Boca Raton, FL: CRC Press; 2015.

3. Ciray HN, Campbell A, Agerholm IE, Aguilar J, Chamayou S, Esbert M, Sayed S. Proposed guidelines on the nomenclature and annotation of dynamic human embryo monitoring by a time-lapse user group. *Human Reprod.* 2014;29(12):2650–60.

4. Basile N, Vime P, Florensa M, Aparicio Ruiz B, Garcia Velasco JA, Remohi J, Meseguer M. The use of morphokinetics as a predictor of implantation: a multicentric study to define and validate an algorithm for embryo selection. *Human Reprod.* 2014;30 (2):276–83.

5. Peterson BM, Boel M, Montag M, Gardner DK. Development of a generally applicable morphokinetic algorithm capable of predicting the implantation potential of embryos transferred on day 3. *Hum Reprod.* 2016;31:2231–44.

6. Fishel S, Campbell A, Foad F, Davies L, Best L, Davis N, et al. Evolution of embryo selection for IVF from subjective morphology assessment to objective time-lapse algorithms improves chance of live birth. *Reprod Biomed Online.* 2020;40(1):61–70.

7. Pribenszky C, Nilselid AM, Montag M. Time-lapse culture with morphokinetic embryo selection improves pregnancy and live birth chances and reduces early pregnancy loss: a meta-analysis. *Reprod Biomed Online.* 2017;35(5):511–20.

8. Armstrong S, Bhide P, Jordan V, Pacey A, Farquhar C. Time-lapse systems for ART. *Reprod Biomed Online.* 2018;1(36):288–9.

9. Tran D, Cooke S, Illingworth PJ, Gardner DK. Deep learning as a predictive tool for fetal heart pregnancy following time-lapse incubation and blastocyst transfer. *Hum Reprod.* 2019;34 (6):1011–18.

10. Chavez SL, Loewke KE, Han J, Moussavi F, Colls P, Munne S, et al. Dynamic blastomere behaviour reflects human embryo ploidy by the four-cell stage. *Nature Comms.* 2012;3:1251.

11. Reignier A, Lammers J. Barriere P, Freour T. Can time-lapse parameters predict embryo ploidy? A systematic review. *Reprod Biomed Online.* 2018;26:380–7.

12. Swain JE. Controversies in ART: can the IVF laboratory influence preimplantation embryo aneuploidy? *Reprod Biomed Online.* 2019;39(4):599–607.

13. Campbell A. Noninvasive techniques: embryo selection by time lapse imaging. In: Markus Montag, editor. *A practical guide to selecting gametes and embryos.* Boca Raton, FL: CRC Press; 2014. p. 177–89.

Noninvasive Analysis of Embryo Nutrient Utilization for Embryo Selection

David K. Gardner, Laura Ferrick, Rebecca L. Kelley, and Yee Shan Lisa Lee

12.1 Introduction

Over the past 40 years, we have become proficient in assessing human embryo morphology as it develops from a fertilized oocyte to the blastocyst stage, thanks to the creation of numerous grading systems to define the development of the embryo at each successive stage [1]. Such an approach has greatly facilitated the identification of embryos with high developmental potential within a cohort, but has been hampered by the subjectivity associated with human visual assessment. With the advent of time-lapse microscopy, we have been provided with a detailed and continuous insight into preimplantation embryo development, and can now determine hitherto unknown variables, such as the precise time of first cleavage, and the initiation and duration of blastocyst formation. The availability of such new data has facilitated the creation of algorithms based on key developmental events in order to rank embryos in terms of their developmental potential [2]. However, the assessment of embryos is still undertaken by an embryologist, and therefore a degree of subjectivity remains. Excitingly, artificial intelligence (AI), capable of maximizing all available information made possible through images captured every few minutes and the use of machine learning [3], has alleviated the issue of subjectivity. Evident advantages of the latter approach include the elimination of variability inherent between embryologists in assessing morphological events, and the dramatic reduction in time required to analyze developmental competency (it takes less than a minute for AI to analyze the entire patient's cohort of embryos). Although the ability of AI to rank and select the most viable embryo looks promising, the full potential of AI in embryo selection now awaits prospective randomized trials.

While morphological analysis of an embryo using conventional light microscopy, whether by an embryologist or computer, has proved to be of value in embryo selection, morphologically similar embryos can still have different implantation potential. Significantly, morphological assessment reveals little regarding the physiological status and health of the embryo. Sibling human blastocysts of the same grade have been shown to differ considerably in their nutrient utilization (Figure 12.1) [4]. It is beyond the scope of this chapter to elaborate on the elegant regulation of human preimplantation embryo metabolism as it develops and differentiates [5, 6]. Rather, the relationship between metabolic functions and embryo health and viability is considered in this chapter. Further, this chapter discusses how metabolism and epigenetic state are coupled through the metaboloepigenetic axis, and subsequently to embryo/fetal health [7, 8].

12.2 How Metabolism and Viability of the Preimplantation Embryo Are Related

A relationship between metabolism and embryo viability (as determined through embryo transfer) was established over 30 years ago in both the cow and mouse, where glucose uptake by the blastocyst was positively related to subsequent pregnancy outcome [9, 10]. This relationship between glucose uptake and viability was subsequently confirmed in the human embryo (Figure 12.2) [11, 12]. Further research on the mouse blastocyst revealed that not only was the amount of glucose consumed important, but also the fate of glucose consumed, in this case the production of lactate, as an indirect measure of glycolytic activity. A benefit from animal studies is that one can assess embryos developed in vivo (as a gold standard) and consequently compare their metabolic activity to embryos developed in culture. With regards to glycolytic activity, a mouse blastocyst developed in vivo converts ~40–50% of glucose to lactate. It was subsequently determined that if a mouse blastocyst developed in vitro had a glycolytic rate of ~50%, that

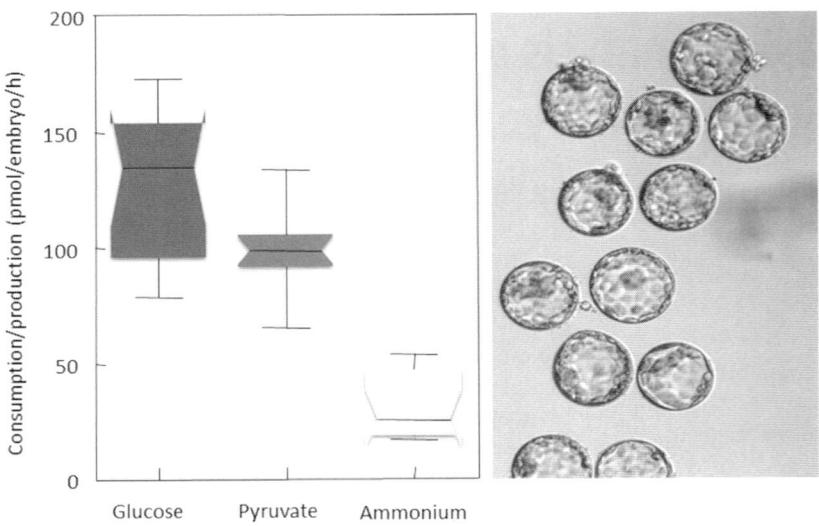

Figure 12.1 Nutrient uptake and ammonium production by individual human blastocysts from the same patient
Thirteen human blastocysts from an oocyte donor were donated to research [4]. These embryos had not undergone cryopreservation. Data are in the form of a notched box plot where the notches represent the interquartile range, therefore including 50% of the data points. Whiskers represent 5% and 95% quartiles. The line across the box represents the median. The spread of glucose uptake is ~100 pmol/embryo/h, a wide spread of nutrient utilization. Pyruvate is not a major nutrient of the blastocyst and does not appear to differ between embryos. The ammonium produced by the blastocysts reflects amino acid turnover. The image of the blastocysts from which the metabolic data were extracted reveals how difficult it can be to select them based on their morphology.

a)

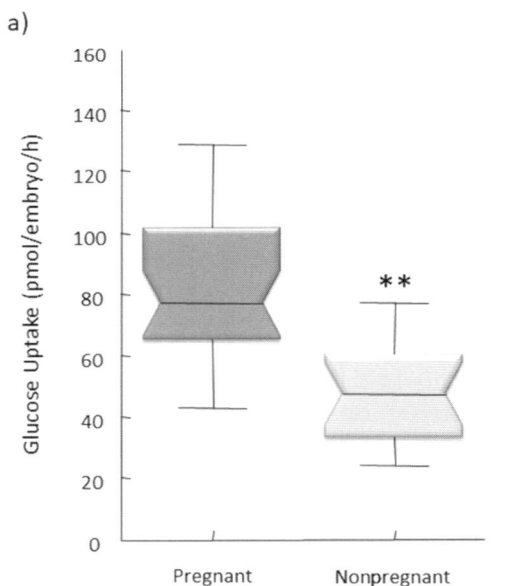

b)

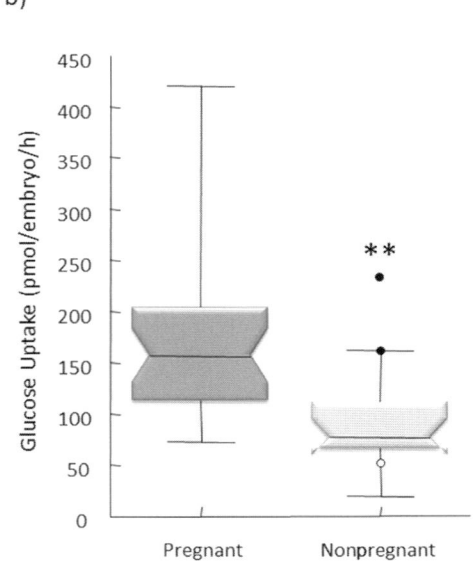

Figure 12.2a Glucose uptake on day 4 of embryonic development and pregnancy outcome (positive fetal heartbeat)
Notches represent the interquartile range (50% of the data), whiskers represent the 5% and 95% quartiles. The line across the box is the median glucose consumption.
Note: **, significantly different from pregnant (P<0.01).

Figure 12.2b Glucose uptake on day 5 of embryonic development and pregnancy outcome (positive fetal heartbeat)
Notches represent the interquartile range (50% of the data), whiskers represent the 5% and 95% quartiles. The line across the box is the median glucose consumption.
Note: **, significantly different from pregnant (P<0.01).
Closed circles represent the two blastocysts that gave rise to a positive fetal sac, but no subsequent fetal heart. The open circle represents the blastocyst that resulted in a positive hCG but not fetal sac.

is, similar to that of an embryo developed in vivo, then viability was high. However, if a blastocyst produced excessive lactate, reflecting an excessive glycolytic rate (close to or above 100%) and hence a loss of metabolic control, then viability was significantly diminished [13]. These data led to the "rate and fate" hypothesis, which proposed that the amount of a nutrient consumed, together with information on how this nutrient was metabolized, provides a measure of embryonic viability [5]. What is fascinating about this hypothesis is that it predicts that when culture conditions are manipulated, they will affect metabolism and in turn affect viability. For example, Lane and Gardner determined that both amino acids and vitamins regulate the glycolytic activity of the mouse blastocyst by decreasing the levels of glycolysis compared to a medium that lacked them, and that if both were removed from the culture environment, the blastocyst rapidly lost control of its metabolic activity and viability was significantly compromised as a result [14].

As well as being regulators of carbohydrate metabolism, amino acids are themselves used as energy metabolites, and also serve numerous important functions during embryo development including pH regulation, osmotic control, biosynthetic precursors, antioxidants, regulation of differentiation, and signaling molecules [15]. Hence analyzing their utilization by the preimplantation embryo has significant physiological merit. Indeed, the use of amino acids by human embryos has been linked to both development in vitro, to subsequent viability post-transfer and possibly to chromosomal complement [12, 16, 17, 18].

12.3 Impact of Culture Conditions on Metabolism

Given the relationship between metabolism and embryo viability, it is not surprising that culture conditions known to adversely affect embryonic development can have a profound effect on metabolic function. One of the most significant regulators of metabolic function is oxygen. It has been documented in all mammalian species studied to date (including humans) that physiological levels of oxygen (~5%) support higher levels of embryo development and viability compared to the use of atmospheric oxygen [19]. Analysis of the impact of oxygen concentration on embryo metabolism determined that not only does

20% oxygen significantly impair the utilization of glucose and amino acids in the mouse embryo [20], it also compromises the ability of the embryo to regulate other functions, such as the transamination of ammonium [21].

Initial studies on human embryo metabolism were performed on cleavage-stage embryos developed in suboptimal culture conditions, that is, no amino acids [22, 23], and/or the embryos were cultured in the presence of 20% oxygen [16]. Importantly, recent studies have employed more physiological conditions [11, 12, 24]. From such works it has been confirmed that glucose uptake is a biomarker of human embryonic viability independent of morphology [11] and both glucose uptake and amino utilization correlate with the Gardner Grade, developmental algorithms, and embryo analysis by AI [12]. Further, we propose that analysis of embryo physiology will not only help identify the most viable embryo for transfer but could also be linked to the subsequent health of the child through the relationship between metabolism and epigenetic programming [7, 8, 25]. Here we describe some of the technologies that can be used to quantitate the dynamic metabolic activity of the preimplantation human embryo, and how such data can assist in selecting the healthiest embryo for transfer.

12.4 Assessment of Embryo Metabolism

Analysis of embryo metabolism comes with technical difficulties (addressed in detail in the following sections), and also the challenge that the preimplantation embryo changes its physiology and metabolic profile at each successive stage of development. Prior to compaction the embryo is primarily dependent upon pyruvate as a main energy source, while after morula formation the embryo becomes increasingly dependent upon glucose [5]. Notably, the overall metabolic activity increases as the embryo progresses from the pronucleate oocyte to the blastocyst stage, and as the embryo develops there is an increasing variation of metabolic activities (Figure 12.3). Consequently, analysis of embryo metabolism is not only more readily quantitated at the blastocyst stage due to its higher metabolic rate, but there exists a greater variability between the metabolic rates at each successive stage of development. With the adoption of single blastocyst transfer as the standard of care in

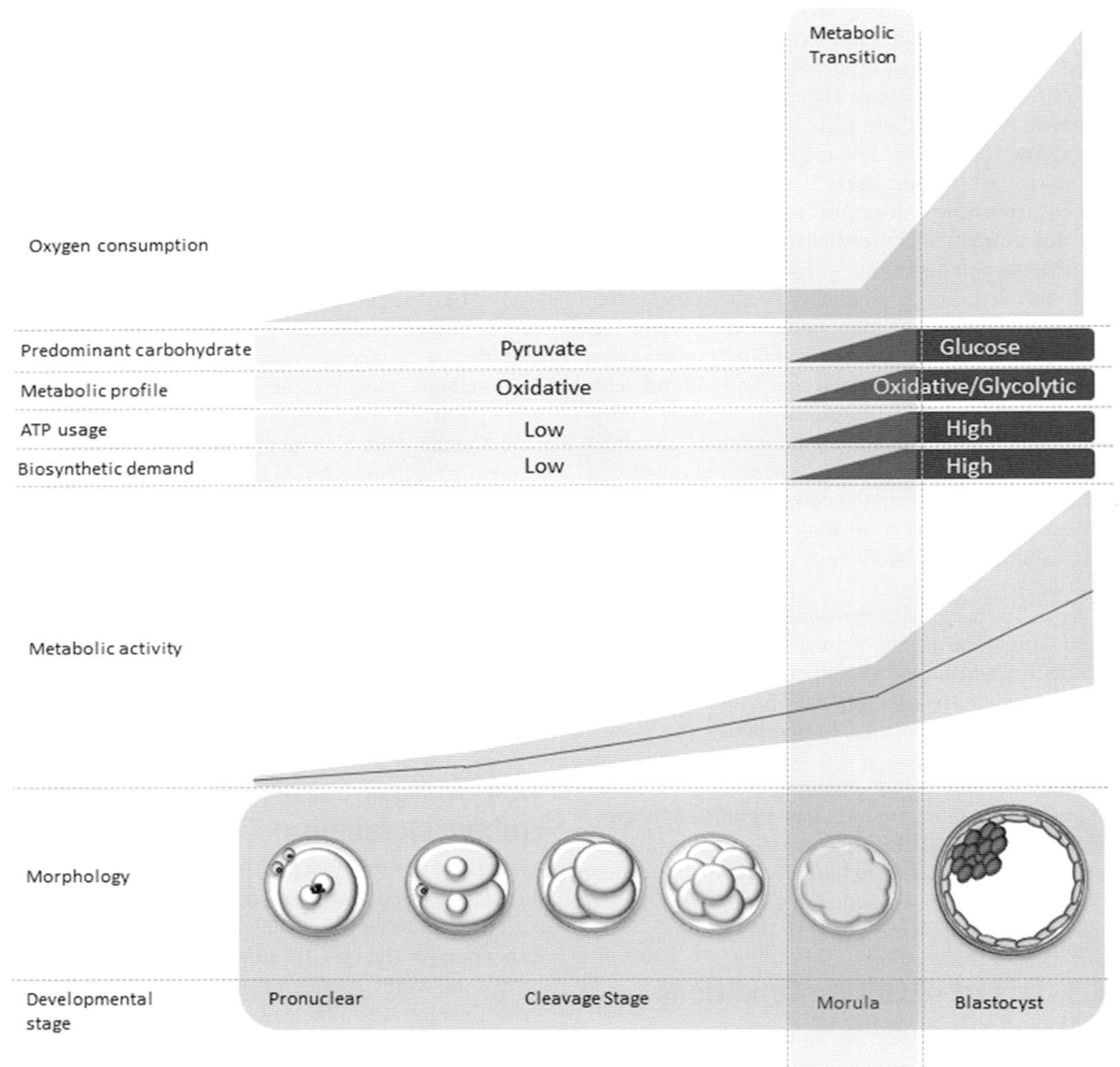

Figure 12.3 Metabolic changes during mammalian preimplantation development
Prior to compaction, the pronucleate oocyte and cleavage-stage embryo predominantly consume pyruvate, and through oxidative metabolism produce appropriate levels of ATP required to support cellular division. After compaction, the embryo exhibits exponential growth, requiring higher levels of ATP synthesis and biosynthetic precursors. This increase in activity is supported by an increase in the overall oxidative capacity of the embryo and also a transition to a highly glycolytic metabolism, whereby higher levels of glucose are consumed and converted to lactate in the presence of oxygen. As overall metabolic activity increases as development proceeds, so does the variation (represented by the shading) around the mean (represented by the solid line).

most clinics worldwide, it is feasible to assess aspects of metabolic activity of individual blastocysts prior to transfer, for example utilization of glucose and amino acids [12, 24]. Interestingly, as noninvasive analysis of cell-free DNA (cfDNA) is being discussed as a potential means of determining embryo ploidy, the incubation of embryos individually, required for such genetic analysis, are the same conditions as currently

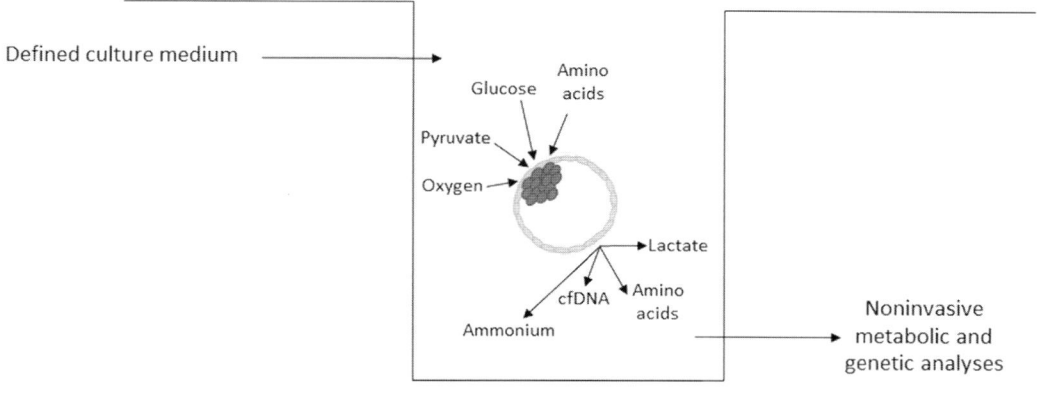

Figure 12.4 Noninvasive analysis of human embryo nutrient consumption and metabolite production, and/or cell-free DNA release into the surrounding medium
Individual embryos can be incubated in 10–15 μl volumes of medium in a microdrop or in a chamber such as in an EmbryoSlide. Samples of medium can then be analyzed by the methods outlined in this chapter.

required to assess metabolic analysis, and hence it will be possible to obtain samples of media for both cfDNA and metabolite analysis (Figure 12.4). Until recently, it was standard practice at most clinics to culture embryos in groups, preventing spent culture media analysis, but the widespread use of time-lapse incubators has necessitated a move toward single-embryo culture, which also facilitates analysis of individual embryo physiology.

A major contributor to the relative paucity of data on the metabolism of individual human embryos has been the sparsity of technologies able to accurately quantitate single embryos, thereby putting the analysis of metabolism out of reach for most IVF clinics. As a result, the majority of data has come from a few specialized laboratories. However, as new technologies develop, there is renewed interest in this area and here we describe the assays and platforms that have been used.

There are two distinct approaches that have been used to assess embryonic metabolic activity; targeted assays to quantitate individual metabolites (which is advantageous if you know which metabolite you wish to measure), and metabolomic platforms able to detect multiple metabolites (which is advantageous if you have no prior hypothesis and wish to perform a broader search). The former category typically includes enzyme-based assays. The latter category typically involves platform-based approaches such as high-performance liquid chromatography (HPLC)

and mass spectrometry, which are usually only available in core facilities, beyond the reach of an IVF laboratory.

Of note, a key to success in any form of analysis is the accuracy of the volumes dispensed. This applies not only to those used in assays, but also the volumes of culture media used for incubation. Even a small percentage variation in volumes can have a significant effect on the assay results [26].

12.5 Assays and Platforms for Individual Metabolic Analyses

12.5.1 Enzyme-Linked Assays for Individual Carbohydrate and Amino Acids

It is feasible to link many metabolites, including carbohydrates and amino acids, to coupled enzymatic reactions that include pyridine nucleotides, NAD(P)H, which fluoresce when excited at 340 nm and emit at 459 nm and above when in the reduced form. When oxidized these nucleotides do not fluoresce. Hence, by quantitating the fluorescence of reactions one can measure the concentration of metabolites. The reactions and assay conditions for pyruvate, lactate, glucose, aspartate, and glutamine are detailed below.

12.5.1.1 Glucose Assay

$$Glucose + ATP \xrightarrow{Hexokinase} Glucose\text{-}6\text{-}phosphate + ADP$$

$$Glucose\text{-}6\text{-}phosphate + NADP^+ \xrightarrow{Glucose\text{-}6\text{-}phosphate\ dehydrogenase}$$
$$6\text{-}phosphogluconate + NADPH + H^+$$

Glucose concentration is proportional to fluorescence.

Reagents for glucose assay: 3.7 mM $MgSO_4.7H_2O$, 0.6 mM $NADP^+$, 0.5 mM ATP, 0.5 mM dithiothreitol, 12 U/ml hexokinase, 6 U/ml glucose-6-phosphate dehydrogenase, in EPPS buffer, pH 8.0.

EPPS buffer: 2.25 g EPPS (4-(2-hydroxyethyl)-1-piperazine propane-sulphonic acid), 10 mg penicillin, 10 mg Streptomycin, made up to 200 ml in water and pH to 8.0 with 1 M NaOH.

12.5.1.2 Lactate Assay

$$Lactate + NAD^+ \xrightarrow{Lactate\ dehydrogenase} Pyruvate + NADH + H^+$$

Lactate concentration is proportional to fluorescence.

Reagents for lactate assay: 4.76 mM NAD^+, 100 U/ml lactate dehydrogenase, 2.6 mM EDTA in glycine-hydrazine buffer, pH 9.4.

Glycine-hydrazine buffer: 7.5 g glycine, 5.2 g hydrazine, 0.2 g EDTA in 50 ml of water, and pH to 9.0 or 9.4 with 2 M NaOH. In this case the reaction facilitated by LDH is effectively nonequilibrium, as the pyruvate is trapped by hydrazine in the form of pyruvate hydrazone, and so the reaction favors the formation of NADH.

12.5.1.3 Pyruvate Assay

$$Pyruvate + NADH + H^+ \xrightarrow{Lactate dehydrogenase} Lactate + NAD^+$$

Pyruvate concentration is inversely proportional to fluorescence.

Reagents for pyruvate assay: 0.12 mM NADH, 28 U/ml lactate dehydrogense in EPPS buffer, pH 8.0.

EPPS buffer: 2.25 g EPPS (4-(2-hydroxyethyl)-1-piperazine propane-sulphonic acid), 10 mg penicillin, 10 mg Streptomycin, made up to 200 ml in water and pH to 8.0 with 1 M NaOH.

12.5.1.4 Aspartate Assay

$$Aspartate + \alpha\text{-}ketoglutarate \xrightarrow{Glutamic\ oxaloacetic\ transaminase}$$
$$Oxaloacetate + Glutamate$$

$$Oxaloacetate + NADH + H^+ \xrightarrow{Malate\ dehydrogenase} Malate + NAD^+$$

Aspartate concentration is inversely proportional to fluorescence.

Reagents for aspartate assay: 0.12 mM α-ketoglutarate, 0.15 mM NADH, 3.5 U/ml malate dehydrogenase, 20 U/ml glutamic oxaloacetic transaminase in imidazole buffer.

Imidazole buffer: 0.2042 g imidazole, 0.4192 g imidazole-HCL, pH 7.0.

12.5.1.5 Glutamine Assay

$$Glutamine + H_2O \xrightarrow{Glutaminase} Glutamate + NH_3$$

$$Glutamate + H_2O + NAD^+ \xrightarrow{Glutamate\ dehydrogenase}$$
$$2\text{-}oxoglutarate + NH_4^+ + NADH$$

Reagents for the glutamine reaction: 50 U/ml glutaminase in acetate buffer, pH 5.0.

Reagents for glutamate reaction: 1.6 mM NAD^+, 1.0 mM ADP, 100 U/ml glutamate dehydrogenase in glycine-hydrazine buffer, pH 9.0.

Unlike the two-step reaction for glucose that can take place in one drop, the glutamine assay has to be carried out in two separate drops as the reactions require different pH optima. Further, the second reaction produces ammonium, and hence by changing the reaction conditions to favor the formation of glutamate and using a triethanolamine buffer at pH 8.0, one can quantitate ammonium [27].

12.5.1.6 Platforms
Ultramicrofluorescence

Ultramicrofluorescence (UMF) is a miniaturization of conventional methods of enzymatic analysis, which uses an inverted fluorescence microscope with photomultiplier or charge-coupled device camera attachments to quantitate the fluorescence associated with coupled reactions. The assays are housed in submicroliter droplets on siliconized microscope slides under heavy mineral oil, rather than in cuvettes as per a standard fluorimeter. Typically, 10–20 nl drops of this reagent cocktail are pipetted using specially constructed constriction pipettes onto a siliconized slide under mineral oil to prevent evaporation (see Gardner [28] for detail on pipette fabrication). Such micropipettes require a micromanipulator and pneumatic control in order to deliver accurately the nanoliter volumes.

The fluorescence of each droplet is measured in turn by exposing the pyridine nucleotides in the assay to a UV light source. Drops are measured using a x20 or x40 objective and are routinely exposed for up to 0.5 seconds, since there is no detectable photooxidation of NADH or NADPH during this time. Following this initial determination of fluorescence, a sample of the culture media (1–5 nl) is added to the reagent cocktail drop. The addition of the substrate initiates the reaction. The drops on the slide are then left until the reaction has gone to completion. This time can vary between three minutes to one hour depending on the substrate being analyzed (which must be determined for each assay by taking readings over time to determine when the reaction has reached completion). The fluorescence of the drops is again quantitated. The change in fluorescence in arbitrary units represents the amount of metabolites. A fresh set of standards are required each day of an experiment in order to relate metabolite concentration to fluorescence. A linear regression value is typically $R > 0.99$. Once a linear standard curve has been established, the concentration of metabolites from samples can be calculated. To measure the production and consumption of embryos within a spent media sample, samples are compared to "no-embryo" control media from drops/wells incubated at the same time as the embryo.

Nanodrop

Nanodrop technology provides a means of adapting enzymatic-based assays to benchtop assays [29]. Similar to UMF, known standards of the metabolite in question are analyzed first to determine a standard, but instead of using constriction pipettes to deliver nanolitre volumes, a commercially available pipette system (eVol positive displacement pipette, SGE Analytical Science) is used to deliver accurately microliter volumes. One microliter of standard or sample is added to 4–9 μl of reagent cocktail in an Eppendorf tube, mixed, and reactions are kept in the dark until it reaches completion as components are light sensitive (generally 20–60 minutes, dependent on the substrate being tested). To measure standards, 2 μl of each reaction is pipetted onto nanodrop platform and the arm of the nanodrop lowered for measurement. This is repeated three times for each standard to produce triplicate readings and then averaged for final fluorescent value to produce a standard curve. Between each measurement the pedestal is wiped down and washed with ultrapure milliQ water.

Once an acceptable linear regression is measured, these steps can then be repeated for samples.

Plate Reader

Plate reader technology is a rapid high-throughput benchtop technology [30] that assists in the rapid detection of metabolites within spent media samples. Typically, 1–5 μl of standard is added to ~50 μl enzymatic cocktail for analysis (dependent on the substrate being analyzed). These reactions can be set up in Eppendorf tubes and kept in the dark until the reaction goes to completion. As the plate reader requires larger volumes, the time to completion is generally longer than using lower volumes in UMF and nanodrop, and reactions may require anywhere from 30 minutes to a few hours.

Following completion of the reactions, triplicates of ~15 μl are pipetted into a microplate and inserted into the plate reader. Multiple reactions can be set up at one time and simultaneously measured as the plate reader can typically measure up to 128 reactions in triplicate using a 384-well plate. Excitation and emission wave lengths can be preset in computer software and analysis takes a matter of minutes. A linear standard curve run with the samples is used to calculate mM concentrations for spent media samples and "no-embryo" control media.

Given the speed of measuring multiple samples simultaneously, the plate reader has greater potential for clinical use compared to the other methods discussed above. Spent culture medium from embryos of an individual's cohort could be removed from culture dishes and analyzed for metabolic biomarkers within a matter of hours to assist in the selection of blastocysts for transfer. The sensitivity of the plate reader, as with all fluorescent platforms, is reliant on incubation time and the concentration of metabolites in media. It is less technically demanding than both UMF and nanodrop, but currently less accurate than UMF.

Microfluidics (Lab-on-a-Chip)

Microfluidics technologies are capable of high throughput and high sensitivity analysis of media samples, and as such make an ideal platform for the analysis of low volumes of sample, such as that obtained from individually cultured embryos. Such devices can readily accommodate a standard enzymatic analysis approach or be coupled with spectroscopies [31]. A microfluidic device capable of accurately measuring volumes in the nanoliter range was developed specifically for this purpose and proved to be an order of magnitude more sensitive than ultramicrofluorescence [32] (Figure 12.5). It is the authors' opinion that microfluidic devices will be available as one of the standard platforms for culture media analysis in the next few years [33].

12.6 Metabolomic Platforms

A distinct advantage of individual targeted assays is their accuracy and affordability, but this is only helpful if you already know which metabolite you wish to measure. From a discovery perspective, metabolomic platforms may be used, such as HPLC, liquid chromatography-mass spectrometry (LC-MS), nuclear magnetic resonance (NMR), and Raman and near-infrared (NIR) spectroscopies.

Both HPLC and LC-MS have been utilized successfully to quantitate amino acids in spent human embryo culture media for several years [12, 16, 24] and remain the platforms of choice for analysis of overall amino acid usage. However, once an amino acid of interest is identified, it is feasible to perform targeted analysis, hereby negating the need for expensive platform-based technology. Other platforms such as nuclear magnetic resonance (NMR) imaging do not appear to possess the sensitivity or resolution to work at the single-embryo level. Raman and NIR spectroscopies have been used to analyze human embryo culture media [34]; however, NIR spectroscopy is not able to quantitate the levels of specific nutrients, but rather creates spectra reflecting the relative abundance of metabolites. Although the latter approach was utilized to create a viability index of human embryos [35], this approach was not able to identify viable embryos in a prospective manner [36]. However, as such technologies rapidly advance research continues in spectroscopy [37].

12.7 Novel Microscopies

Developments in fluorophore-mediated and autofluorescence microscopy have focused on distinguishing very subtle differences in the fluorescence properties of closely related molecules. For example, small differences in fluorescence of bound- and free-NADH can be measured using fluorescence lifetime imaging microscopy (FLIM). The ratio between bound- and free-NADH is indicative of glycolytic or oxidative phosphorylation activity. FLIM was used to demonstrate the differences between mural granulosa and cumulus cell metabolism compared to oocyte metabolism within ovarian follicles in situ [38] and the effects of hypoxia on mouse embryos [39]. Another novel fluorescence-based technique is hyperspectral autofluorescence microscopy. Most fluorescence microscopes utilize no more than four different excitation light wavelengths (colors), generated by different lasers or LEDs. With the development of lasers that generate continuously tunable excitation light from UV to near-infrared spectral range, or the use of multiple LEDs, a broad range of autofluorescence signals can be investigated. This approach has enabled new insights into the heterogeneity of cellular metabolism between individual oocytes and embryos and has been used to distinguish between embryos cultured in different oxygen concentrations [40, 41].

12.8 Concluding Thoughts

The relationship between blastocyst metabolism and viability has been established in several species including the human. The primary reason why this approach has not been adopted more widely has been a limitation of technologies, combined with the need for single-embryo incubations for at least 24 hours from the morula stage on day 4. Importantly, techniques for media analysis are becoming more readily available, and the move to single-embryo culture has been facilitated by the increasing use of both time-lapse and preimplantation genetic testing. Hence, now is the time to focus on analysis of human embryo physiology as an adjunct to current technologies, including algorithms and AI (Figure 12.6). Indeed, we have now shown that although there exists a tight correlation between glucose uptake and amino acid utilization by individual human embryos and their blastocyst grade, morphokinetics, and AI analysis, there exists within each grade/score a wide range of metabolic activities, indicating that metabolism is relevant as a biomarker of embryo health [12].

A further reason for the failure to adopt analysis of metabolism as a biomarker of embryo health and viability has been conflicts within the literature. Two issues stand out: (a) the need to ensure accuracy of volume delivery for the assays and for embryo incubations, and (b) the need to use physiological oxygen

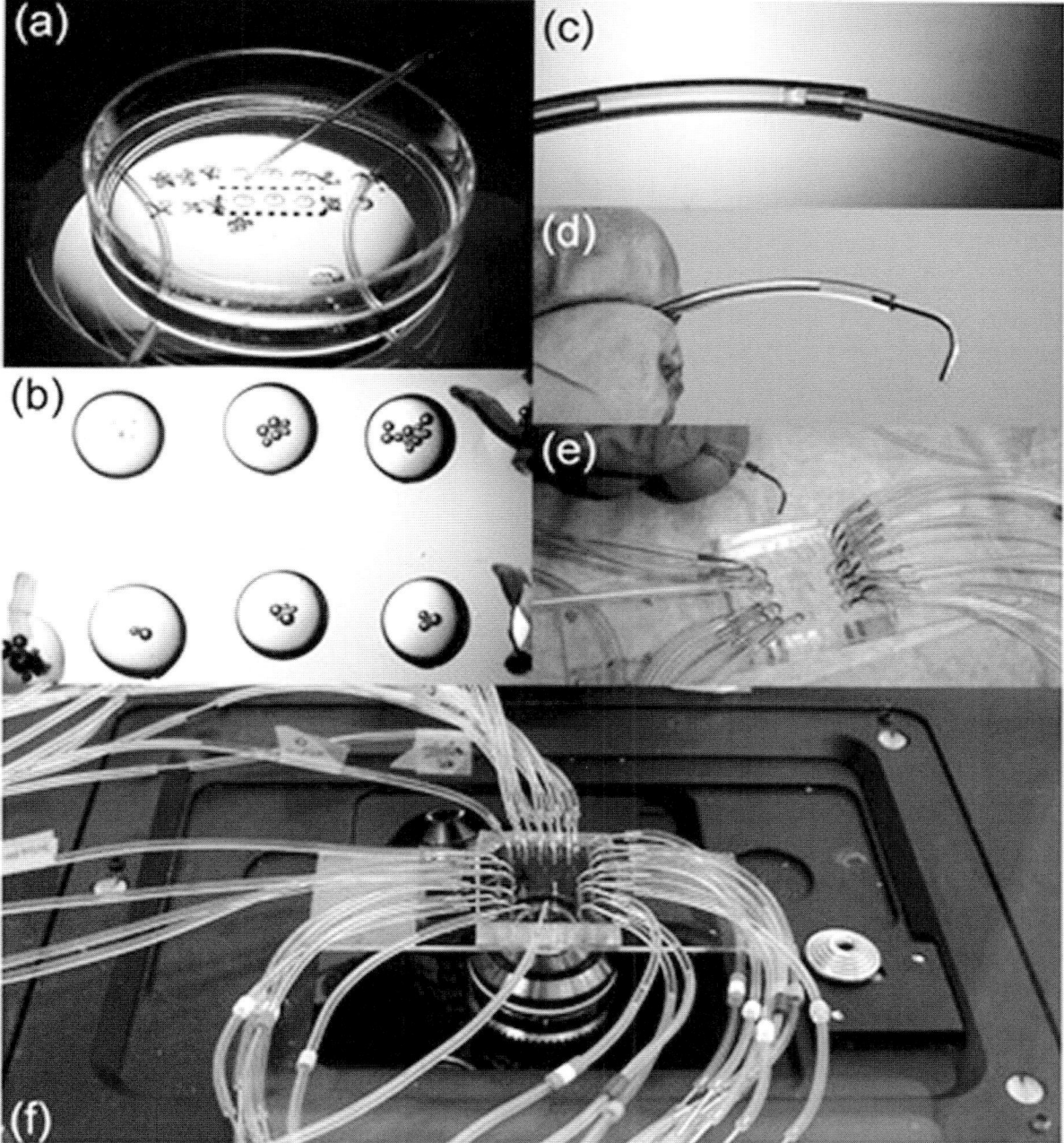

Figure 12.5 **An example of a microfluidic chip for the analysis of the culture medium surrounding an individual embryo**
Sample loading sequence: (a, b) Spent embryo media samples are stored in a Petri dish (35 mm) under oil to prevent evaporation. (c) A gel-loading pipette tip is recommended for transfer of individual media samples (typically 1–5 μL working volume) directly into a length of 500 μm i.d. Tygon tubing. (d) The end of the tubing may be cut to prevent the carryover of any oil prior to adding a sterilized pin. (e) All samples and reagent lines are connected to a detector chip that already is connected to the control manifold, then (f) mounted on an inverted microscope for the experiment. Taken from [32] with permission.

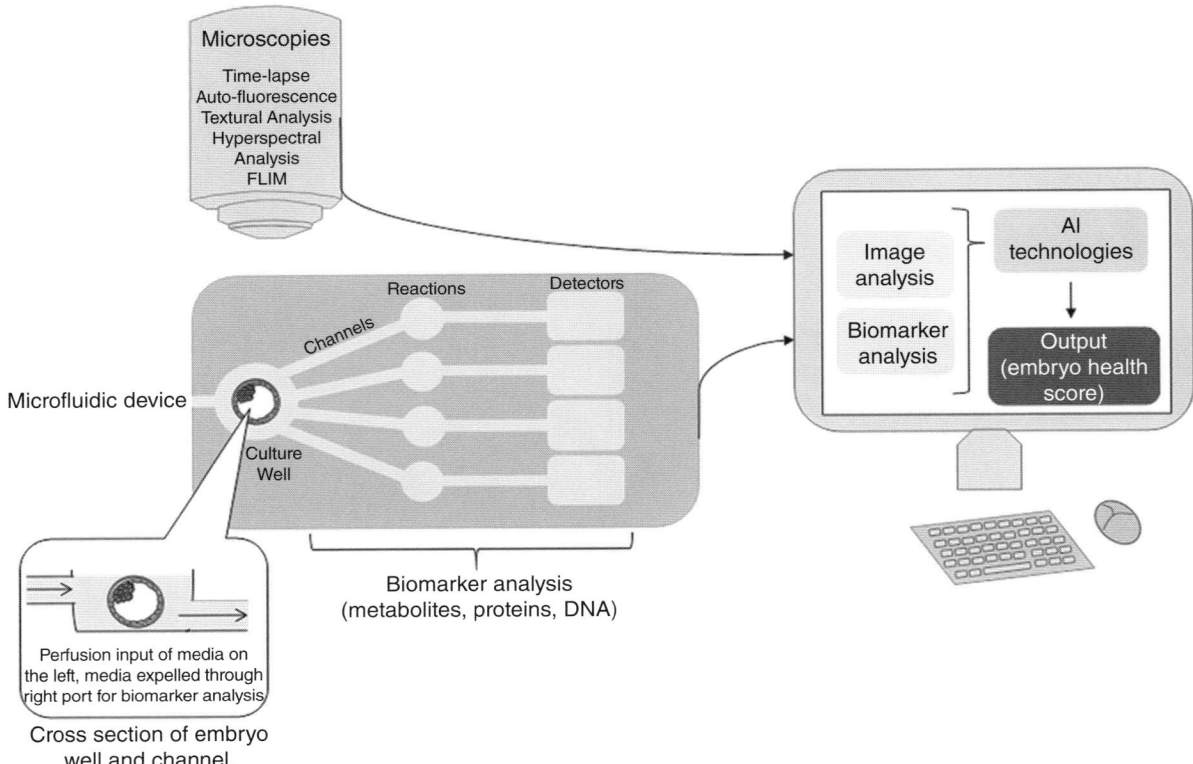

Figure 12.6 Integration of microscopies and microfluidics to quantitate embryo physiology and health in a clinical setting
Embryos are cultured in microfluidic devices where media flow is regulated to facilitate sampling. Concomitantly, data from microscopy technologies are acquired and together these data are sent to a central computer system where AI could be used to help create a health score for each individual embryo.

concentrations. For several years the "quiet hypothesis" [42] that proposed a viable human embryo should have a low or "quiet" metabolism, has been prominent in human embryology. However, the data upon which this hypothesis was established were from experiments using 20% oxygen, which is known to suppress metabolism. Gardner and Wale countered this hypothesis with data obtained at 5% oxygen, which showed that glucose uptake was positively correlated with human blastocyst viability. It was proposed that a higher rate of metabolism was consistent with embryo viability, and that there would be a range of normality. Should metabolism become too high or too low, viability will be compromised [5]. The "quiet hypothesis" has subsequently been reconsidered and has been replaced with the "Goldilocks principle" [43]. What is clearly evident is that when physiological oxygen (5%) is used for culture and

analysis, then metabolic functions are positively related to embryo viability post-transfer. Hence, such analyses of biomarkers may be of immense value in not only selecting the most viable embryo for transfer, but also to identify the healthiest embryo, that is, those that will give rise to a healthy child and resultant adult [12, 19, 25].

> **Key Messages**
> - Embryo viability is related to amino acid utilization, and positively correlated to glucose uptake.
> - Combinations of biomarkers will provide a more accurate analysis of viability and health.
> - Culture conditions affect metabolism, especially oxygen concentration.
> - The "quiet hypothesis" was established using data from incubations at 20% oxygen and

reflects metabolic stress of embryos and not their viability.

- Successful analysis requires accuracy in both pipetting the incubation volume for the embryo and ensuring the embryo is washed well and moved in and out of incubation drops in minimal volume.
- Accurate analysis requires precision in pipetting the assay and media samples (a positive displacement pipette is recommended).

References

1. Gardner DK, Balaban B. Assessment of human embryo development using morphological criteria in an era of time-lapse, algorithms and 'OMICS': is looking good still important? *Mol Hum Reprod.* 2016;22:704–18.

2. Basile N, Vime P, Florensa M, Aparicio Ruiz B, Garcia Velasco JA, Remohi J, et al. The use of morphokinetics as a predictor of implantation: a multicentric study to define and validate an algorithm for embryo selection. *Hum Reprod.* 2015;30:276–83.

3. Tran D, Cooke S, Illingworth PJ, Gardner DK. Deep learning as a predictive tool for fetal heart pregnancy following time-lapse incubation and blastocyst transfer. *Hum Reprod.* 2019;34:1011–18.

4. Gardner DK, Lane M, Stevens J, Schoolcraft WB. Noninvasive assessment of human embryo nutrient consumption as a measure of developmental potential. *Fertil Steril.* 2001;76:1175–80.

5. Gardner DK, Wale PL. Analysis of metabolism to select viable human embryos for transfer. *Fertil Steril.* 2013;99:1062–72.

6. Gardner DK, Harvey AJ. Blastocyst metabolism. *Reprod Fertil Dev.* 2015;27:638–54.

7. Donohoe DR, Bultman SJ. Metaboloepigenetics: interrelationships between energy metabolism and epigenetic control of gene expression. *J Cell Physiol.* 2012;227:3169–77.

8. Harvey AJ, Rathjen J, Gardner DK. Metaboloepigenetic regulation of pluripotent stem cells. *Stem Cells Int.* 2016;1816525.

9. Renard JP, Philippon A, Menezo Y. In-vitro uptake of glucose by bovine blastocysts. *J Reprod Fertil.* 1980;58:161–4.

10. Gardner DK, Leese HJ. Assessment of embryo viability prior to transfer by the noninvasive measurement of glucose uptake. *J Exp Zool.* 1987;242:103–5.

11. Gardner DK, Wale PL, Collins R, Lane M. Glucose consumption of single post-compaction human embryos is predictive of embryo sex and live birth outcome. *Hum Reprod.* 2011;26:1981–6.

12. Ferrick L, Lee YSL, Gardner DK. Metabolic activity of human blastocysts correlates with their morphokinetics, morphological grade, KIDScore and artificial intelligence ranking. *Hum Reprod.* 2020;35:2004–16.

13. Lane M, Gardner DK. Selection of viable mouse blastocysts prior to transfer using a metabolic criterion. *Hum Reprod.* 1996;11:1975–8.

14. Lane M, Gardner DK. Amino acids and vitamins prevent culture-induced metabolic perturbations and associated loss of viability of mouse blastocysts. *Hum Reprod.* 1998;13:991–7.

15. Gardner DK. Dissection of culture media for embryos: the most important and less important components and characteristics. *Reprod Fertil Dev.* 2008;20:9–18.

16. Houghton FD, Hawkhead JA, Humpherson PG, Hogg JE, Balen AH, Rutherford AJ, et al. Non-invasive amino acid turnover predicts human embryo developmental capacity. *Hum Reprod.* 2002;17:999–1005.

17. Brison DR, Houghton FD, Falconer D, Roberts SA, Hawkhead J, Humpherson PG, et al. Identification of viable embryos in IVF by non-invasive measurement of amino acid turnover. *Hum Reprod.* 2004;19:2319–24.

18. Picton HM, Elder K, Houghton FD, Hawkhead JA, Rutherford AJ, Hogg JE, et al. Association between amino acid turnover and chromosome aneuploidy during human preimplantation embryo development in vitro. *Mol Hum Reprod.* 2010;16:557–69.

19. Gardner DK, Kelley RL. Impact of the IVF laboratory environment on human preimplantation embryo phenotype. *J Dev Orig Health Dis.* 2017;8:418–35.

20. Wale PL, Gardner DK. Oxygen regulates amino acid turnover and carbohydrate uptake during the preimplantation period of mouse embryo development. *Biol Reprod.* 2012;87:24.

21. Wale PL, Gardner DK. Oxygen affects the ability of mouse blastocysts to regulate ammonium. *Biol Reprod.* 2013;89:75.

22. Conaghan J, Hardy K, Handyside AH, Winston RM, Leese HJ. Selection criteria for human embryo transfer: a comparison of pyruvate uptake and morphology. *J Assist Reprod Genet.* 1993;10:21–30.

23. Leese HJ, Hooper MA, Edwards RG, Ashwood-Smith MJ. Uptake of pyruvate by early human

embryos determined by a non-invasive technique. *Hum Reprod.* 1986;1:181–2.

24. Leary C, Sturmey RG. Metabolic profile of in vitro derived human embryos is not affected by the mode of fertilization. *Mol Hum Reprod.* 2020;26:277–87.

25. Ferrick L, Lee YSL, Gardner DK. Reducing time to pregnancy and facilitating the birth of healthy children through functional analysis of embryo physiology. *Biol Reprod.* 2019;101:1124–39.

26. Jalas C, Seli E, Scott RT, Jr. Key metrics and processes for validating embryo diagnostics. *Fertil Steril.* 2020;114:16–23.

27. Gardner DK, Lane M. Amino acids and ammonium regulate mouse embryo development in culture. *Biol Reprod.* 1993;48:377–85.

28. Gardner DK. Non-invasive metabolic assessment of single cells. *Methods Mol Med.* 2007;132:1–9.

29. Choi BI, Harvey AJ, Green MP. Bisphenol A affects early bovine embryo development and metabolism that is negated by an oestrogen receptor inhibitor. *Sci Rep.* 2016;6:29318.

30. Guerif F, McKeegan P, Leese HJ, Sturmey RG. A simple approach for COnsumption and RElease (CORE) analysis of metabolic activity in single mammalian embryos. *PLoS One.* 2013;8: e67834.

31. Thouas GA, Potter DL, Gardner DK. Microfluidic devices for the analysis of gamete and embryo physiology. In: Gardner DK, Sakkas D, Seli E, Wells D, editors. *Human gametes and preimplantation embryos:*

assessment and diagnosis. New York: Springer; 2013. p. 281–99.

32. Urbanski JP, Johnson MT, Craig DD, Potter DL, Gardner DK, Thorsen T. Noninvasive metabolic profiling using microfluidics for analysis of single preimplantation embryos. *Anal Chem.* 2008;80:6500–7.

33. Gardner DK, Reineck P, Gibson BC, Thompson JG. Microfluidics and microanalytics to facilitate quantitative assessment of human embryo physiology. In: Agarwal A, Varghese A, Nagy ZP, editors. *Practical manual of in vitro fertilization: advanced methods and novel devices.* 2nd ed. New Jersey: Humana Press; 2019. p. 557–66.

34. Seli E, Sakkas D, Scott R, Kwok SC, Rosendahl SM, Burns DH. Noninvasive metabolomic profiling of embryo culture media using Raman and near-infrared spectroscopy correlates with reproductive potential of embryos in women undergoing in vitro fertilization. *Fertil Steril.* 2007;88:1350–7.

35. Seli E, Bruce C, Botros L, Henson M, Roos P, Judge K, et al. Receiver operating characteristic (ROC) analysis of day 5 morphology grading and metabolomic Viability Score on predicting implantation outcome. *J Assist Reprod Genet.* 2011;28:137–44.

36. Hardarson T, Ahlstrom A, Rogberg L, Botros L, Hillensjo T, Westlander G, et al. Non-invasive metabolomic profiling of day 2 and 5 embryo culture medium: a prospective randomized trial. *Hum Reprod.* 2012;27:89–96.

37. Krisher RL, Heuberger AL, Paczkowski M, Stevens J, Pospisil C, Prather RS, et al. Applying

metabolomic analyses to the practice of embryology: physiology, development and assisted reproductive technology. *Reprod Fertil Dev.* 2015;27:602–20.

38. Cinco R, Digman MA, Gratton E, Luderer U. Spatial characterization of bioenergetics and metabolism of primordial to preovulatory follicles in whole ex vivo murine ovary. *Biol Reprod.* 2016;95:129.

39. Seidler EA, Sanchez T, Venturas M, Sakkas D, Needleman DJ. Non-invasive imaging of mouse embryo metabolism in response to induced hypoxia. *J Assist Reprod Genet.* 2020;37:1797–805.

40. Gosnell ME, Anwer AG, Mahbub SB, Menon Perinchery S, Inglis DW, Adhikary PP, et al. Quantitative non-invasive cell characterisation and discrimination based on multispectral autofluorescence features. *Sci Rep.* 2016;6:23453.

41. Sutton-McDowall ML, Gosnell M, Anwer AG, White M, Purdey M, Abell AD, et al. Hyperspectral microscopy can detect metabolic heterogeneity within bovine post-compaction embryos incubated under two oxygen concentrations (7% versus 20%). *Hum Reprod.* 2017;32:2016–25.

42. Leese HJ. Quiet please, do not disturb: a hypothesis of embryo metabolism and viability. *Bioessays.* 2002;24:845–9.

43. Leese HJ, Guerif F, Allgar V, Brison DR, Lundin K, Sturmey RG. Biological optimization, the Goldilocks principle, and how much is lagom in the preimplantation embryo. *Mol Reprod Dev.* 2016;83:748–54.

Timeline of the Most Notable Advances in Clinical IVF

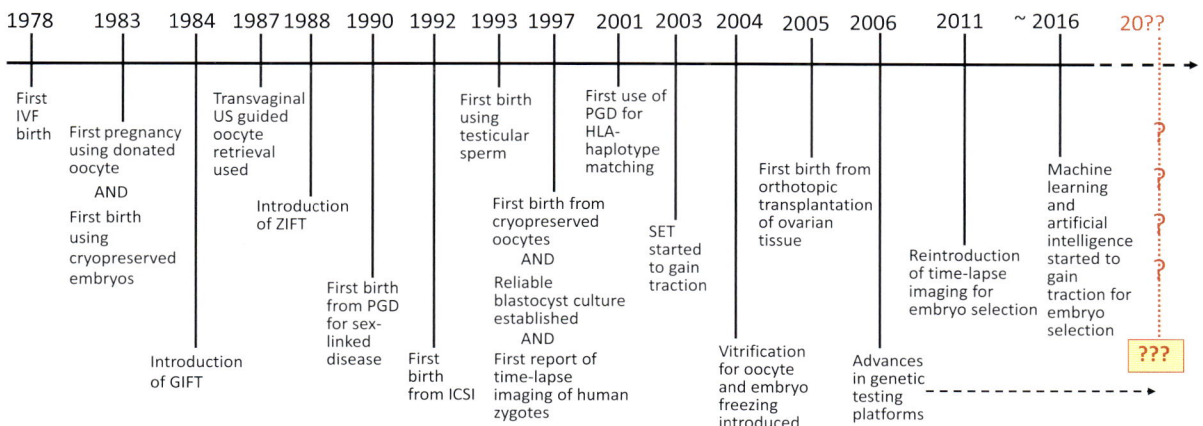

Figure 1.1 Timeline of the most notable advances in clinical IVF (Courtesy of Dr. Catherine Racowsky)

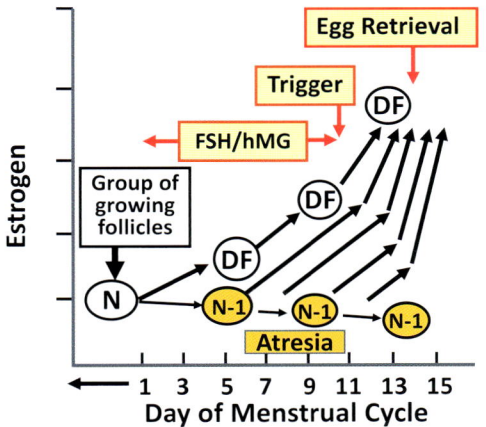

- The cohort is typically heterogeneous in quality
- Only ~75% oocytes are mature
- Only ~75% of mature oocytes fertilize
- Not all mature oocytes are euploid
- Not all euploid embryos are developmentally competent
- Not all aneuploid embryos are developmentally incompetent

Ovarian stimulation typically leads to a cohort of embryos of varying developmental potential

hCG = human chorionic gonadotropin; DF = dominant follicle; N = number of follicles in the cohort
FSH = follicle-stimulating hormone; hMG = human menopausal gonadotropin

Figure 1.2 Follicular maturation
Growth and maturation of human follicles is a complex process that takes over 180 days. The majority of the growing follicles will arrest and become atretic. Only 1 in 1 000 follicles in an ovary of a newborn will ever reach ovulation. Despite this seemingly strong selection of growing follicles, the frequency of aneuploid human oocytes is from 25% to 80% depending on the age of the woman. (Adapted from [7], with permission).

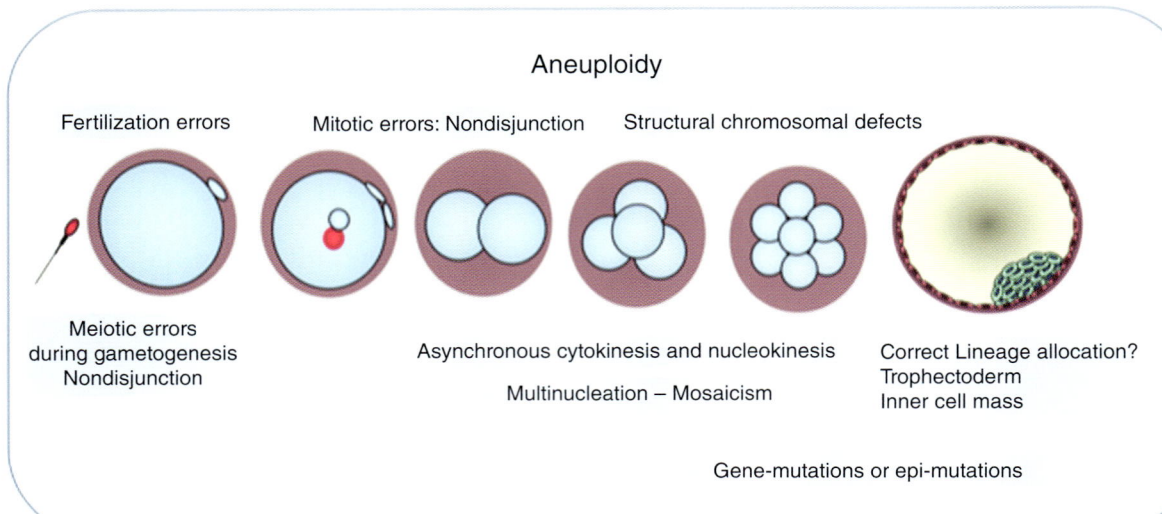

Figure 1.3 Errors in embryo development
Human gametogenesis is far from perfect and mature gametes may contain the wrong number of chromosomes (aneuploid). Fertilization and early cleavage may introduce new errors during mitosis (nondisjunction) frequently leading to embryos where at least one blastomere is aneuploid. Culture conditions may also have an influence on embryo viability. The embryologist working in clinical IVF is therefore faced with a situation where the embryos obtained may vary greatly with respect to implantation potential. The challenge therefore is to rank embryos so the best ones may be selected for fresh transfer and for cryopreservation.

1978	Defining the developmental timeline
1980s	Conventional morphology selection – cleavage stage
1990s	Conventional morphology selection – blastocyst stage
1990	PGT-M with FISH for X-linked disorder
1997	Time-lapse imaging of human zygotes
2001	PGT with blastomere biopsy
2005	PGT with trophectoderm biopsy and advanced sequencing platforms
2007	Metabolomics
2011	Time-lapse imaging reintroduced
2016	Machine learning and artificial intelligence started to gain traction
2016	PGT-A with cell-free DNA analyses
20??	........? ? ?

Courtesy of Dr Catherine Racowsky

Figure 1.4 Where are we with embryo selection going forward? (Courtesy of Dr. Catherine Racowsky)

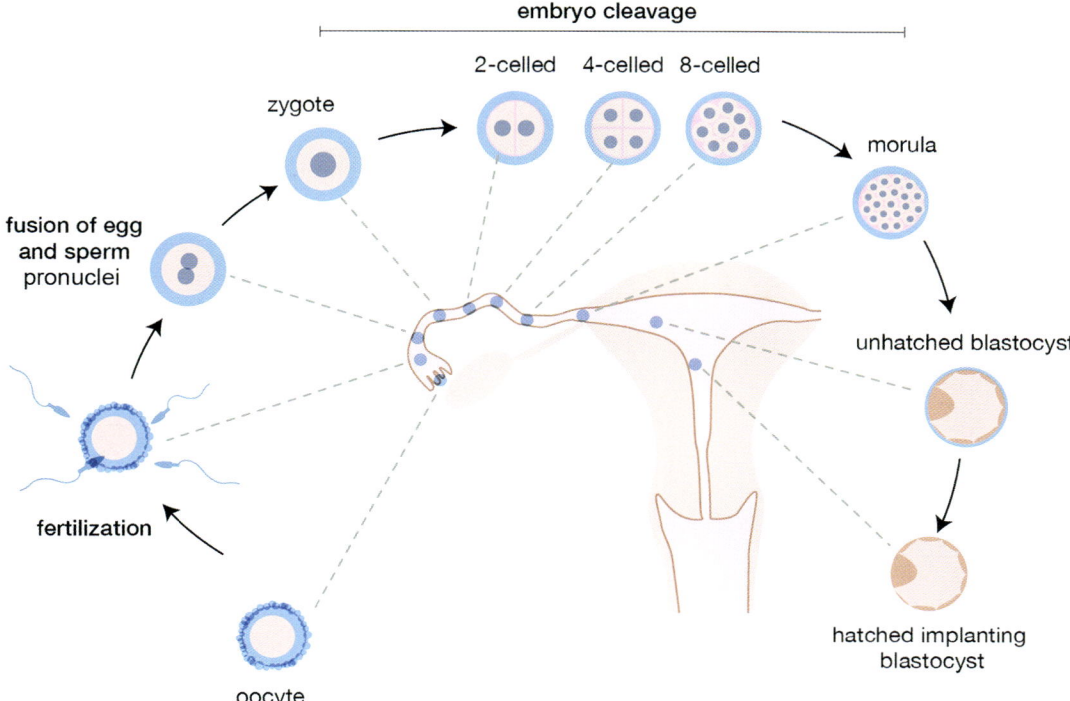

Figure 3.1 The pathway of normal embryo development
The oocyte released from the dominant ovarian follicle enters the fallopian tube, where it is fertilized to form a zygote, then undergoes a series of cell divisions to form 2-, 4-, and 8-cell embryos. A morula/early blastocyst is the embryonic stage of entry into the uterine cavity. It is within this microenvironment that the blastocyst hatches and prepares for attachment to and invasion between the endometrial epithelial cells, in the process of implantation.

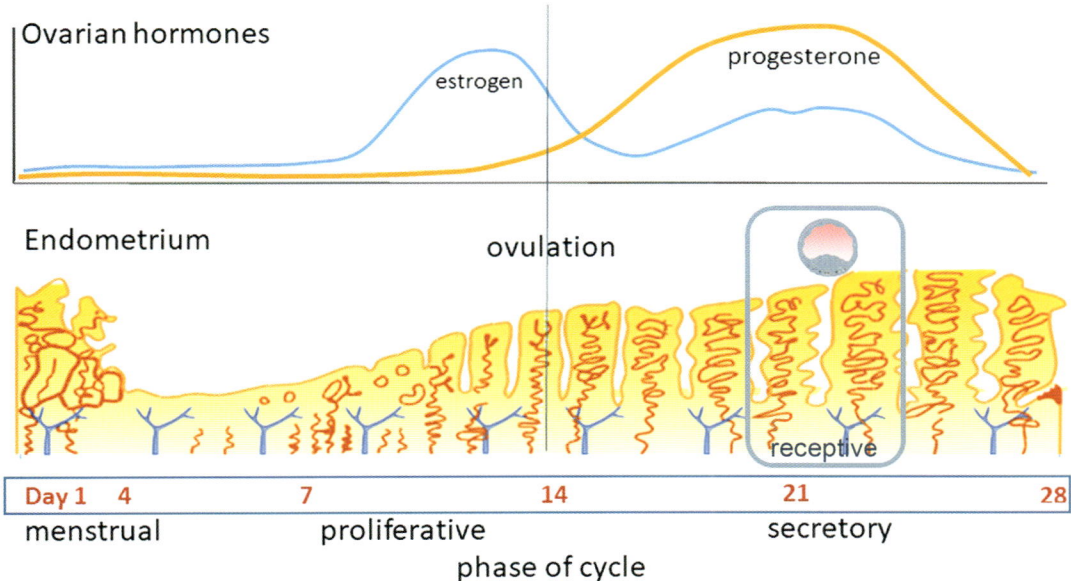

Figure 3.2 Cyclical endometrial changes are normally driven by hormones
Following endometrial shedding at menstruation, the tissue is restored during the proliferative phase of the cycle under the stimulus of rising estrogen from the dominant follicle. Following ovulation, all the cells undergo differentiation under the influence of progesterone in the presence of estrogen. This results in the endometrium becoming "receptive" to embryo implantation. In the absence of an embryo, falling estrogen and progesterone levels result in menstruation.

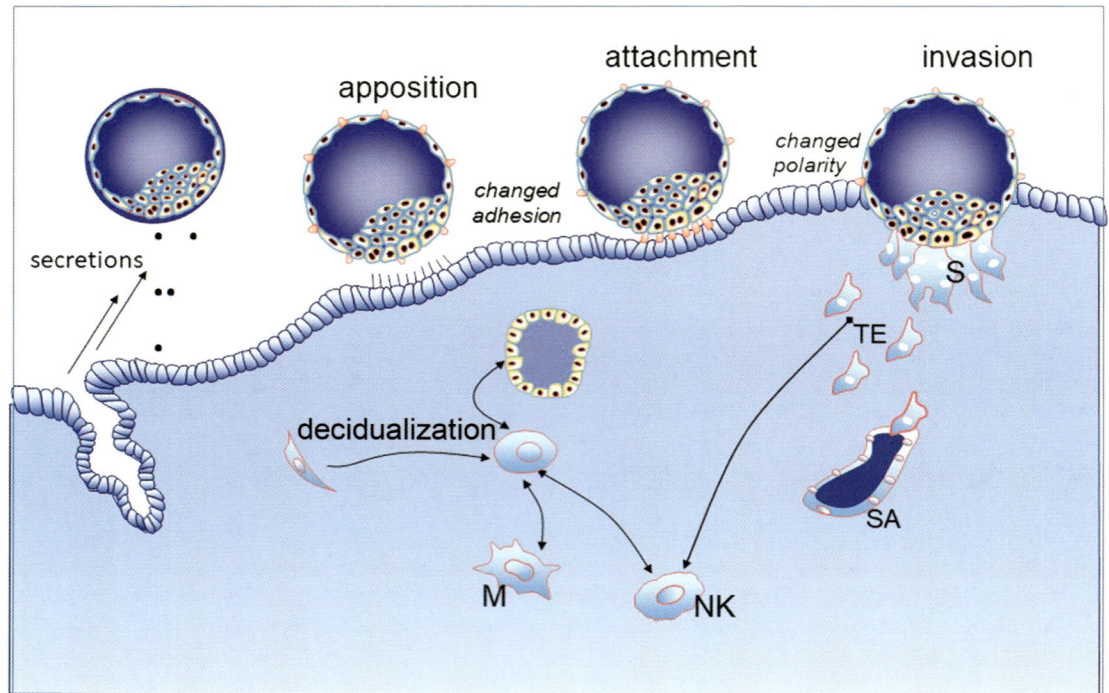

Figure 3.3 Processes leading to successful implantation and early placentation

The embryo as a blastocyst undergoes preimplantation development within the microenvironment of the uterine cavity. This enables it to become apposed to, then attach to the receptive luminal epithelium of the endometrium. The trophectodermal cells then penetrate between the epithelial cells that transiently lose their polarity. The trophectoderm forms a syncytium (S) beneath the epithelium, from which invasive trophoblast cells (TE) invade through the decidual compartment to reach the spiral arterioles (SA). Simultaneously, endometrial stromal fibroblasts undergo decidualization. The resultant decidual cells release chemokines and other factors that attract macrophages (M) and uterine natural killer cells (NK) into the decidua. Straight arrows represent soluble secretions. • represent extracellular vesicles.

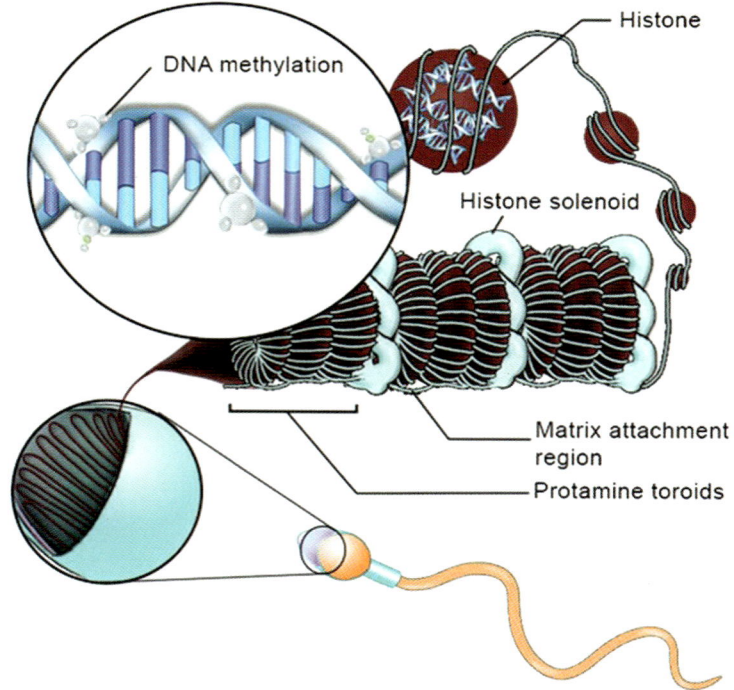

Figure 4.1 DNA chromatin remodeling and packaging

Schematic depicting chromatin remodeling and DNA packaging including histone modifications, protamine toroid structure, and connection with the matrix attachment regions.

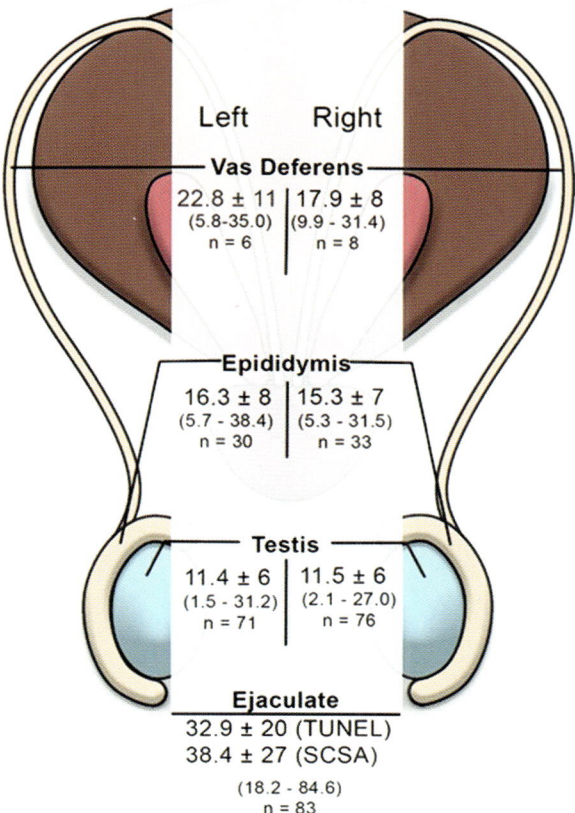

Left   Right

Vas Deferens

22.8 ± 11	17.9 ± 8
(5.8-35.0)	(9.9 - 31.4)
n = 6	n = 8

Epididymis

16.3 ± 8	15.3 ± 7
(5.7 - 38.4)	(5.3 - 31.5)
n = 30	n = 33

Testis

11.4 ± 6	11.5 ± 6
(1.5 - 31.2)	(2.1 - 27.0)
n = 71	n = 76

Ejaculate
32.9 ± 20 (TUNEL)
38.4 ± 27 (SCSA)
(18.2 - 84.6)
n = 83

Figure 4.2 DNA fragmentation throughout the male reproductive tract
Schematic showing measurements of DNA fragmentation in the male reproductive tract, from the lowest levels in the testis, followed by the epididymis and then vas deferens, with the highest levels in the ejaculate. Measurement data are adapted from Xie et al. [11].

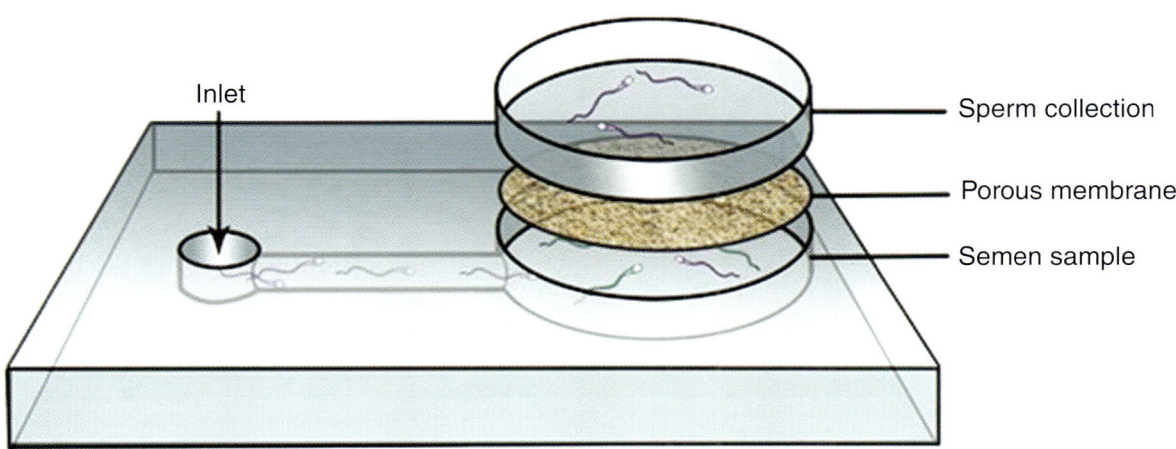

Inlet

Sperm collection

Porous membrane

Semen sample

Figure 4.3 A microfluidic technique for isolating the highest-quality sperm
Schematic of a microfluidic technique demonstrating that the highest-quality sperm (high motility and low DNA fragmentation levels) are able to traverse through the porous membrane into the upper chamber.

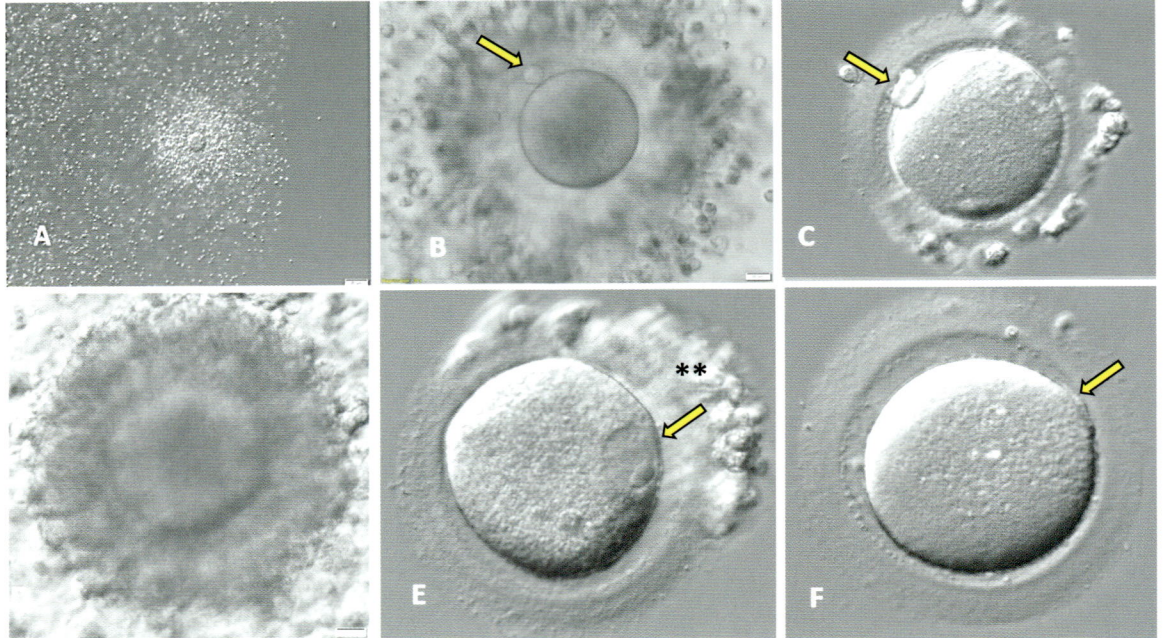

Figure 5.1 Human oocyte morphology following controlled ovarian stimulation
A: low-magnification image of cumulus–oocyte complex shortly after retrieval illustrating monodispersed nature of expanded cumulus and disposition of corona cells surrounding the oocyte. B: intact corona with enclosed metaphase-2 oocyte with polar body (arrow); note radially oriented striations formed by corona cell transzonal projections. C: metaphase-2 stage oocyte with polar body (arrow) following removal of cumulus corona; note abundance of vesicles within perivitelline space. D: compact, unexpanded corona enclosing immature, germinal vesicle (GV) stage oocyte; GV (arrow) shown in E following hyaluronidase and mechanical stripping, although some corona radiata cells remain (**). F: presumed aged metaphase-2 oocyte with flattened first polar body at 2 o'clock (arrow); cytoplasm lacks homogeneity. Hoffmann modulation optics (A, C, E, and F); polarization optics (B, D).

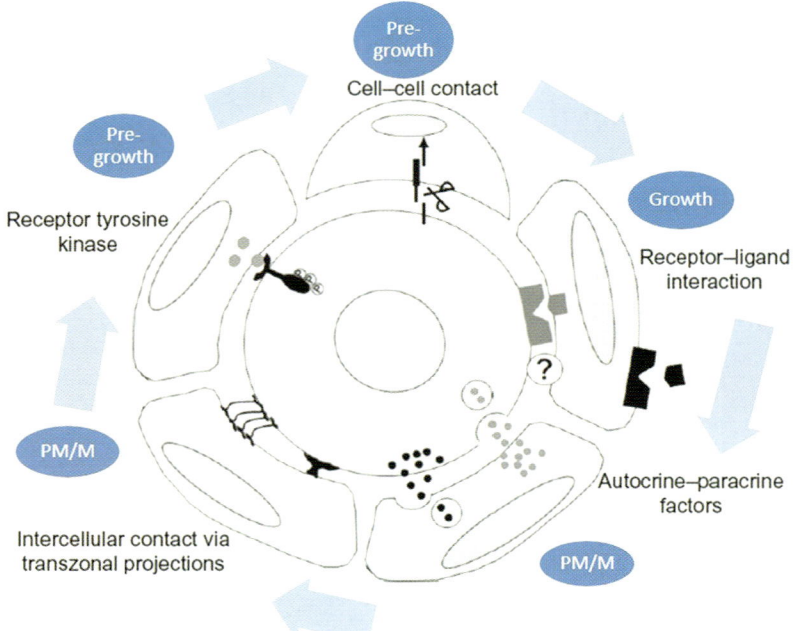

Figure 5.2 Schematic illustrating the sequence of signaling interactions known to occur between granulosa/cumulus cells and the oocyte during the course of folliculogenesis
In dormant primordial follicles (top), cell contact and receptor tyrosine kinases maintain oocytes in an arrested state. Upon follicle activation, a series of signaling systems develops at the cumulus–oocyte interface that regulate the growth phase of oogenesis (G) and the pre and maturation phases (PM/M). Image redrawn from reference [2].

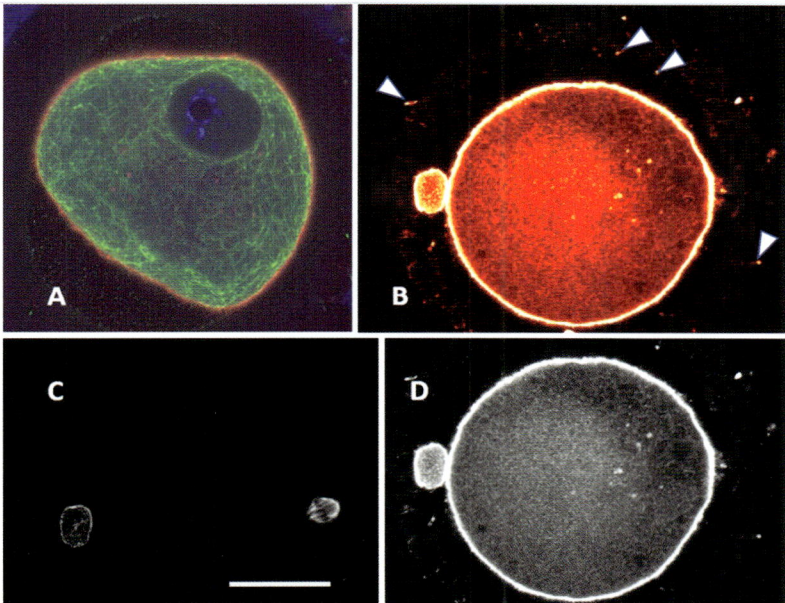

Figure 5.3 Comparison of immature GV stage oocyte (A) and mature metaphase-2 oocyte with spindle positioned 180 degrees opposite the first polar body (B, C, and D). Note transzonal projection remnants within the zona pellucida (arrow heads, B), perpendicular orientation of metaphase-2 spindle with respect to the polar body (C), and gradient of filamentous actin from left to right, with lowest density apparent at pole demarcated by meiotic spindle (B, D). All images are single optical planes obtained with laser scanning light microscope after labeling with antitubulin antibodies (A, green; C, white) or red phalloidin (B, D). Scale bar = 50 microns.

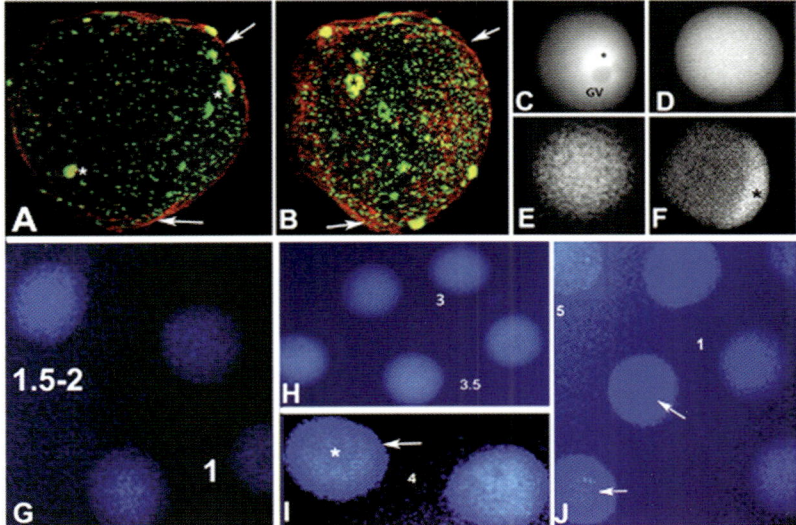

Figure 9.3 Panels A and B are images of a hemisphere of human MII oocytes showing differential intracellular temperatures revealed with a cell-permeable chemical intracellular thermometer whose fluorescent emission wavelength is a function of temperature. The temperature in the subplasmalemmal cytoplasm where a circumferential domain of high polarized mitochondria reside is slightly higher (arrows, red) than mitochondria in small clusters within the cytoplasm (green). The asterisks indicate larger mitochondrial aggregates that appear slightly warmer than those in smaller clusters. The oocyte in panel A was cultured in an atmosphere of 5% oxygen while the one in panel B was cultured in room air (~20% oxygen). The effect of the higher oxygen concentration is evident by the occurrence of red fluorescent mitochondria within the cytoplasm indicating that a higher intracellular availability of oxygen may upregulate mitochondrial respiratory activity and ATP production that would seem to be manifested by increases in temperature.

Panels C–J: Autofluorescent detection of NADH/NADPH in cohorts of human MII oocytes indicates differential intensities that can be related to ATP content and provide an indication of relative bioenergetic state. Panels C–D show typical autofluorescent phenotypes from a relatively uniform distribution (D) to one with numerous aggregates (E), or asymmetric localization (asterisk, F). The asterisk in panel C shows the typical pregerminal vesicle breakdown perinuclear accumulation of mitochondria.

Panels G–J indicate relative autofluorescent intensities in unfertilized human oocytes on a scale of 1 to 5 where 1 is the least intense and 5 the highest. These intensities were correlated with net ATP content and developmental performance in vitro after artificial (parthenogenetic) activation (see text for details). The arrows in panel J indicate small clusters/aggregates of mitochondria that can be detected by this autofluorescence method.

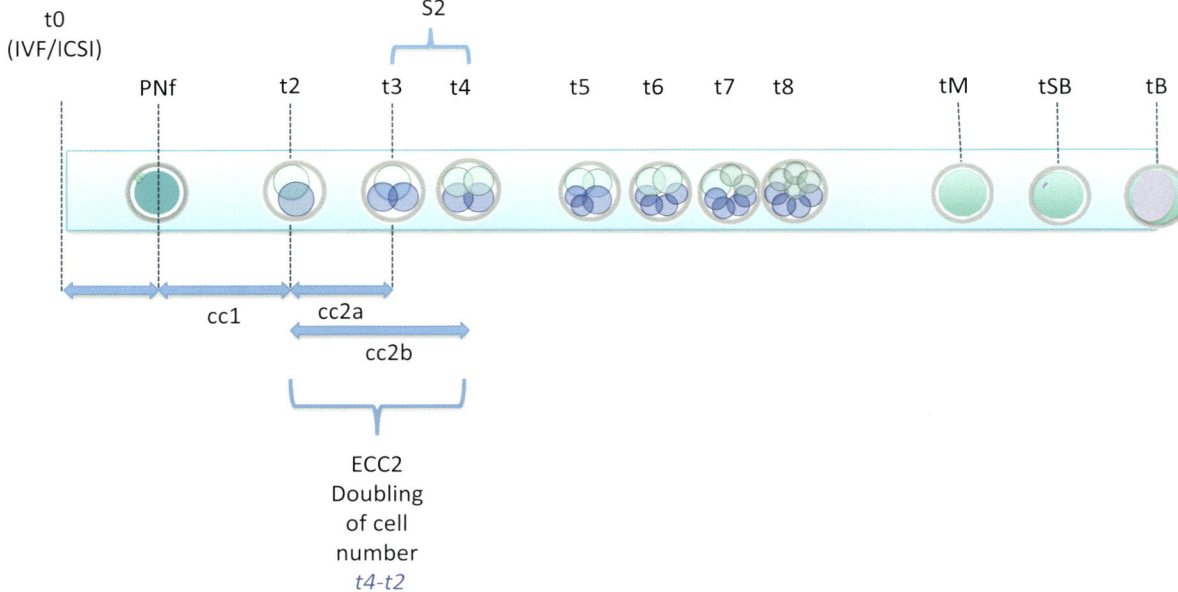

Figure 11.1 Schematic of time-lapse nomenclature. Adapted from Campbell A, Fishel S, editors. Atlas of time lapse embryology. Boca Raton, FL: CRC Press; 2015.

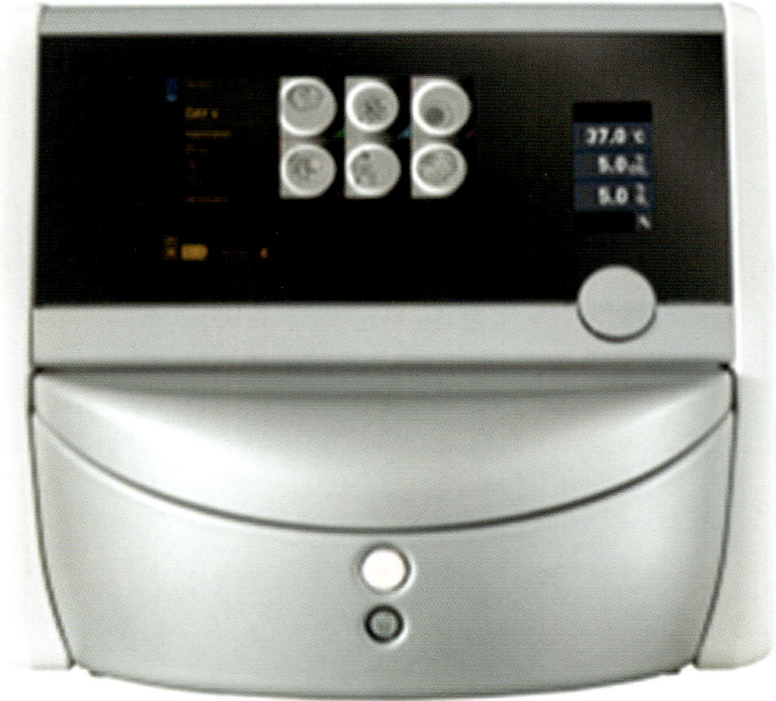

Figure 11.2 Example of a time-lapse imaging device. EmbryoScope Flex (image provided by Vitrolife, Sweden).

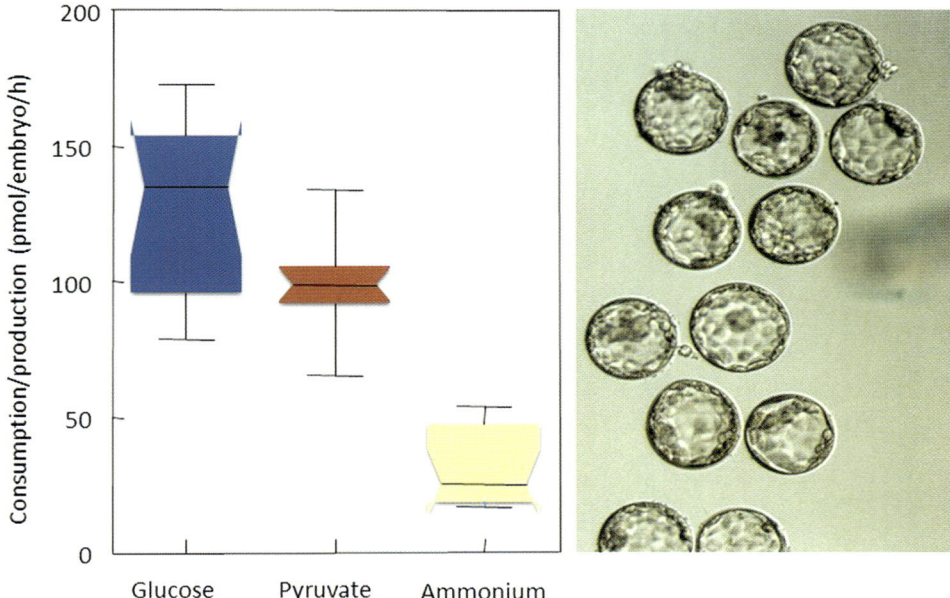

Figure 12.1 Nutrient uptake and ammonium production by individual human blastocysts from the same patient
Thirteen human blastocysts from an oocyte donor were donated to research [4]. These embryos had not undergone cryopreservation. Data are in the form of a notched box plot where the notches represent the interquartile range, therefore including 50% of the data points. Whiskers represent 5% and 95% quartiles. The line across the box represents the median. The spread of glucose uptake is ~100 pmol/embryo/h, a wide spread of nutrient utilization. Pyruvate is not a major nutrient of the blastocyst and does not appear to differ between embryos. The ammonium produced by the blastocysts reflects amino acid turnover. The image of the blastocysts from which the metabolic data were extracted reveals how difficult it can be to select them based on their morphology.

a)

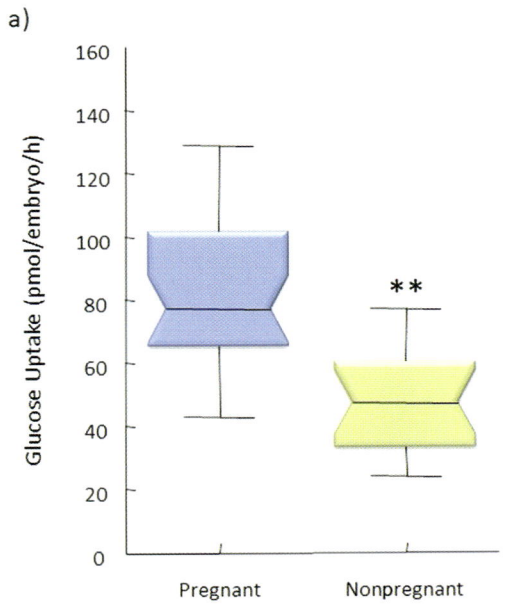

b)

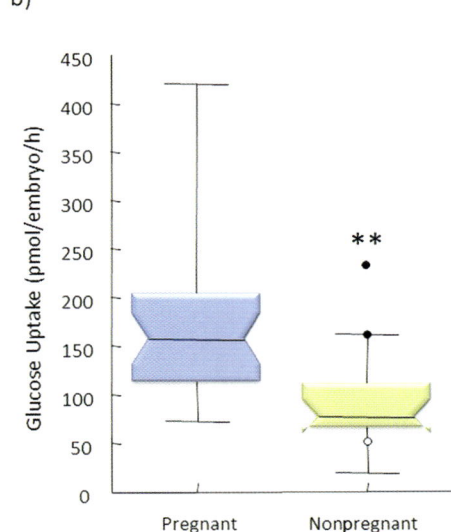

Figure 12.2a Glucose uptake on day 4 of embryonic development and pregnancy outcome (positive fetal heartbeat)
Notches represent the interquartile range (50% of the data), whiskers represent the 5% and 95% quartiles. The line across the box is the median glucose consumption.
Note: **, significantly different from pregnant (P<0.01).

Figure 12.2b Glucose uptake on day 5 of embryonic development and pregnancy outcome (positive fetal heartbeat)
Notches represent the interquartile range (50% of the data), whiskers represent the 5% and 95% quartiles. The line across the box is the median glucose consumption.
Note: **, significantly different from pregnant (P<0.01).
Closed circles represent the two blastocysts that gave rise to a positive fetal sac, but no subsequent fetal heart. The open circle represents the blastocyst that resulted in a positive hCG but not fetal sac.

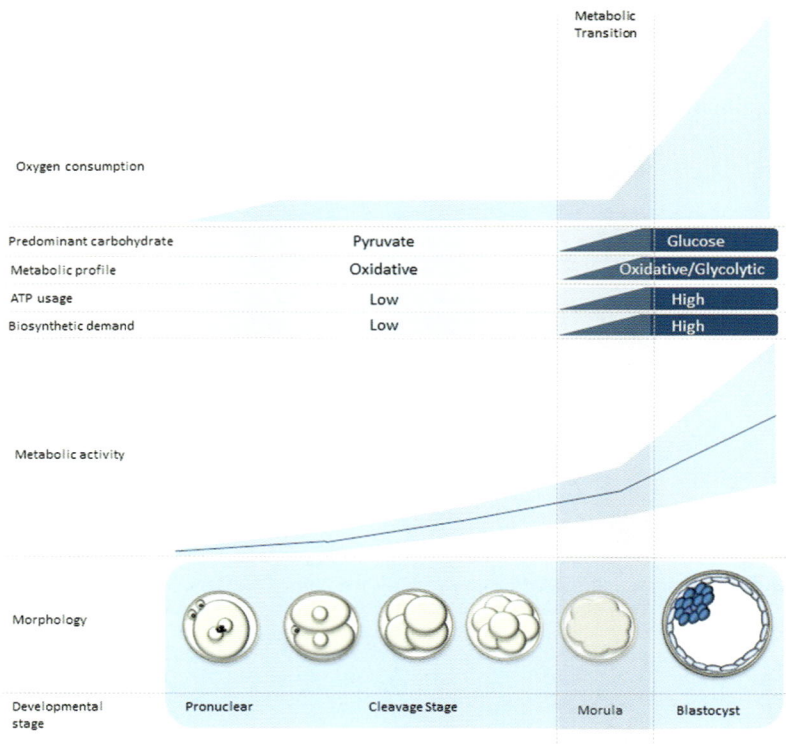

Figure 12.3 Metabolic changes during mammalian preimplantation development

Prior to compaction, the pronucleate oocyte and cleavage-stage embryo predominantly consume pyruvate, and through oxidative metabolism produce appropriate levels of ATP required to support cellular division. After compaction, the embryo exhibits exponential growth, requiring higher levels of ATP synthesis and biosynthetic precursors. This increase in activity is supported by an increase in the overall oxidative capacity of the embryo and also a transition to a highly glycolytic metabolism, whereby higher levels of glucose are consumed and converted to lactate in the presence of oxygen. As overall metabolic activity increases as development proceeds, so does the variation (represented by the shading) around the mean (represented by the solid line).

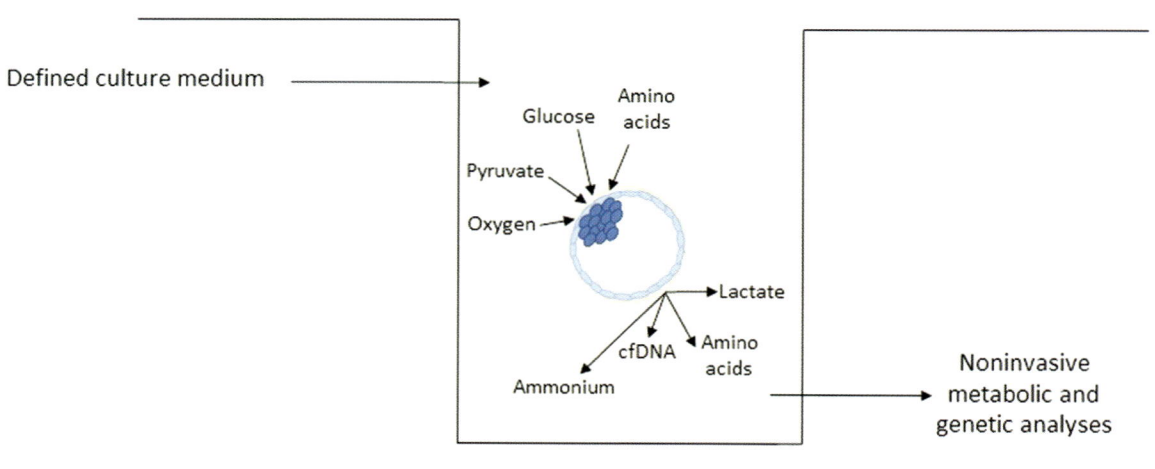

Figure 12.4 Noninvasive analysis of human embryo nutrient consumption and metabolite production, and/or cell-free DNA release into the surrounding medium

Individual embryos can be incubated in 10–15 µl volumes of medium in a microdrop or in a chamber such as in an EmbryoSlide. Samples of medium can then be analyzed by the methods outlined in this chapter.

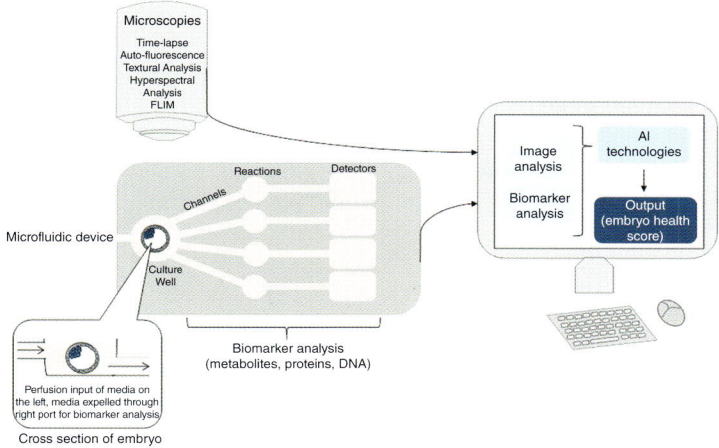

Figure 12.6 Integration of microscopies and microfluidics to quantitate embryo physiology and health in a clinical setting
Embryos are cultured in microfluidic devices where media flow is regulated to facilitate sampling. Concomitantly, data from microscopy technologies are acquired and together these data are sent to a central computer system where AI could be used to help create a health score for each individual embryo.

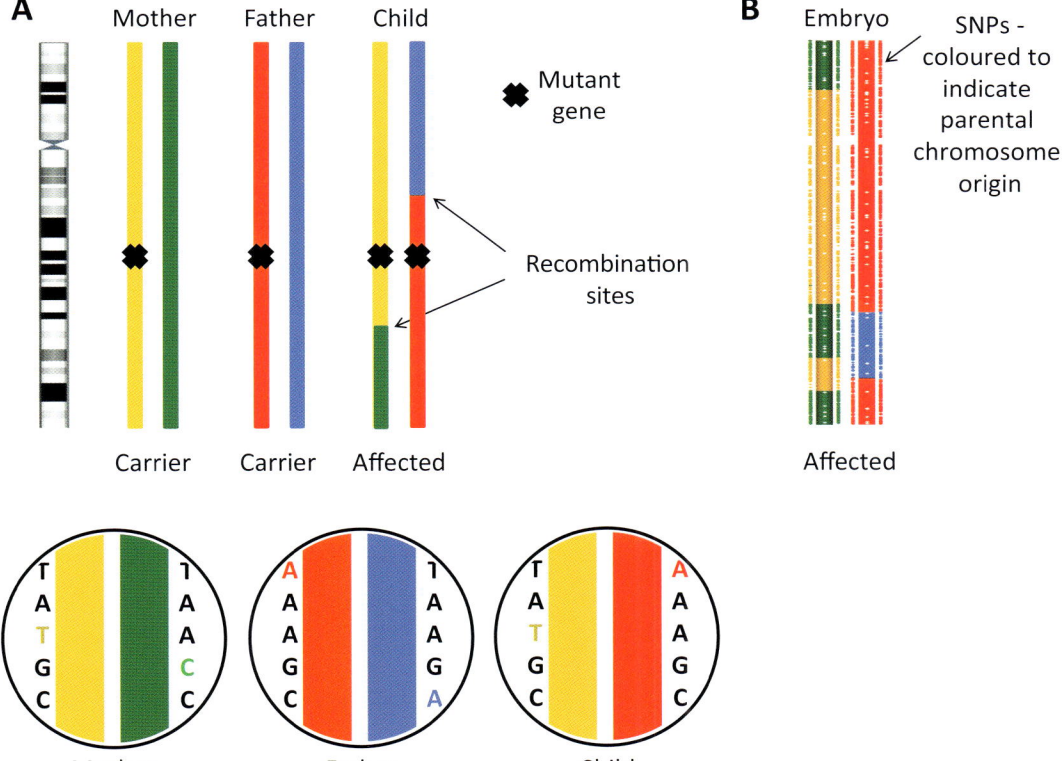

Figure 13.1 Karyomapping
Both parents and an additional family member (most often an affected child of the couple) are assessed using a microarray, providing genotype information for ~300 000 SNPs scattered across the genome. SNP alleles close to the mutant gene are inherited along with it and consequently provide an indirect indication of the presence of the mutation. Each parental chromosome has a unique pattern of SNP alleles, which serves as a genetic fingerprint, identifying that chromosome. Examples of allele combinations that allow individual chromosomes to be distinguished are shown at the foot of the figure. Based on the SNP results obtained, parental chromosomes are color-coded (A). This allows easy visualization of the chromosomes inherited by embryos, even revealing sites where meiotic recombination occurred. Multiple informative SNPs are present on each chromosome as shown in this example of a karyomapping result (B). Each spot flanking the graphical representation of the chromosome corresponds to an informative SNP, colored in order to show the parental chromosome for which that particular SNP provides evidence.

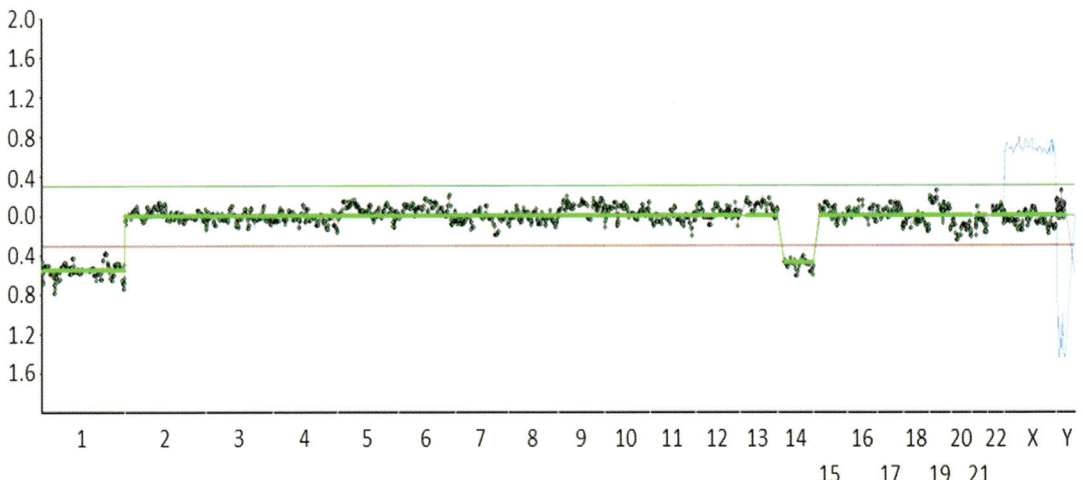

Figure 13.2 Microarray comparative genomic hybridization (aCGH)
The image shows an aCGH result for a trophectoderm biopsy sample with an apparent loss of chromosomes 1 and 14. The embryo was therefore predicted to have monosomy 1 and monosomy 14, a lethal abnormality. The z-axis represents the relative amount of red fluorescence (normal control DNA) and green fluorescence (embryo DNA) detected on chromosome specific probes situated on the microarray. On the scale, 0.0 equates to an equal quantity of red and green fluorescence. Values toward the foot of the image indicate increasing red, whereas those toward the top of the page indicate more green.

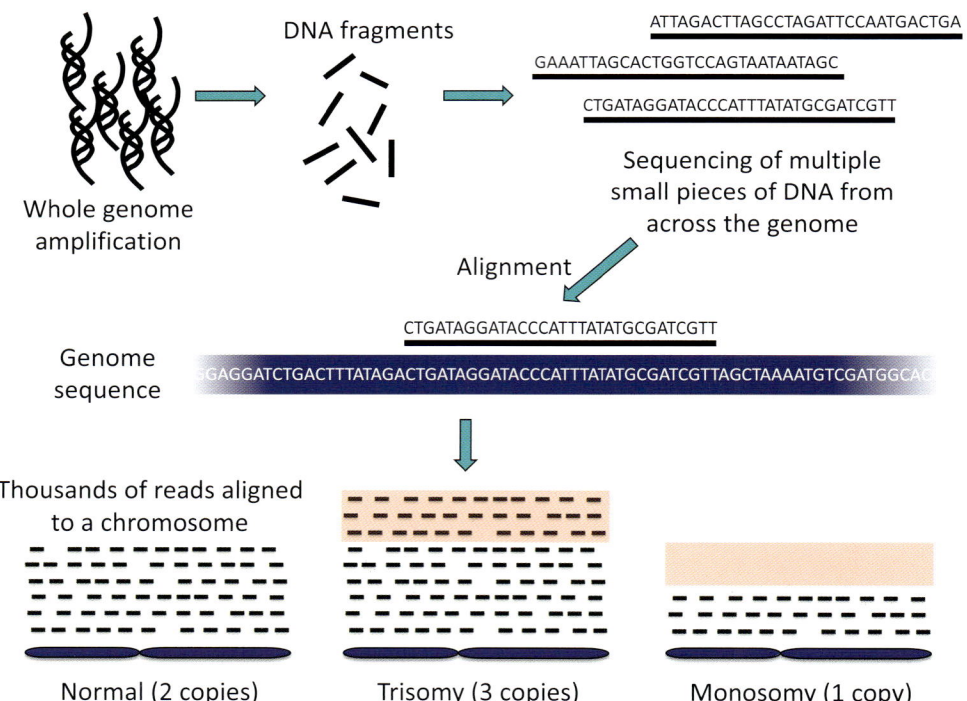

Figure 13.3 Next-generation sequencing (NGS)
For NGS, the DNA contained within the embryo biopsy specimen is first subjected to whole-genome amplification. The resulting DNA is prepared for sequencing that results in the production of millions of DNA fragments. Sequencing of these fragments reveals the order of DNA bases (G, A, T, and C) along their length. The fragments of DNA sequence thus obtained are known as "reads." The DNA sequence of each fragment can then be compared to the sequence of the human genome in order to determine the location it originally came from, a computer-driven process known as alignment. The relative proportion of "reads" aligned to each chromosome is identical for all samples with a normal number of chromosomes. Extra chromosomal material (e.g. a trisomy) causes an overrepresentation in the amount of reads from the affected chromosomes, whereas a monosomy is associated with a reduction in the relative number of reads from the abnormal chromosome.

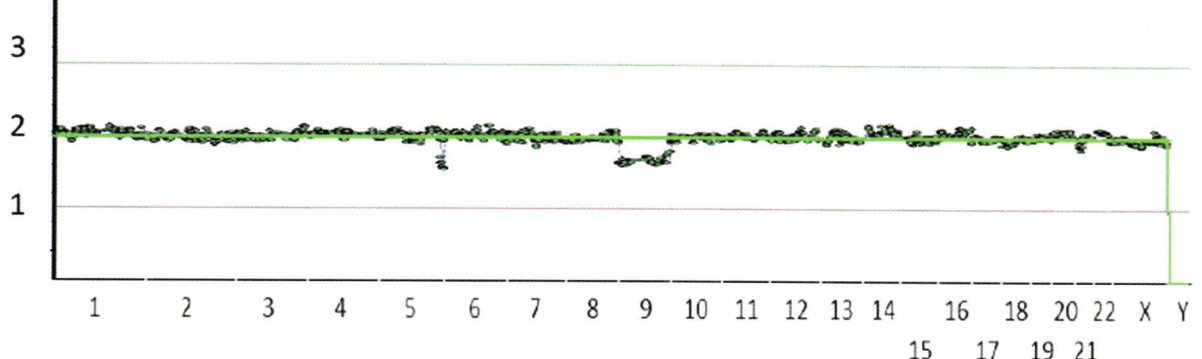

Figure 13.4 NGS result from an embryo biopsy specimen
For NGS analysis of chromosome abnormalities, the genome is divided into segments, referred to as "bins." Analysis focuses on determining the proportion of the total sequence "reads" aligning within each bin. After comparing the results to those obtained from chromosomally normal "reference" samples, it is possible to deduce how much of the embryo DNA was derived from each area of the genome. Each data point in the figure represents a result from one bin, arranged in their respective order along the length of each chromosome. The y-axis indicates the predicted copy number of each chromosome. In this case, an intermediate value, falling midway between 1 and 2 copies, is shown for chromosome 9 and also for a small segment at the end of the long arm of chromosome 5. This result is interpreted as meaning that the TE biopsy specimen was mosaic, likely containing a mixture of euploid cells and cells monosomic for chromosome 9 and with a segmental loss on chromosome 5q.

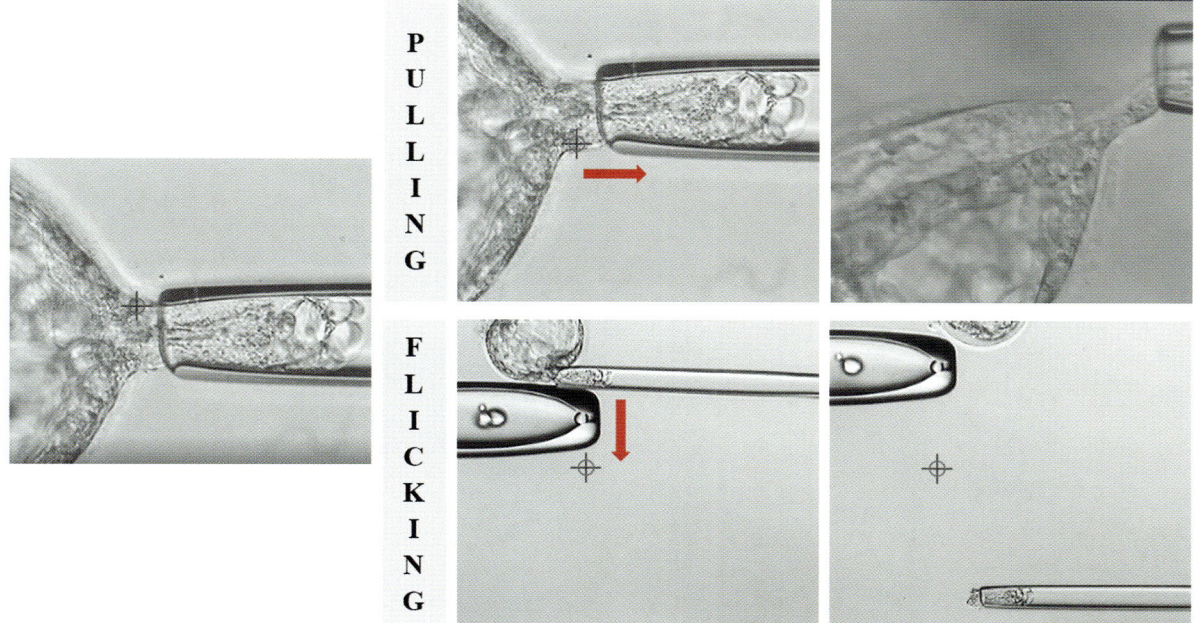

Figure 14.1 The pulling and flicking methods to remove a fragment of the trophectoderm during blastocyst biopsy

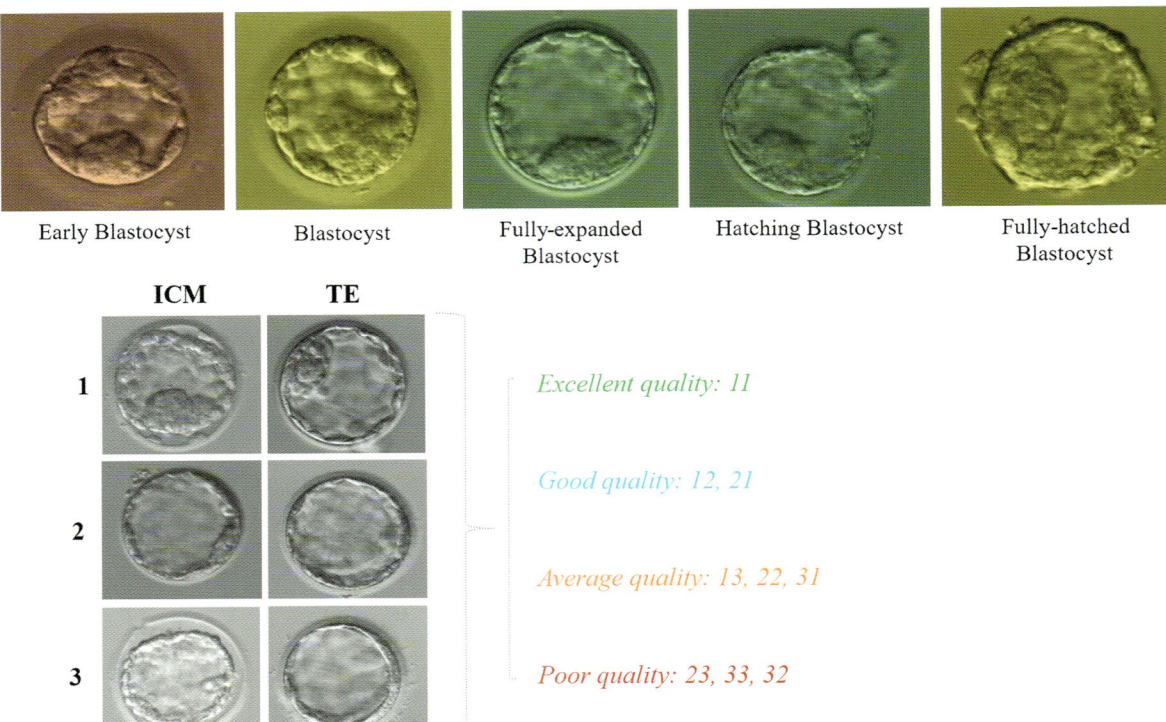

| Early Blastocyst | Blastocyst | Fully-expanded Blastocyst | Hatching Blastocyst | Fully-hatched Blastocyst |

ICM   **TE**

Excellent quality: 11

Good quality: 12, 21

Average quality: 13, 22, 31

Poor quality: 23, 33, 32

Figure 14.2 The conventional scheme for blastocyst morphological evaluation

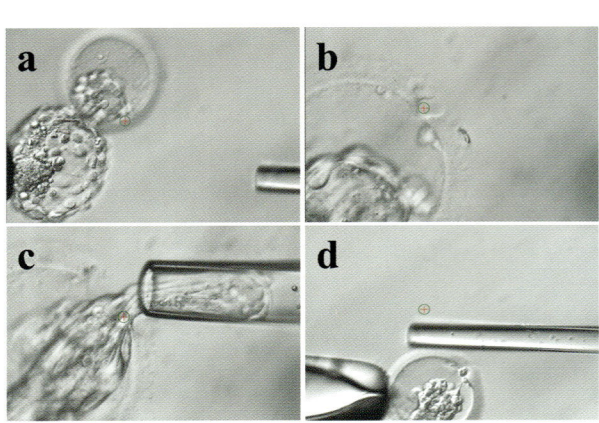

Figure 14.3 Biopsy of an embryo hatching from the inner cell mass after a laser-assisted zona opening at the cleavage stage
a) embryo before the biopsy; b) ZP opening on the opposite side of the former hole; c) the selected trophectoderm cells are sucked into the biopsy pipette and cut with a few laser shots; d) the biopsy is finalized.

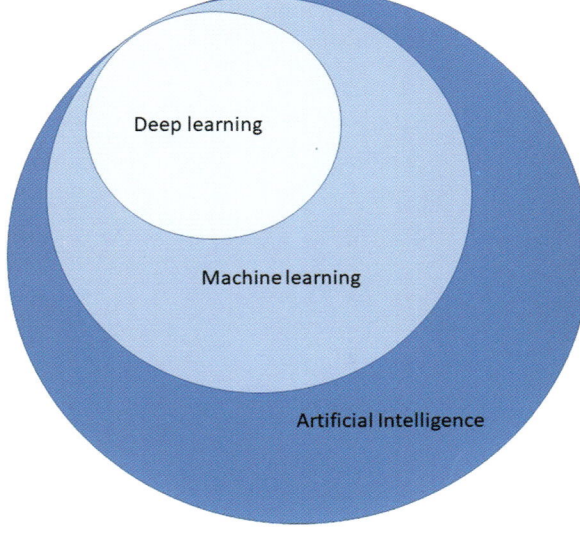

Figure 16.1 Relationship between artificial intelligence, machine learning, and deep learning
AI encompasses the science and engineering of creating human-like intelligence in computer systems. Machine learning is a type of AI, while deep learning is a further subdivision of machine learning based on artificial neural networks.

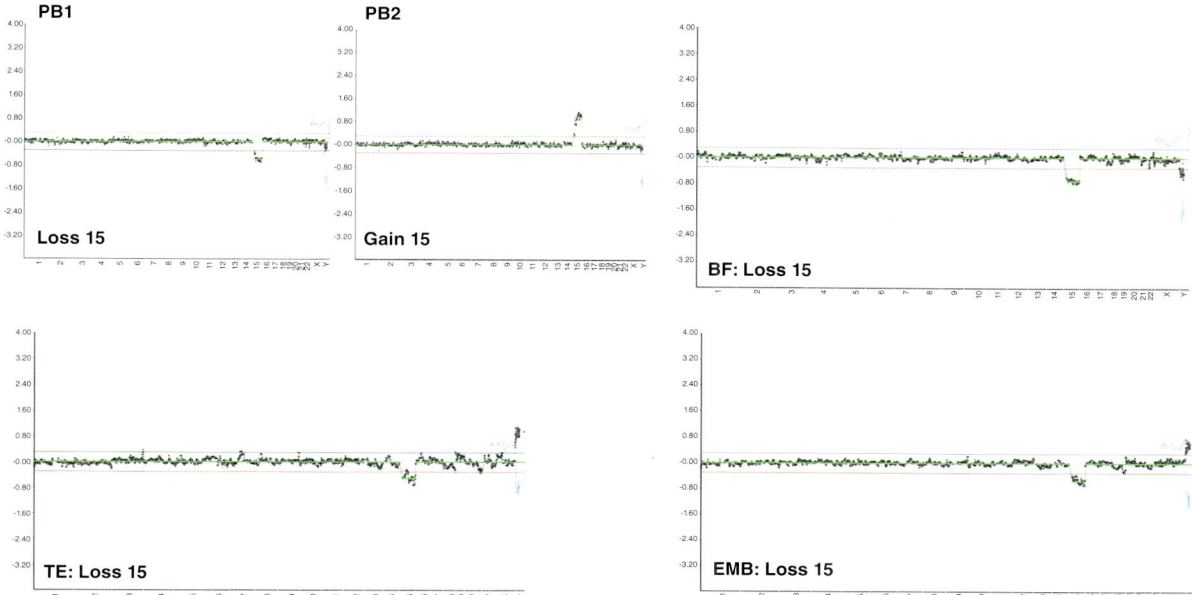

Figure 15.2 Concordance between PB1 and PB2 chromosomal results and those from the corresponding BF, TE, and whole-embryo analyses. Following PB analysis, the embryo is predicted to be monosomic for chromosome 15 as proven by BF, TE biopsy, and by the analysis of the whole embryo.

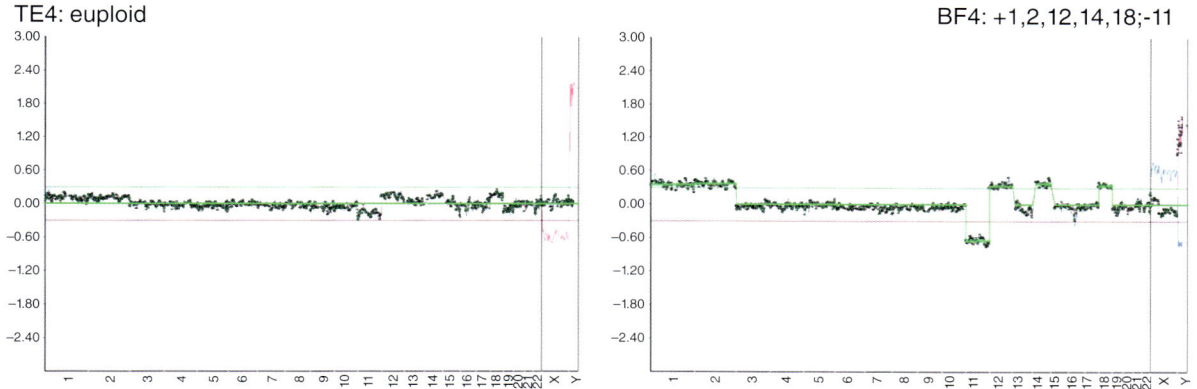

Figure 15.3 Chromosome analysis by a-CGH in the TE biopsy and corresponding BF
The blastocyst is called euploid by the software analyzing the TE biopsy, although a modest grade of mosaicism is identified for chromosome 1, 2, 11, 12, 14, and 18. The analysis of the BF reveals a clear aneuploid status by calling an extra copy for chromosomes 1, 2, 12, 14, and 18, and a single copy for chromosome 11. This result supports the role of BF as the collector of aneuploid cells in an attempt by the mosaic embryo to restore an euploid condition.

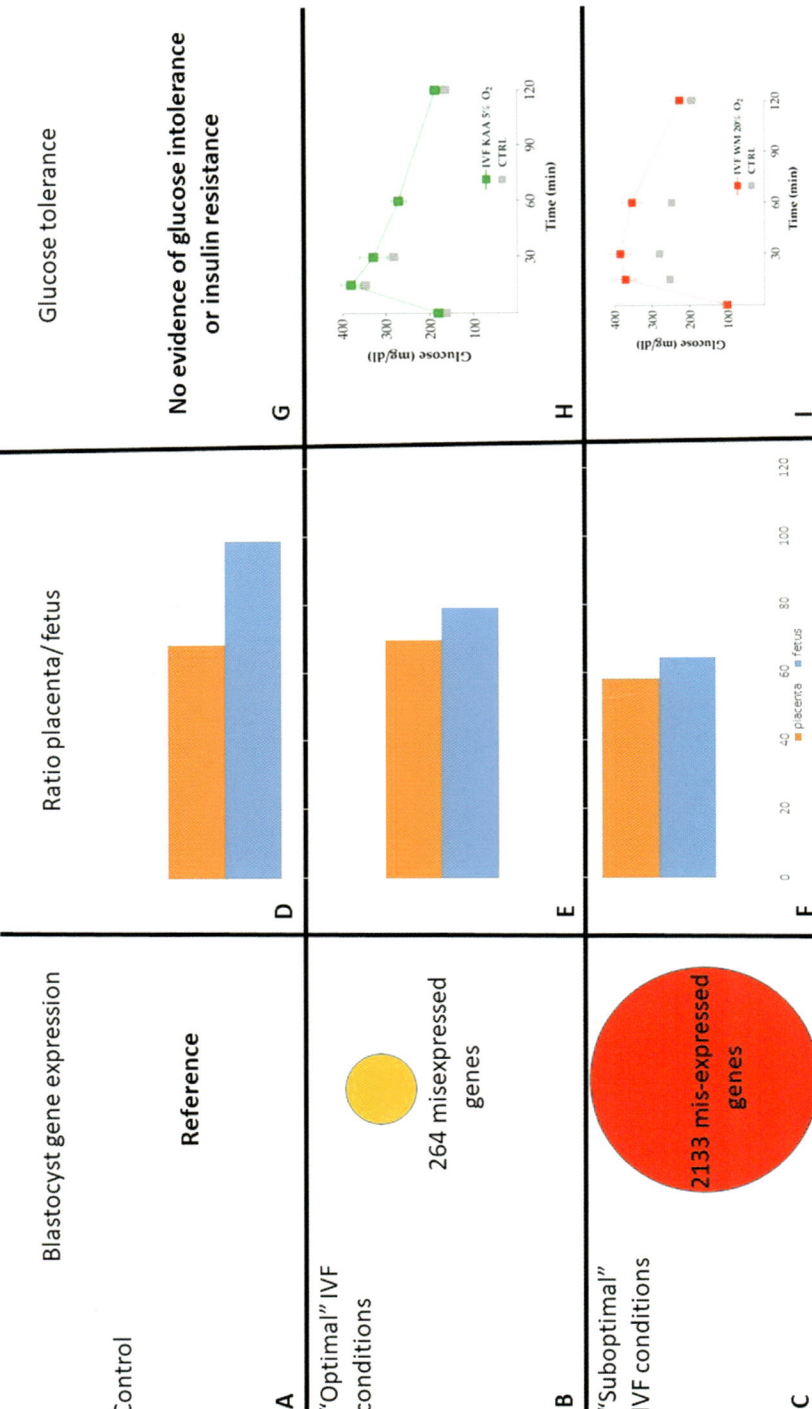

Figure 16.2 Selecting embryos with less stress might result in healthier offspring

To measure embryonic stress, blastocyst gene expression was measured by microarray technology. Compared to control mouse embryos flushed out of the uterus at the blastocyst stage (**A**), blastocysts generated by IVF and cultured in optimal conditions have 264 misexpressed genes (**B**). Blastocysts that were cultured in suboptimal conditions have nearly 10-fold misexpressed genes (n = 2 133, **C**). The size of the circle is proportional to the number of abnormal genes. (Data are from Feuer SK et al., *Reprod*. 2016;153:107–22.) Importantly, the embryonic stress is memorized: at mid-gestation (day 12.5 in mice), fetuses generated in vitro in optimal conditions have lower weight and larger and heavier placentae (**E**) when compared to in vivo embryos (**D**); this effect is even more evident in embryos that were cultured in suboptimal conditions (**F**). (Data are from Delle Piane L et al., *Hum Reprod*. 2010;25:2039).

Finally, adult mice generated by IVF in optimal conditions have normal glucose levels when tested with a glucose tolerance test (GTT) (**H**), although they have higher fasting insulin levels (indicating insulin resistance – data not shown). On the contrary, mice generated by IVF in stressful conditions are glucose intolerant when tested by GTT (**I**). Data are from Feuer SK et al., *Endocrin*. 2014;155:1956.

These data suggest that limiting stress to embryos (for example by minimizing the number of procedures done to gametes and embryos) might benefit the future health of the individual.

Genomics for Embryo Selection

Elpida Fragouli and Dagan Wells

13.1 Introduction

There are two main reasons why a genetic selection of embryos may take place during an IVF cycle:

1. To reduce the risks that a genetic abnormality will be transmitted to the next generation. This can involve the identification of embryos with a dominant gene mutation inherited from the male or female partner, recessive gene mutations carried by both male and female parents, X-linked mutations inherited from the female, or chromosome imbalances caused by a structural chromosome rearrangement carried by either partner.

2. To improve the efficiency of the IVF process by distinguishing embryos of high potential from those that are unlikely to be viable due to the presence of genetic defects, most notably aneuploidy.

The process of embryo selection taking place due to a specific genetic issue is widely known as preimplantation genetic testing (PGT), although the term used to describe this procedure up until recently was preimplantation genetic diagnosis. PGT aims to identify among a cohort of embryos generated by a couple with a known genetic disorder, those that are free of the condition. With the transfer of embryos predicted to be "unaffected," it is hoped that any clinical pregnancies established will ultimately lead to the birth of a healthy child. Hence, PGT is increasingly being considered as an alternative to routine prenatal diagnosis, having the added advantage of greatly reducing the number of pregnancy terminations. PGT carried out due to the presence of inherited mutations affecting the function of a gene is known as PGT-M, where the M stands for "monogenic" disorders. PGT performed for the detection of chromosomal deletions or duplications associated with parental chromosome rearrangements, such

as inversions and reciprocal or Robertsonian translocations, is known as PGT-SR, where SR stands for "structural rearrangement." In addition to an increased likelihood of establishing a healthy clinical pregnancy and avoiding terminations, PGT often has the capacity to eliminate an inherited genetic disorder that has been present in a family for many generations.

An IVF cycle including PGT involves the removal of a few cells from each of the embryos being tested via a process of embryo biopsy. Currently, the most common type of embryo biopsy takes place 5–6 days after fertilization, at the blastocyst stage of preimplantation development. At this stage the embryo has undergone its first cellular differentiation and consists of an external cellular layer, the trophectoderm (TE), and an internal cluster of cells referred to as the inner cell mass (ICM). After embryo implantation, the TE will give rise to the placenta and a subset of cells in the ICM will generate the fetus. During blastocyst biopsy, a few (usually approximately five) cells are taken from the TE and the DNA they contain is subjected to genetic testing. Various diagnostic methodologies can be employed, and these differ depending on the type of genetic testing that is being undertaken.

Embryo selection for the purpose of improving IVF outcomes, used for infertile couples without any specific gene mutation or chromosome rearrangement, focuses on the detection of chromosome losses and gains. This form of testing is termed preimplantation genetic testing for aneuploidy, or PGT-A. It has been known for many years that numerical chromosome abnormalities (aneuploidy) are common during the early stages of human embryo development [1, 2]. Chromosomally abnormal embryos are very likely to stop developing, fail to implant, or miscarry early in gestation. It has therefore been hypothesized that the detection of chromosome errors in IVF-generated embryos, and the preferential selection and transfer of those that are normal (euploid) could assist infertile couples by improving various aspects of IVF, including helping them to become pregnant with fewer embryo transfers, a lower incidence of miscarriage, and less risk of aneuploid syndromes (e.g. Down syndrome) [3]. Currently, the most common indication for PGT-A is advanced female reproductive age, although other patient groups such as those with recurrent pregnancy losses (RPL), repeated implantation failure (RIF), or male factor infertility are also often referred. The clinical processes involved during PGT-A are very similar to those taking place for other forms of PGT. Hence, embryos are biopsied at the blastocyst stage, and the cells removed undergo a genetic test, in this case to determine chromosome number. In the following sections we will cover technical aspects of PGT-M, PGT-SR, and PGT-A, including challenges and troubleshooting. The potential clinical value of different forms of PGT for patients that request these tests in order to achieve a pregnancy will also be discussed.

13.2 Preimplantation Genetic Testing for Monogenic Disorders

Couples where one or both partners are carriers of an inherited mutation affecting gene function, and who seek PGT-M to achieve a healthy live birth, are generally reproductively younger and fertile. The absence of a defect in fertility and, most importantly of all, the younger age in comparison with most other patients undergoing IVF treatment, means that the chances of achieving a pregnancy for this patient cohort could be expected to be relatively high in comparison with other IVF patient groups. However, the loss of embryos due to an unfavorable diagnosis works to reduce the chances of a successful cycle, since the embryos considered most likely to deliver a viable pregnancy are sometimes among those found to be affected and are therefore excluded from transfer. Overall, pregnancy rates following PGT-M are not dissimilar to those obtained during routine IVF. For example, Gutierrez-Mateo and colleagues [4] reported clinical outcome results after PGT-M for 46 different disorders. The transfer of 414 embryos led to a pregnancy rate per transfer of 51%, with 43% of these progressing to the presence of a gestational sac and a heartbeat during ultrasound assessment.

For many years the polymerase chain reaction (PCR) was the basis for all PGT-M diagnostic strategies. Specifically, a PCR approach was applied to the biopsied cell(s), amplifying a fragment of the DNA that encompasses the mutation causing the inherited disorder. Initial PGT-M diagnostic strategies examined only the mutation site [5], but protocols evolved to include the assessment of additional polymorphic markers closely linked to the affected locus [6, 7]. Such multiplex PCR approaches are still frequently used for PGT-M today.

The amplification of DNA from single or low numbers of cells can be technically challenging. One technical problem associated with such amplifications is allele dropout (ADO). ADO can be defined as failure of DNA amplification affecting one of the two alleles in a heterozygous cell. This amplification failure can potentially cause the heterozygous cell to appear homozygous at the locus affected by ADO, increasing the risk of inaccurate genotyping and misdiagnosis. Multiplex PCR approaches used for PGT-M are employed to address this issue. DNA polymorphisms closely linked to the locus affected by the mutation are inherited along with it. Therefore, the use of PCR primer sets that allow amplification and interrogation of not only the mutation site, but also a few closely linked polymorphic markers, enables utilization of direct (mutation site) and an indirect (linked markers) diagnostic strategies in parallel [8], thus increasing the accuracy of PGT-M.

Primer sets targeting hypervariable polymorphisms have often been chosen for multiplex PCR protocols used for PGT-M. Short tandem repeat (STR) polymorphisms have been particularly popular as multiple alleles may exist for each locus, increasing the likelihood of finding an "informative" polymorphism (i.e. a polymorphic site where the combination of alleles present allows individual chromosomes to be differentiated). The hypervariable nature of STRs has also led to their frequent use in the context of DNA fingerprinting [9]. The ability of STRs to distinguish DNA from different individuals is also helpful for the detection of DNA contamination in tubes containing biopsied cells, another source of possible misdiagnosis during PGT-M. When examining an embryo biopsy specimen, the embryo is expected to inherit one allele from each parent. The presence of an STR allele that is not present in either of the parents is indicative of an external contaminant having been introduced in the sample tube, while the presence of more than one allele from a single parent can indicate contamination from a parental source. For example, the detection of two maternal alleles plus one paternal allele could be the result of detecting embryonic DNA plus genetic material from a cumulus cell or other maternal source. It should be noted that the design and optimization of traditional PGT-M strategies frequently requires a high degree of customization, necessitating significant effort in the laboratory. It is therefore not unusual for patients requesting PGT-M to have to wait for several weeks before beginning their IVF cycle.

Recently an alternative PGT-M approach was developed, termed karyomapping [10]. Karyomapping relies on an assessment of whether a mutant gene has been inherited based upon analysis of approximately 300 000 single nucleotide polymorphisms (SNPs), scattered across the genome using a microarray. For the purpose of PGT-M, analysis is focused on the genotypes of groups of SNPs that are in close proximity to the gene of interest. The genotypes of the mother, father and other family member(s) are analyzed by software, revealing the characteristic groups of linked SNP alleles (haplotype) that accompany the mutation [10, 11]. As karyomapping simultaneously examines numerous sites in the genome, informative SNPs can be identified in the vicinity of virtually any gene of interest. Thus, karyomapping provides a universal protocol for the PGT-M of different inherited monogenic conditions. Karyomapping has the added advantage, over conventional PGT-M approaches, of enabling the detection of certain types of chromosome abnormalities, such as monosomies (revealed by apparent homozygosity for all SNPs on the affected chromosome), as well as trisomies of meiotic origin (SNP alleles characteristic of three distinct chromosome copies are detected). The parental origin of meiotic trisomies (i.e. whether they are derived from the sperm or the oocyte) can also be determined. In their study, Ben-Nagi and colleagues [12] found that 30% of embryos that underwent karyomapping had detectable chromosome abnormalities of types likely to impact the chances of a viable pregnancy. Figure 13.1 provides a summary of the karyomapping technique.

Since its development, PGT-M via karyomapping has found wide clinical application, and has shown promising outcome results. Konstantinidis et al. [11] in their investigation reported on clinical outcomes after PGT-M carried out either via karyomapping or

conventional mutation analysis. The study summarized data obtained from PGT-M for 35 different autosomal dominant, autosomal recessive, and X-linked diseases. PGT-M took place at the blastocyst stage, and karyomapping led to successful diagnosis of 99.6% of embryos assessed and a 70% ongoing pregnancy rate for cycles that had an embryo transfer, although this figure was based on only 20 transfers. Another study [12], yielded similar results with 81 embryo transfers following karyomapping resulting in a 63% ongoing pregnancy rate. More recently, genome sequencing technologies have been used to reveal the same sort of SNP genotype information as obtained using karyomapping, an approach termed haplarithmisis [13], allowing combined PGT-M and aneuploidy detection. Table 13.1 summarizes the technical details and compares the most commonly used PGT-M strategies.

13.3 Preimplantation Genetic Testing for Structural Rearrangements

Balanced carriers of structural chromosome rearrangements, such as Robertsonian or reciprocal translocations, are phenotypically normal, but are at risk of generating genetically abnormal (unbalanced) gametes, due to the way that the normal and derivative (rearranged) chromosomes pair during meiosis. It is not uncommon for balanced carriers of structural chromosome rearrangements to experience reproductive problems, such as recurrent miscarriage, or the birth of unbalanced offspring. Data suggest that 0.5–5% of all infertile couples carry a balanced structural chromosome rearrangement [14].

For many years fluorescent in situ hybridization (FISH) was the method used for PGT of structural rearrangements. The most common FISH diagnostic strategy for PGT-SR involved the use of a total of three probes that were specific for the chromosomes involved in the structural rearrangement. Cells were biopsied, usually at the cleavage stage of preimplantation development, then fixed on microscope slides, and subsequently analyzed with FISH. In cases of reciprocal translocations, two FISH probes would hybridize to chromosomal sites flanking the breakpoint on one of the chromosomes involved in the translocation (often one probe located at the centromere and the other in the subtelomeric region), while the third probe would target a site on the other chromosome, typically the centromere. Diagnosis

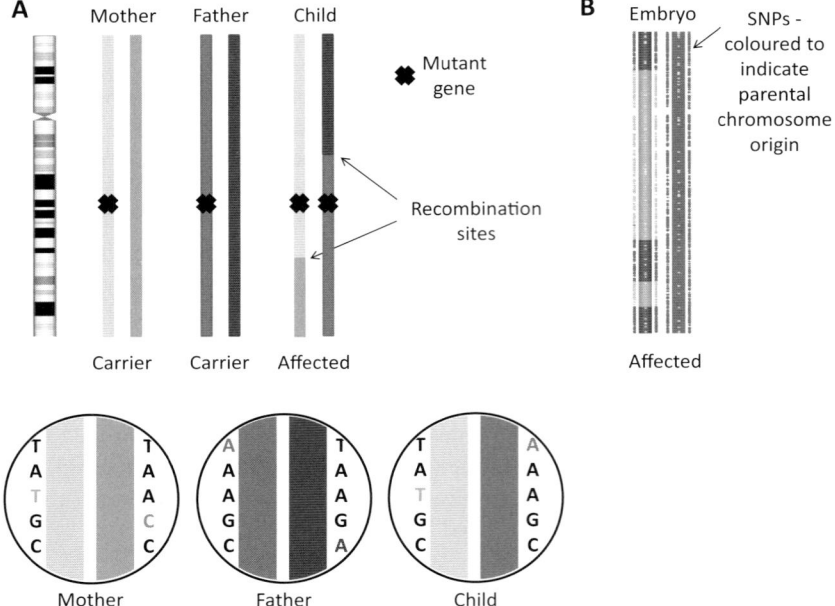

Figure 13.1 Karyomapping

Both parents and an additional family member (most often an affected child of the couple) are assessed using a microarray, providing genotype information for ~300 000 SNPs scattered across the genome. SNP alleles close to the mutant gene are inherited along with it and consequently provide an indirect indication of the presence of the mutation. Each parental chromosome has a unique pattern of SNP alleles, which serves as a genetic fingerprint, identifying that chromosome. Examples of allele combinations that allow individual chromosomes to be distinguished are shown at the foot of the figure. Based on the SNP results obtained, parental chromosomes are color-coded (A). This allows easy visualization of the chromosomes inherited by embryos, even revealing sites where meiotic recombination occurred. Multiple informative SNPs are present on each chromosome as shown in this example of a karyomapping result (B). Each spot flanking the graphical representation of the chromosome corresponds to an informative SNP, colored in order to show the parental chromosome for which that particular SNP provides evidence.

was based on the fact that any abnormal chromosome segregation patterns associated with the translocation would result in a deviation from the normal number of copies (two) of each probe. The use of FISH was associated with some technical challenges, especially in relation to the spreading of cells onto slides and the interpretation of the FISH signals observed under the microscope. Additionally, the method was unable to assess the entire chromosome complement of the biopsied cells.

The optimization and subsequent validation of new molecular cytogenetic methodologies, with the ability to assess all of the chromosomes within single cells, led to their clinical application for the purpose of PGT-SR. The first molecular cytogenetic method to be used for the clinical analysis of embryonic samples was metaphase comparative genomic hybridization (CGH) [2]. The initial step in the procedure involved DNA amplification of the embryonic biopsy sample.

This took place via PCR approaches that used random or semidegenerate primers capable of amplifying the majority of the genome of the biopsied cells. These techniques are typically referred to as whole genome amplification (WGA). The second step involved a simultaneous hybridization of two differentially labeled DNAs, one which was chromosomally normal (reference sample) and another composed of the amplified DNA from the embryonic sample, to metaphase chromosomes on a microscope slide. The metaphase spreads were karyotyped in order to distinguish one chromosome from another and the relative amount of fluorescence attributable to hybridized DNA from the reference sample and the embryo sample was measured for each chromosome. If the cytogenetic constitution of the test sample was identical to the reference sample, that is, the test sample was normal, then all chromosomes would display a similar amount of fluorescence for each of the two

Table 13.1. Diagnostic strategies currently used for preimplantation genetic testing for monogenic disorders (PGT-M)

Diagnostic strategy	Method used	Additional technical information	Protocol design required?	Detection of chromosome errors?
Conventional	Multiplex PCR	Multiple sets of primers are used to target the site of the mutation, along with linked and other polymorphisms to detect allele dropout and contamination	Yes, the diagnostic strategy is usually uniquely designed for the mutation in question. Parental DNAs are required during protocol optimization. Protocol design and optimization can be lengthy	Conventional PGT-M strategies are not able to detect chromosome errors, unless the chromosome affect happens to be the one targeted during amplification
Karyomapping	Whole genome amplification followed by analysis using array interrogating over 300 000 single nucleotide polymorphisms across the human genome	Karyomapping can be combined with conventional mutation detection analysis via some form of multiplex PCR. The diagnostic approach will depend on the mutation for which PGT-M will be carried out	Yes, if a conventional mutation detection step is added to the diagnostic strategy. Parental DNAs as well as DNA from an affected relative are also required during protocol optimization. Generally, protocol design is not as lengthy as conventional PGT-M approaches	Yes, karyomapping is capable of detecting all meiotic monosomies and trisomies, all mitotic monosomies and some mitotic trisomies

differentially labeled DNA samples. If, on the other hand, the test sample had an extra chromosome compared to the reference sample (i.e. a trisomy), then the affected chromosome would display a greater intensity of fluorescence in the color in which the embryo DNA had been labeled. A monosomy would also show a change in the relative fluorescence associated with the reference and test/embryo DNAs, but in the opposite direction. Metaphase CGH provided, for the first time, an overview of the entire chromosome complement of the biopsied embryonic samples. It was, however, technically demanding, time-consuming and labor-intensive, precluding its use for high-throughput applications.

Metaphase CGH was rapidly superseded by microarray CGH (aCGH), a similar method that employed slides (arrays) spotted with DNA probes corresponding to multiple distinct regions along the length of each of the chromosomes. These probes, rather than metaphase chromosomes, served as targets for the hybridization of the differentially labeled embryo and reference DNA samples [15]. Analysis occurred by placing the microarray slides through a scanner, rather than capturing metaphase images under the microscope, followed by the use of specialized software that would determine the test sample chromosome constitution. As with metaphase CGH, differences in the relative fluorescence attributable to the two labeled DNA samples revealed losses and duplications of chromosomal regions. A clinical result after the use of aCGH is shown in Figure 13.2.

aCGH found wide application for the purposes of PGT-SR [e.g. 16], but in recent years has been largely replaced by another technology known as next-generation sequencing (NGS). The term NGS encompasses several different methods that enable the massive parallel sequencing of small DNA fragments [17]. Hundreds of thousands of fragments are sequenced from each sample and are "mapped," revealing the region of the genome from which they were derived. By determining the proportion of sequenced fragments from each chromosome, losses and duplications

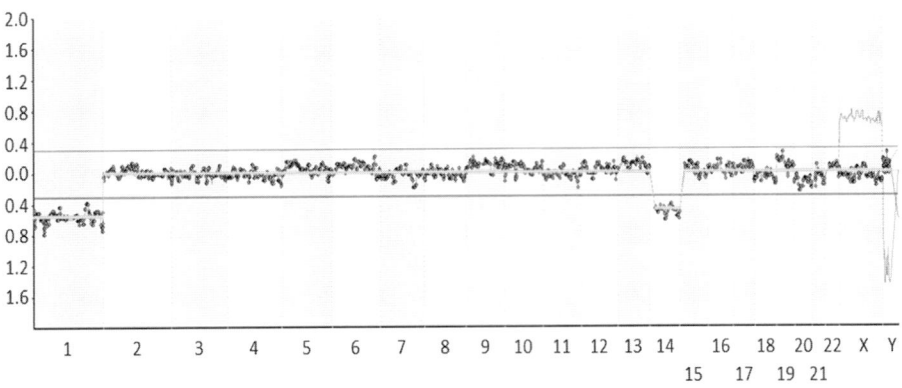

Figure 13.2 Microarray comparative genomic hybridization (aCGH)
The image shows an aCGH result for a trophectoderm biopsy sample with an apparent loss of chromosomes 1 and 14. The embryo was therefore predicted to have monosomy 1 and monosomy 14, a lethal abnormality. The z-axis represents the relative amount of red fluorescence (normal control DNA) and green fluorescence (embryo DNA) detected on chromosome specific probes situated on the microarray. On the scale L, 0.0 equates to an equal quantity of red and green fluorescence. Values toward the foot of the image indicate increasing red, whereas those toward the top of the page indicate more green.

of chromosomal material can be revealed. NGS is currently the main method used for both PGT-SR and PGT-A, as it has several advantages over array-based methodologies, including its ability to simultaneously test samples biopsied from multiple embryos, increasing throughput and reducing the cost of diagnosis. Additionally, NGS is more sensitive than array-based approaches, and is capable of detecting mosaic chromosome abnormalities affecting a minority of cells in the biopsied embryonic sample. Both WGA and targeted PCR, simultaneously amplifying large numbers of specific DNA sequences across the 24 chromosomes, can be used as the initial step, providing sufficient DNA for subsequent NGS [18, 19]. A technical overview of NGS is given in Figure 13.3.

Clinical outcomes after PGT-SR using comprehensive cytogenetic approaches have generally been encouraging, with studies reporting pregnancy rates ranging between 26% and 38% per cycle [16, 20, 21]. Similar to the use of karyomapping for PGT-M, comprehensive cytogenetic approaches deployed for PGT-SR have revealed secondary findings in embryonic samples, presenting in the form of aneuploidies unrelated to the structural rearrangement. Data analysis obtained during the PGT-SR of 498 blastocysts via aCGH demonstrated that 24% were normal/balanced for the structural rearrangement, but had other unrelated chromosome errors [21]. As is the case with PGT-M via karyomapping, avoiding the transfer of embryos affected by these additional unrelated

aneuploidies is expected to decrease spontaneous miscarriages and improve the rate of births per transfer, but will also lead to a greater number of cycles with no transfer due to all embryos being classified abnormal, especially for couples where the female partner is of advanced reproductive age. Table 13.2 summarizes the technical details of the PGT-SR and PGT-A methods.

13.4 Preimplantation Genetic Testing for Aneuploidy

Several indications for PGT-A have been proposed, including advanced female reproductive age, repeated unexplained implantation failure or recurrent pregnancy loss (RIF and RPL, respectively), male factor infertility, or previous aneuploid conceptions with both partners having a normal karyotype. The reason for considering PGT-A for patients in these categories is the suspicion that they might have elevated levels of aneuploidy in their embryos, although for some of these indications the evidence for an increased abnormality rate is weak. Nonetheless, given the fact that embryo aneuploidy is seen at an appreciable frequency for all patients undergoing IVF, including young patients and egg donations cycles, it is possible that PGT-A would be beneficial in most cycles.

Ever since its initial clinical application in the early 1990s, a principal aim of PGT-A has been to

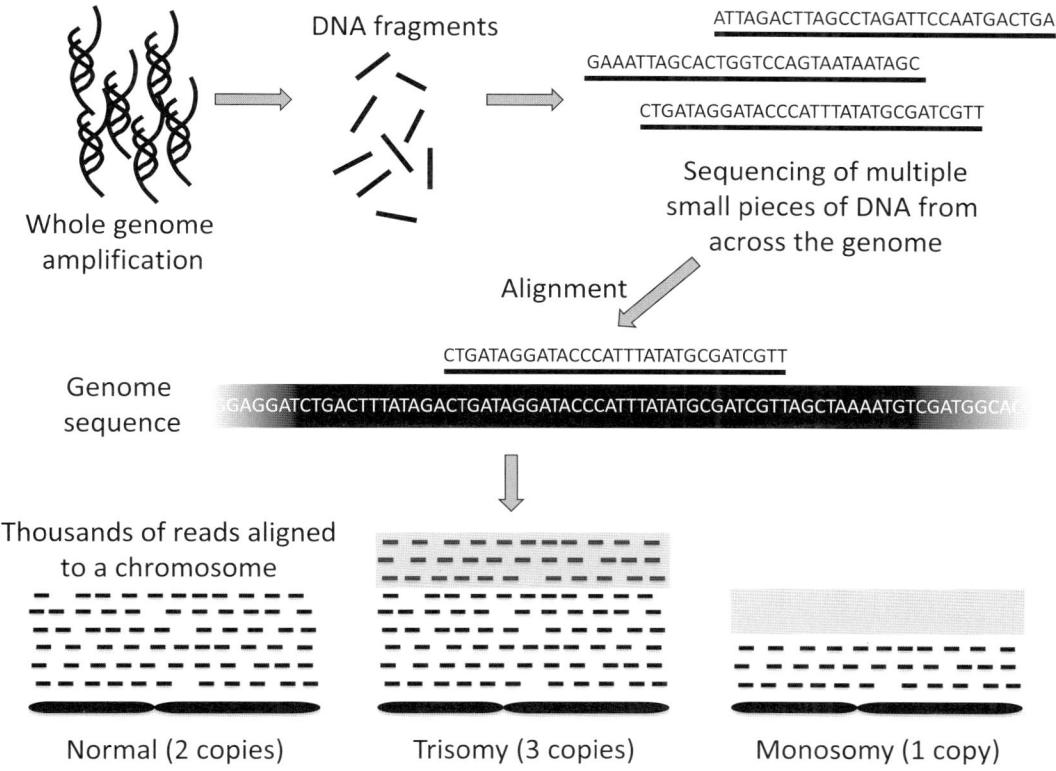

Figure 13.3 Next-generation sequencing (NGS)

For NGS, the DNA contained within the embryo biopsy specimen is first subjected to whole-genome amplification. The resulting DNA is prepared for sequencing that results in the production of millions of DNA fragments. Sequencing of these fragments reveals the order of DNA bases (G, A, T, and C) along their length. The fragments of DNA sequence thus obtained are known as "reads." The DNA sequence of each fragment can then be compared to the sequence of the human genome in order to determine the location it originally came from, a computer-driven process known as alignment. The relative proportion of "reads" aligned to each chromosome is identical for all samples with a normal number of chromosomes. Extra chromosomal material (e.g. a trisomy) causes an overrepresentation in the amount of reads from the affected chromosomes, whereas a monosomy is associated with a reduction in the relative number of reads from the abnormal chromosome.

improve certain clinical outcomes after IVF. In theory, avoiding the transfer of aneuploid embryos, predicted to have reduced viability, should improve the chances of pregnancy per embryo transfer, reduce the time taken to achieve a viable pregnancy, and decrease miscarriage rates and the incidence of aneuploid syndromes. Currently, PGT-A is the most widely used of all PGT approaches, due to its relative simplicity and the larger populations of patients to which it is considered applicable.

Similar to PGT-SR, FISH was the first method used for PGT-A. FISH strategies employed for PGT-A involved the analysis of 5–12 chromosomes, most often applied to single blastomeres biopsied from cleavage-stage embryos. However, several randomized clinical trials (RCTs) failed to demonstrate that this approach was capable of improving clinical

outcomes [22]. This failure was attributed to FISH's inability to assess the entire chromosome complement of biopsied cells, the high rate of chromosomal mosaicism during the cleavage stage of preimplantation development [23], and the negative impact that the removal of a single blastomere had on the viability of the corresponding embryos [24].

The optimization of more comprehensive molecular cytogenetic approaches and the improvement of IVF culture systems meant that the way that PGT-A was performed changed dramatically in the mid-2000s. Specifically, extended culture of embryos until they reached the blastocyst stage became routine, allowing safe sampling of several cells. Our group [25] were the first to report on clinical data obtained by employing CGH for the cytogenetic analysis of TE samples biopsied from blastocyst stage embryos. It

Table 13.2. Diagnostic strategies that have been used for detection of structural (PGT-SR) and numerical (PGT-A) chromosome abnormalities

Method	Additional technical information	Protocol design required?	Aneuploidy types detected	Method currently in use?
FISH	Fluorescently labeled DNA probes employed that hybridize either on the chromosome centromeres, or on loci on the long or short arm. Several FISH rounds can be performed to increase number of chromosomes examined	Yes, for reciprocal translocations, inversions, insertion, etc.	Abnormalities only detected for the specific chromosomes tested	No
CGH	Requires whole genome amplification of biopsied embryo sample as initial step. Competitive hybridization of two differentially labeled DNA samples, a test DNA (embryo sample) labeled in green, and a chromosomally normal reference DNA labeled in red to a microscope slide of normal metaphase chromosomes. Comparison of the ratio of green:red fluorescence along the length of each chromosome determines the relative chromosome copy number in the test sample compared to the reference.	No, the protocol is universal irrespective of the type of diagnosis required	Whole or partial abnormalities affecting all 46 chromosomes	No
aCGH	Requires whole genome amplification of biopsied embryo sample as initial step. Competitive hybridization of two differentially labeled DNA samples, a test DNA (embryo sample) labeled in green, and a chromosomally normal reference DNA labeled in red to a microscope slide (array) spotted with DNA probes from multiple sites along the length of the 24 chromosomes. Comparison of the ratio of green:red fluorescence along the length of each chromosome determines the relative chromosome copy number in the test sample compared to the reference.	No, the protocol is universal irrespective of the type of diagnosis required	Whole or partial abnormalities affecting all 46 chromosomes	No
NGS	Biopsied embryo sample is amplified either via whole genome amplification or a targeted PCR strategy. The amplified product is then fragmented into pieces of 100–200 base pairs. Sequencing of fragments follows. The data obtained after the sequencing is compared with a reference human genome, and counted to determine chromosome copy number of the biopsied embryo sample.	No, the protocol is universal irrespective of the type of diagnosis required	Whole or partial abnormalities affecting all 46 chromosomes. Abnormalities of meiotic and postfertilization mitotic (mosaic) origin are identified	Yes

was clear from this dataset that aneuploidy persisted to the final stage of preimplantation development, and affected all chromosomes. As was the case with PGT-SR, CGH was initially replaced by approaches such as aCGH, SNP arrays, or quantitative real-time PCR, and eventually NGS. With the exception of quantitative real-time PCR, all molecular cytogenetic strategies were not capable of yielding results in a time frame compatible with a fresh embryo transfer. It is therefore common practice that all blastocysts generated by couples going through PGT-A are vitrified once TE biopsy has taken place. If any embryos are found to have a normal chromosome complement after PGT-A analysis, they can be warmed and prioritized for transfer in a subsequent cycle.

The clinical efficacy of PGT-A via the use of comprehensive molecular cytogenetic strategies has been the subject of several RCTs, most of which have reported promising results. A recent meta-analysis including some of these RCTs [26] concluded that PGT-A is capable of improving clinical outcomes for couples where the female partner has a normal ovarian reserve, but it was unclear if the test offered the same benefits for poorer-prognosis patients. An additional two RCTs that were published in the past two years yielded conflicting results. Specifically, Munné et al. [27] used NGS to examine TE samples biopsied from embryos generated by patients with a wide female age range (25–40 years). The RCT included IVF clinics in the USA and Europe, and only couples capable of producing at least two good-quality blastocysts participated. The results obtained during this RCT were indicative of a potential improvement in clinical outcomes for women of advanced reproductive age. Such an improvement was not observed in the RCT carried out by Verpoest and colleagues [28]. Similar to the Munné et al. [27] study, several European IVF clinics participated in this RCT. Unlike the Munné et al. [27] RCT, however, the results obtained by Verpoest and colleagues did not show a difference in clinical pregnancy rates between their test and control patient groups, irrespective of female age. It should be noted that this RCT involved analysis of the first and second polar body (PB) using aCGH analysis, a strategy rarely used for PGT-A, which is of questionable accuracy and is unable to detect paternally derived or postfertilization chromosome abnormalities. Furthermore, while the two polar bodies are often considered biproducts of female meiosis, superfluous

to embryonic development, it has not yet been demonstrated that their removal is truly neutral in terms of subsequent embryo viability. The difference in embryo assessment stage, and the methodology used, could be causative of the variation in clinical outcomes seen between these two recent RCTs.

There are two main issues that raise questions over the clinical efficacy of PGT-A: the potential impact of the biopsy procedure, and uncertainty over the extent to which a result from a single TE sample is representative of the rest of the embryo. Irrespective of the developmental stage during which the biopsy occurs, it requires a lengthy training period for the embryologists performing it to ensure that embryo viability is not compromised. Additionally, IVF clinics that are considering offering any type of PGT need to purchase expensive laser equipment, in order to perform the biopsy. Importantly, the biopsy procedure itself is not standardized. Multiple aspects of the technique vary between individual embryologists, including the number of laser pulses and the number of TE cells removed from the embryo. While existing data suggests there is little if any impact on the embryo when TE biopsy is carried out by experienced personnel [29], it is conceivable that suboptimal practice could reduce embryo viability.

Uncertainty over the extent to which a single TE sample is representative of the rest of the embryo could be caused by inadequacies of genetic testing methods or due to a biological phenomenon known as mosaicism. Mosaicism can be defined as the presence of two or more chromosomally distinct cell lines within the same embryo. Mosaicism arises from chromosome malsegregation taking place during the mitotic divisions after fertilization, and leads to the formation of embryos containing a mixture of euploid and abnormal cells, or embryos that have different aneuploidies affecting individual cells in the absence of any euploid cells.

The optimization and application of molecular cytogenetic methodologies capable of examining the entire embryonic chromosome complement, demonstrated that mosaic chromosome abnormalities are common during preimplantation development, but decrease in frequency between the cleavage and blastocyst stages [23, 25]. However, mitotically derived aneuploidy and mosaicism only recently became readily detectable during PGT-A , due to the increasing use of NGS for the purposes of PGT-A. NGS is much more sensitive compared to previously employed PGT-A strategies, such as aCGH, and is able to detect chromosome errors present either in all or part of the biopsied TE cells. Mosaic chromosome abnormalities carry the possibility of negatively impacting the diagnostic accuracy of PGT-A, and there has been some confusion about the best way to clinically manage embryos that are an apparent mixture of euploid and abnormal cells, termed "mosaic diploid-aneuploid." An example of a mosaic TE sample, as identified after NGS analysis, is illustrated in Figure 13.4.

Several datasets have recently been published concerning the viability and implantation capacity of mosaic diploid-aneuploid embryos [30–37] (see Table 13.3 for a summary). Most of these investigations were retrospective and conclude that mosaic diploid-aneuploid blastocysts have significantly lower implantation and pregnancy rates (some also indicating higher miscarriage rates) compared to embryos that have an entirely euploid trophectoderm biopsy sample. However, most recently, a well-designed prospective trial has indicated that there may be little if any difference between the viability of euploid and mosaic embryos [37]. Thus, while there is general agreement that many mosaic embryos are capable of producing a viable, healthy pregnancy, there remains some uncertainty about whether they should be considered equivalent to embryos with a euploid TE

biopsy, or whether they should be given a lower priority for transfer to the uterus. Guidelines to aid the clinical management of blastocyst stage embryos with different types of PGT-A results have been published by the Preimplantation Genetic Diagnosis International Society, and were recently updated to reflect new data concerning the impact of mosaic chromosomal abnormalities [38].

Some studies have suggested that mosaicism affects more than 20% of blastocyst stage embryos. However, recent research has indicated that the true rate may be much lower [39]. Errors in the classification of embryos can occur due to suboptimal PGT-A methods, or as a result of problems such as DNA contamination, which can cause fully aneuploid embryos to appear mosaic. For this reason, it is important to use well-validated methods, shown to be highly accurate and capable of detecting DNA contamination when it occurs [39]. Furthermore, it should be demonstrated that embryos classified as "aneuploid" have little or no chance of producing a child. Surprisingly, very few of the commercially available PGT-A methods have been subjected to this important level of validation [29].

13.5 Conclusion

Preimplantation genetics is a rapidly evolving field that has succeeded in helping many patients and

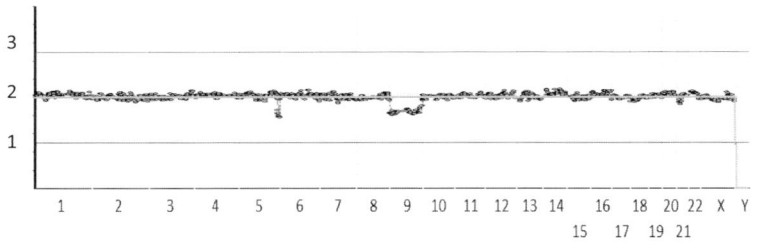

Figure 13.4 NGS result from an embryo biopsy specimen

For NGS analysis of chromosome abnormalities, the genome is divided into segments, referred to as "bins." Analysis focuses on determining the proportion of the total sequence "reads" aligning within each bin. After comparing the results to those obtained from chromosomally normal "reference" samples, it is possible to deduce how much of the embryo DNA was derived from each area of the genome. Each data point in the figure represents a result from one bin, arranged in their respective order along the length of each chromosome. The y-axis indicates the predicted copy number of each chromosome. In this case, an intermediate value, falling midway between 1 and 2 copies, is shown for chromosome 9 and also for a small segment at the end of the long arm of chromosome 5. This result is interpreted as meaning that the TE biopsy specimen was mosaic, likely containing a mixture of euploid cells and cells monosomic for chromosome 9 and with a segmental loss on chromosome 5q.

Table 13.3. Studies examining the developmental potential of mosaic embryos

Study	Implantation rate after mosaic embryo transfer	Ongoing pregnancy rate after mosaic embryo transfer	Implantation rate after euploid embryo transfer	Ongoing pregnancy/live birth rate after euploid embryo transfer
Greco et al., 2015	44%	33%	-	-
Fragouli et al., 2017	30%	15%	56%	46%
Munné et al., 2017	53%	41%	71%	63%
Spinella et al., 2018	38%	30%	54%	46%
Victor et al., 2019	38%	30%	50%	47%
Munné et al., 2019	49%	37%	83%	77%
Viotti et al., 2021	47%	37%	57%	52%
Capalbo et al., 2021	55–56%*	42–43%*	56%	43%

Note: *Embryos having results consistent with low levels of aneuploid cells in the ranges 20–30% and 30–50% were transferred. Embryos with apparent mosaicism involving higher levels of aneuploid cells (>50% in the biopsy specimen) were not transferred in this study.

holds much promise for the future. Innovations in the delivery of PGT-M have led to accurate tests, involving the simultaneous analysis of multiple informative sites in the genome in order to boost reliability. Modern methods typically require less patient-specific customization than early PGT-M strategies, shortening waiting times. Additionally, it is now common to detect aneuploidy and certain other incidental genetic abnormalities of relevance to health and embryo viability at the same time as performing PGT-M, potentially improving treatment outcomes. While most disorders assessed using PGT-M are similar to those that have traditionally been subject to prenatal testing, there is a relative increase in the proportion of late onset and incomplete penetrance disorders tested at the preimplantation stage of development. More controversially, PGT-M technology has also been applied to determine whether healthy embryos are HLA-compatible with seriously ill siblings in need of stem cell transplantation to cure their condition [40]. Stem cells can be harvested from the umbilical cord of the resulting children at birth and provided to the affected sibling. Recently, preimplantation testing has also been applied to polygenic disorders, generating relative risk scores for certain

conditions rather than a more definitive diagnosis [41]. It is not yet clear whether this latest expansion of PGT-M has significant clinical value or whether it complicates an already challenging process with relatively little gain. With the cost of DNA sequencing continuing to decline, and methods applicable to single cells being developed, the analysis of entire embryo genomes may soon become a viable prospect. Whether this is desirable, given ethical concerns over the use of the data produced, clinical problems interpreting the information, and difficulties counseling patients, remains a subject of debate.

Despite the fact that PGT-A has been used clinically for almost 30 years, its efficacy remains controversial. It seems obvious that patients having PGT-A will benefit from reduced risks of Down syndrome birth, aneuploid pregnancy, and miscarriage, but unfortunately most studies have not been adequately powered to provide conclusive proof. Although several RCTs have demonstrated improvements in pregnancy rate per embryo transfer, and in some cases increased live birth rates, debate over the value of PGT-A continues. It is therefore of the utmost importance that more well-designed RCTs are performed. Given the potential impact of embryo biopsy and the challenges of analyzing the small number of cells in a TE biopsy specimen, such studies should only be carried out by well-trained embryologists, in collaboration with experienced genetics laboratories, using highly validated methods. Of course, this also means that the findings will only be applicable in situations where a similar array of skills can be deployed, however, it is naive to think that a high-complexity procedure such as PGT-A can fulfil its potential without rigorous optimization and attention to detail. Noninvasive methods of PGT-A (niPGT-A), focusing on analysis of embryonic DNA found in the culture medium or blastocoel cavity, may allow the embryo sampling procedure to be "deskilled" and should, theoretically, have no impact on the embryo [42]. However, to date the reported niPGT-A methods fail to give a result from ~10% of samples and are associated with high false positive and false negative rates. For PGT-A results to be managed appropriately, a full understanding of the mosaicism phenomenon is also urgently needed. In particular, information concerning the degree to which mosaic embryos can normalize – ejecting, arresting, or destroying aneuploid cells – is currently missing. It seems likely that most embryos classified as mosaic are potentially viable, are highly unlikely to produce an abnormal pregnancy, and should not therefore be excluded from transfer.

Key Messages

- Preimplantation genetic testing is a well-established and valuable reproductive option for patients at high risk of transmitting an inherited disorder.
- Using modern PGT-M methods, such as trophectoderm biopsy combined with analysis of multiple relevant genomic sites (e.g. mutation sites and linked polymorphisms) test accuracies frequently exceed 99%.
- It is widely accepted that PGT-A is likely to reduce risks of aneuploid syndromes and miscarriage. Furthermore, embryos classified "euploid" or "normal" using PGT-A appear to have better than average chances of producing a viable pregnancy. Nonetheless, the clinical efficacy of PGT-A remains the subject of debate.
- Some PGT-A methods are superior to others in terms of accuracy, adding to confusion in the literature with respect to the efficacy of the method. Given the difference in the performance of PGT-A methods, generalizations about the clinical value of PGT-A are not appropriate.
- It is important to carry out nonselection studies to confirm that viable embryos are not erroneously excluded from transfer after PGT-A. At the time of writing, few PGT-A providers have conducted such a study.
- PGT was initially used for the avoidance of the same sort of genetic conditions for which prenatal testing is routinely employed. Today, a growing number of disorders of late onset are also tested at the preimplantation stage, as well as conditions with incomplete penetrance. Furthermore, PGT has been used to identify tissue matched embryos capable of providing stem cells for seriously ill siblings and, controversially, for the evaluation of polygenic disease risk.

References

1. Delhanty JD, Harper JC, Ao A, Handyside AH, Winston RM. Multicolour FISH detects frequent chromosomal mosaicism and chaotic division in normal preimplantation embryos from fertile patients. *Hum Genet.* 1997;99:755–60.

2. Wells D, Delhanty JD. Comprehensive chromosomal analysis of human preimplantation embryos using whole genome amplification and single cell comparative genomic hybridization. *Mol Hum Reprod.* 2000;6:1055–62.

3. Munné S, Lee A, Rosenwaks Z, Grifo J, Cohen J. Diagnosis of major chromosome aneuploidies in human preimplantation embryos. *Hum Reprod.* 1993;8:2185–91.

4. Gutierrez-Mateo C, Sánchez-García JF, Fischer J, Tormasi S, Cohen J, Munné S, Wells D. Preimplantation genetic diagnosis of single-gene disorders: experience with more than 200 cycles conducted by a reference laboratory in the United States. *Fertil Steril.* 2009;5:1544–56.

5. Handyside AH, Kontogianni EH, Hardy K, Winston RM. Pregnancies from biopsied human preimplantation embryos sexed by Y-specific DNA amplification. *Nature.* 1990;344:768–70.

6. Sermon K, Lissens W, Nagy ZP, Van Steirteghem A, Liebaers I. Simultaneous amplification of the two most frequent mutations of infantile Tay-Sachs disease in

single blastomeres. *Hum Reprod.* 1995;10:2214–17.

7. Findlay I, Urquhart A, Quirke P, Sullivan K, Rutherford AJ, Lilford RJ. Simultaneous DNA 'fingerprinting', diagnosis of sex and single-gene defect status from single cells. *Hum Reprod.* 1995;10:1005–13.

8. Piyamongkol W, Harper JC, Delhanty JD, Wells D. PGD protocols using multiplex fluorescent PCR. *Reprod Biomed Online.* 2001;2:212–14.

9. Tracey M. Short tandem repeat-based identification of individuals and parents. *Croat Med J.* 2001;42:233–8.

10. Natesan SA, Bladon AJ, Coskun S, Qubbaj W, Prates R, Munné S, et al. Genome-wide karyomapping accurately identifies the inheritance of single-gene defects in human preimplantation embryos in vitro. *Genet Med.* 2014;16:838–45.

11. Konstantinidis M, Prates R, Goodall NN, Fischer J, Tecson V, Lemma T, et al. Live births following karyomapping of human blastocysts: experience from clinical application of the method. *Reprod Biomed Online.* 2015;3:394–403.

12. Ben-Nagi J, Wells D, Doye K, Loutradi K, Exeter H, Drew E, et al. Karyomapping: a single centre's experience from application of methodology to ongoing pregnancy and live-birth rates. *Reprod Biomed Online.* 2017;35:264–71.

13. Masset H, Zamani Esteki M, Dimitriadou E, Dreesen J, Debrock S, Derhaag J, et al. Multi-centre evaluation of a comprehensive preimplantation genetic test through haplotyping-by-sequencing. *Hum Reprod.* 2019;34:1608–19.

14. Munné S, Sandalinas M, Escudero T, Fung J, Gianaroli L, Cohen J. Outcome of preimplantation genetic diagnosis of

translocations. *Fertil Steril.* 2000;73:1209–18.

15. Fragouli E, Alfarawati S, Spath K, Jaroudi S, Sarasa J, Enciso M, Wells D. The origin and impact of embryonic aneuploidy. *Hum Genet.* 2013;132:1001–13.

16. Alfarawati S, Fragouli E, Colls P, Wells D. First births after preimplantation genetic diagnosis of structural chromosome abnormalities using comparative genomic hybridization and microarray analysis. *Hum Reprod.* 2011;26:1560–74.

17. Wells D, Kaur K, Grifo J, Glassner M, Taylor JC, Fragouli E, Munné S. Clinical utilization of a rapid low-pass whole genome sequencing technique for the diagnosis of aneuploidy in human embryos prior to implantation. *J Med Genet.* 2014;51:553–62.

18. Fragouli E, Alfarawati S, Spath K, Tarozzi N, Borini A, Wells D. Analysis of implantation and ongoing pregnancy rates following the transfer of mosaic diploid-aneuploid blastocysts. *Hum Genet.* 2017;136:805–19.

19. Zimmerman RS, Tao X, Marin D, Werner MD, Hong KH, Lonczak A, et al. Preclinical validation of a targeted next generation sequencing-based comprehensive chromosome screening methodology in human blastocysts. *Mol Hum Reprod.* 2018;24:37–45.

20. Idowu D, Merrion K, Wemmer N, Mash JG, Pettersen B, Kijacic D, Lathi RB. Pregnancy outcomes following 24-chromosome preimplantation genetic diagnosis in couples with balanced reciprocal or Robertsonian translocations. *Fertil Steril.* 2015;103:1037–42.

21. Tobler KJ, Brezina PR, Benner AT, Du L, Xu X, Kearns WG. Two different microarray technologies for preimplantation genetic diagnosis and screening, due to reciprocal translocation

imbalances, demonstrate equivalent euploidy and clinical pregnancy rates. *J Assist Reprod Genet.* 2014;31:843–50.

22. Mastenbroek S, Twisk M, Veen F, van der Repping S. Preimplantation genetic screening: a systematic review and meta-analysis of RCTs. *Hum Reprod Update.* 2011;17:454–66.

23. Wells D, Delhanty JD. Comprehensive chromosomal analysis of human preimplantation embryos using whole genome amplification and single cell comparative genomic hybridization. *Mol Hum Reprod.* 2000;6:1055–62.

24. Scott RT, Upham KM, Forman EJ, Zhao T, Treff NR. Cleavage-stage biopsy significantly impairs human embryonic implantation potential while blastocyst biopsy does not: a randomized and paired clinical trial. *Fertil Steril.* 2013;100:624–30.

25. Fragouli E, Lenzi M, Ross R, Katz-Jaffe M, Schoolcraft WB, Wells D. Comprehensive molecular cytogenetic analysis of the human blastocyst stage. *Hum Reprod.* 2008;23:2596–608.

26. Dahdouh EM, Balayla J, García-Velasco JA. Comprehensive chromosome screening improves embryo selection: a metaanalysis. *Fertil Steril.* 2015;104:1503–12.

27. Munné S, Kaplan B, Frattarelli J, Gysler M, Child T, Nakhuda G, et al. Global multicenter randomized controlled trial comparing single embryo transfer with embryo selected by preimplantation genetic screening using next-generation sequencing versus morphologic assessment. *Fert Steril.* 2017;108:e19.

28. Verpoest W, Staessen C, Bossuyt PM, Goossens V, Altarescu G, Bonduelle M, et al. Preimplantation genetic testing for aneuploidy by microarray analysis of polar bodies in advanced maternal age: a

147

randomized clinical trial. *Hum Reprod.* 2018;33:1767–76.

29. Tiegs AW, Tao X, Zhan Y, Whitehead C, Kim J, Hanson B, et al. A multicenter, prospective, blinded, nonselection study evaluating the predictive value of an aneuploid diagnosis using a targeted next-generation sequencing-based preimplantation genetic testing for aneuploidy assay and impact of biopsy. *Fertil Steril.* 2021;115:627–37.

30. Greco E, Minasi MG, Fiorentino F. Healthy babies after intrauterine transfer of mosaic aneuploid blastocysts. *N Engl J Med.* 2015;373:2089–90.

31. Fragouli E, Alfarawati S, Spath K, Tarozzi N, Borini A, Wells D. Analysis of implantation and ongoing pregnancy rates following the transfer of mosaic diploid-aneuploid blastocysts. *Hum Genet.* 2017;136:805–19.

32. Munné S, Blazek J, Large M, Martinez-Ortiz PA, Nisson H, Liu E, et al. Detailed investigation into the cytogenetic constitution and pregnancy outcome of replacing mosaic blastocysts detected with the use of high-resolution next-generation sequencing. *Fertil Steril.* 2017;108:62–71.

33. Spinella F, Fiorentino F, Biricik A, Bono S, Ruberti A, Cotroneo E, et al. Extent of chromosomal mosaicism influences the clinical outcome of in vitro fertilization treatments. *Fertil Steril.* 2018;109:77–83.

34. Munné S, Spinella F, Grifo J, Zhang J, Beltran MP, Fragouli E, Fiorentino F. Clinical outcomes after the transfer of blastocysts characterized as mosaic by high resolution Next Generation Sequencing – further insights. *Eur J Med Genet.* 2019;21:103741.

35. Victor AR, Griffin DK, Brake AJ, Tyndall JC, Murphy AE, Lepkowsky LT, et al. Assessment of aneuploidy concordance between clinical trophectoderm biopsy and blastocyst. *Hum Rep.* 2019;34:181–92.

36. Viotti M, Victor AR, Barnes FL, Zouves CG, Besser AG, Grifo JA, et al.. Using outcome data from one thousand mosaic embryo transfers to formulate an embryo ranking system for clinical use. *Fertil Steril.* 2021;115:1212–24.

37. Capalbo A, Poli M, Rienzi L, Girardi L, Patassini C, Fabiani M, et al. Mosaic human preimplantation embryos and their developmental potential in a prospective, non-selection clinical trial. *Am J Hum Genet.* 2021;108:2238–47.

38. Leigh D, Cram DS, Rechitsky L, Handyside A, Wells D, Munne S, et al. PGDIS position statement on the transfer of mosaic embryos 2021. *Reprod Biomed Online.* 2022;S1472–S6483.

39. Kim J, Tao X, Cheng M, Steward A, Guo V, Zhan Y, et al. The concordance rates of an initial trophectoderm biopsy with the rest of the embryo using PGTseq, a targeted next-generation sequencing platform for preimplantation genetic testing-aneuploidy, *Fertil Steril.* 2022;117:315–23.

40. Verlinsky Y, Rechitsky S, Sharapova T, Morris R, Taranissi M, Kuliev A. Preimplantation HLA testing. *JAMA.* 2004;291:2079–85.

41. Treff NR, Zimmerman R, Bechor E, Hsu J, Rana B, Jensen J, et al. Validation of concurrent preimplantation genetic testing for polygenic and monogenic disorders, structural rearrangements, and whole and segmental chromosome aneuploidy with a single universal platform. *Eur J Med Genet.* 2019;62:103647.

42. Leaver M, Wells D. Non-invasive preimplantation genetic testing (niPGT): the next revolution in reproductive genetics? *Hum Reprod Update.* 2020;26:16–42.

Biopsy Techniques from Polar Body to Blastocyst

Danilo Cimadomo, Nicoletta Barnocchi, Letizia Papini, Federica Innocenti, Filippo Maria Ubaldi, and Laura Rienzi

14.1 Introduction

Preimplantation genetic testing (PGT) is adopted in modern IVF to test human embryos for monogenic diseases (PGT-M), structural rearrangements (PGT-SR), and aneuploidies (PGT-A). Across the years from its first clinical application [1], different molecular diagnostic techniques, several stages of embryo preimplantation development, and different protocols have been investigated in order to identify a gold standard approach. Blastomere biopsy at the cleavage stage has represented the most prevalent approach for several years, and it is still widely used nowadays despite the evidence of its possible impact on embryo reproductive potential [2]. At present, instead, mainly trophectoderm (TE) biopsy at the blastocyst stage is conducted, which has been demonstrated as reproducible across different operators [3], as well as safer and more accurate than blastomere biopsy for PGT [2, 4], possibly due to a higher number of cells sampled (5–15 rather than a single cell) from a nonembryonic section of the embryo (the TE gives origin to the embryonic annexes, while the inner cell mass is kept intact). Clearly, implementing TE-based PGT in an IVF clinic requires high expertise at every stage of the treatment from intracytoplasmic sperm injection (ICSI), via extended embryo culture, up to vitrification and warming, as well as a thoughtful patients' counseling.

Three TE biopsy protocols have been described across the years: (a) the first pioneering protocol, which entails zona pellucida (ZP) opening in day 5–6 whenever the blastocyst reaches full expansion [5] (Video 14.1); (b) the most widely used protocol, which is known as the "day 3 ZP opening-based TE biopsy" approach [6, 7] (Video 14.2); (c) and the latest protocol, which does not involve any assisted hatching and has been named the "day 5–7 sequential ZP opening and TE fragment retrieval" approach [8] (Video 14.3).

ZP opening might be conducted through a mechanical protocol, an acidified Tyrode's solution-mediated one, or a laser-assisted one, the latter of which is the most user-friendly, the fastest, and therefore the most widely used one. Two methods are instead available for TE fragment final cutting: the "pulling" method and the "flicking" method (Figure 14.1).

In parallel to both blastomere and TE biopsy, the polar body (PB) biopsy approach has been proposed as an alternative option to embryo biopsy for PGT [9, 10]. Such an approach is still currently used in those counties where embryo biopsy is restricted (e.g. Austria). However, PB biopsy is now rarely used in countries that permit this approach (<3% cycles) because it involves a higher workload, and is limited to the investigation of maternal meiotic errors.

In this chapter, we briefly describe the different biopsy techniques, and then focus on TE biopsy. Some tips and troubleshooting will be provided, along with advice for an efficient and safe implementation of PGT in the workflow of an IVF clinic.

14.2 Considerations for an IVF Clinic Implementing PGT

A successful treatment requires an efficient interaction between embryologists, molecular biologists, and clinicians. All the different professional figures involved in this process must be aware of the whole process and its possible pitfalls, pivotal to guide the couples through the cycle and provide them with suitable counseling.

When choosing the biopsy approach among PBs, blastomere, and TE, it is advisable to ponder safety, validation, reproducibility, reliability, efficiency, and workload. TE biopsy when combined with comprehensive chromosome testing (CCT) techniques (quantitative polymerase chain reaction, array comparative genomic hybridization, array single nucleotide

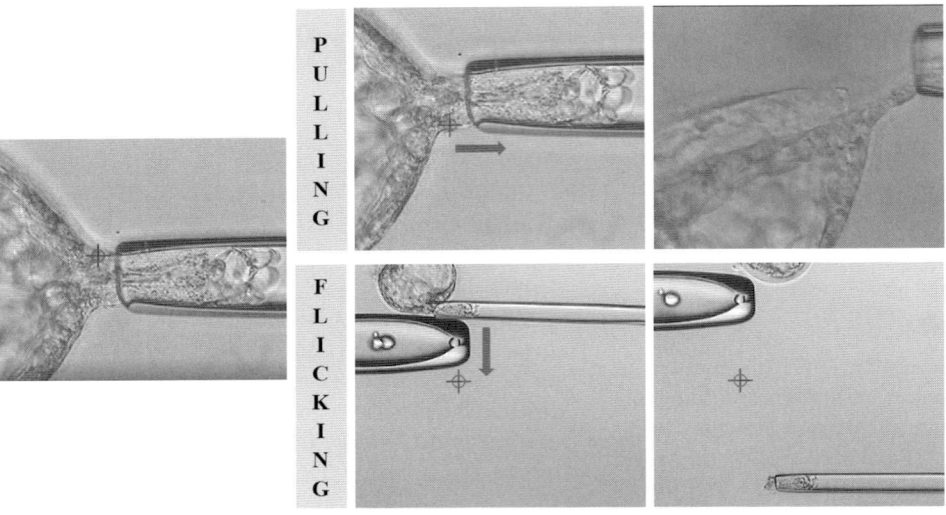

Figure 14.1 The pulling and flicking methods to remove a fragment of the trophectoderm during blastocyst biopsy

polymorphisms, next-generation sequencing) in the PGT workflow, involves (a) the highest predictive power upon euploid embryos' implantation potential [2], (b) the lowest prevalence (~5%) of euploid-aneuploid chromosomal mosaicism (i.e. the presence of cells with different karyotypes within the same embryo) [11], (c) an almost total concordance with the inner cell mass (ICM) [12], (d) clinically relevant false negative error rates equal to 0.1–0.7% per delivery depending on the CCT technique adopted [13, 14], and (e) false positive error rates lower than 3–4% (provided that no diagnosis of mosaicism or of segmental aneuploidies is attempted on a single TE biopsy) [2, 15].

When implementing a TE biopsy approach, particular attention should be given to culture media formulation, incubators, and air quality, aiming at a reduced manipulation of the gametes and embryos. For instance, the use of a continuous culture media and of a time-lapse incubator, although not involving better clinical outcomes per se, might result in a lower number of exposures of the embryos to suboptimal culture conditions as well as a lower workload. In general, low oxygen incubators should be adopted, ICSI may be the elective method for oocyte insemination so to minimize the risk for cumulus cells or sperm DNA contamination, and the vitrification protocol should be used for biopsied embryos' cryopreservation. The results (e.g. fertilization, cleavage, blastocyst, and survival after warming rates) must be constantly monitored and fulfil the competency or

(even better) the benchmark key performance indicators (KPIs) set by scientific societies like the ESHRE (e.g. Vienna consensus [16]).

When it comes to the biopsy and the vitrification procedure, the operators should undergo a supervised practicing and training period [17], and, after being qualified to their clinical application, each embryologist should be monitored for their performance in terms of mean duration of the biopsy procedure, inconclusive diagnosis rate, survival rate after warming, as well as live birth rate [18, 19]. Of note, the number of TE cells retrieved from different operators is comparable, although such a number should be kept roughly below 15, not to impair euploid blastocysts' reproductive competence [20].

An efficient traceability is also crucial for the management of a PGT cycle. In this regard, a failure modes and effect analysis represents a suitable scheme to identify the most dangerous steps along the workflow and adopt effective witnessing and corrective measures [21].

To minimize the risk for exogenous DNA contamination, it is mandatory to use DNA-free materials at any step of the biopsy protocol (from the preparation of the dishes to the tubing) and avoid the use of devices and solutions potentially toxic to the embryo. The tubing procedure must be performed under a laminar flow hood at room temperature, and particular care should be invested also in this step to avoid a DNA amplification failure [19]. Biopsy samples must be stored at −20°C until shipment or analysis in the genetic laboratory.

14.3 Zona Pellucida Opening

In previous years, several approaches have been adopted for the ZP opening procedure in oocytes and embryos (i.e. mechanical dissection, chemical drilling, laser ablation).

The first blastomere biopsy technique was performed using three pipettes: one to hold the embryo, another to drill the ZP with the acidified Tyrode's solution, and the third to aspirate the blastomere [1]. Since then, several other procedures have been developed to conduct ZP opening. The ideal approach should be simple, efficient, and minimize changes in oocyte or embryo microenvironment (i.e. pH and temperature).

14.3.1 Acidified Tyrode's Solution Opening

In 1998, the three-pipettes approach was replaced with the two-pipettes approach developed by Chen and colleagues [22]. In this simplified protocol, the ZP drilling and embryo biopsy procedures were performed through a single larger pipette filled with a small amount of acidified Tyrode's solution. This solution is expelled until a hole is produced in the ZP and then sucked back before removing the selected blastomere with the same pipette. Throughout the following years, the two-pipettes approach was confirmed a valid alternative for blastomere biopsy, due to its simplicity and the short time required for the procedure.

14.3.2 Mechanical Opening

The mechanical ZP opening is conducted through a glass partial zona dissection (PZD) microneedle, which is inserted through the ZP, tangentially to the oocytes/embryos. The continuous rubbing between the PZD microneedle and the holding pipette allows the formation of a slit in the ZP [23, 24]. This method was considered reliable and safer than chemical digestion.

14.3.3 Laser-Assisted Opening

In 1995, Germond and colleagues adopted a diode-laser system for PB biopsy, to perform a microdissection of the ZP of mouse and human oocytes and zygotes [25]. The same year, Licciardi and colleagues adopted it instead for the ablation of mouse ZP aimed at blastomere biopsy [26]. Conventionally, a single laser irradiation is sufficient to create a hole, but a proper irradiation time is necessary to allow the insertion of the biopsy pipette through the hole to conduct the biopsy. Currently, a noncontact diode laser is adopted to drill the ZP and create a single 14–18 μm hole, and normally a 1.2–1.6 mJ irradiation is adopted (12–16 ms of irradiation time) [27]. This ZP opening approach is less time-consuming and easier than the former ones, and it is therefore the preferred protocol. Of note, the correct laser target alignment should be verified before each biopsy procedure. If the laser position appears inaccurate, immediately recalibrate it. The entire system should be routinely serviced at least every six months to check that all optical elements are properly cleaned and proper calibration is assured.

14.4 Polar Body Biopsy

This approach is based on the idea that PBs are waste products of female meiosis; they are not required for fertilization and do not represent embryonic cells, therefore might suit a minimally invasive genetic testing. Secondly, chromosomal mosaicism does not represent an issue at this stage. Lastly, an embryo developing from an oocyte whose PB analysis highlighted a normal gene would be transferred in the same cycle, and no cryopreservation is needed.

The genotype of the 1st PB (PB1) mirrors exactly that of its corresponding oocyte; however, due to recombination, the analysis of PB1 might not allow an accurate diagnosis. Similarly, the aneuploidies deriving from the second meiotic division cannot be detected by analyzing only the PB1, and both PBs are needed. This drawback makes this biopsy approach time-consuming and expensive. Yet, the ESHRE has recently published a randomized controlled trial based on the array-CGH analysis of both PBs versus the standard care in about 200 patients per arm. Interestingly, no difference was reported in the cumulative live birth rate per couple, but such an outcome was achieved with fewer embryo transfers, fewer cryopreserved embryos, and a lower miscarriage rate per clinical pregnancy [28]. In other terms, although PBs-based PGT-A excludes paternal meiotic and postzygotic mitotic errors from the analysis, the selection against maternal meiotic missegregations is sufficient to elicit a higher efficiency after IVF.

PB biopsy might be conducted through a sequential approach on day 0 (from the oocyte) and day 1 (from the zygote), or through a simultaneous approach at 6–9 hours after ICSI. In the latter case, PB1 and PB2 should be distinguished based on their morphology (i.e. PB2 is smaller and regular in shape and it is also connected to the oocyte with a cytoplasmic strand, while PB1 could be dislocated in the perivitelline space) [29].

ZP opening should be better conducted mechanically or through the laser, since the acidified Tyrode's solution is not well tolerated by the oocyte and may interfere with further embryo development [30, 31].

14.5 Blastomere Biopsy

Blastomere biopsy is conducted at day 3 of embryo development, when the 6- to 10-cells cleavage stage is reached. Across the years from its very first experience [1], the protocol has been improved through (a) the introduction of a two-pipettes system [22], (b) the introduction of the $Ca^{[2]+}$-$Mg^{[2]+}$ free medium to decompact the embryo [32], and (c) the introduction of the laser to drill the ZP [33].

Of note, after ZP opening, the blastomere can be removed via either aspiration or displacement, as described by Wang and colleagues in 2009 [34]. Although blastomere aspiration is traditionally performed, it might be tricky not to lyse the cell during the procedure and the embryo might be severely damaged if more than one cell is aspirated. Blastomere displacement is indeed a valuable alternative since the blastomere is simply forced to pop out from the opening in the ZP by expelling some media through the hole or by exerting some pressure onto the embryo.

Blastomere biopsy is fast and compatible with fresh ET, and it has been reported efficient in high-standards IVF clinics when associated with array-CGH to conduct PGT-A in advanced maternal age women [35]. However, (a) blastomere biopsy might be detrimental toward embryo reproductive competence [2], especially when two blastomeres are retrieved; (b) cryopreservation is still required for all surplus embryos; (c) mosaicism reaches its highest prevalence at this stage of preimplantation development, and (d) single-cell analysis is still not as efficient

as multiple TE cells analysis. All these reasons undermine the clinical efficiency of such an approach.

14.6 Trophectoderm Biopsy

14.6.1 Blastocyst Selection and Grading

Embryos can reach the blastocyst stage any time from day 5 to 7 of preimplantation development. Blastocysts can mature in an asynchronous fashion and with heterogeneous morphology. Any blastocyst classification scheme in IVF is adapted from Gardner and Schoolcraft's parameters scoring expansion, ICM and TE morphology (Figure 14.2).

The ideal grade to conduct TE biopsy is represented by a fully expanded blastocyst with a visible and compact ICM and several well-organized small TE cells. Nevertheless, in view of the low correlation between the aneuploidy rate and blastocyst morphological evaluation [8], any kind of blastocyst should be biopsied regardless of its quality.

14.6.2 Workflow of the Different Blastocyst Biopsy Protocols

Three blastocyst biopsy approaches have been described to date that are still currently used: the first one published by Veiga and colleagues in 1997 [5], the mostly used approach described in 2004 by de Boer and colleagues [6], and the latest one described by Capalbo and colleagues in 2014 [8].

14.6.2.1 Day 5–6 ZP Opening-Based Trophectoderm Biopsy Protocol

Laser-assisted ZP drilling is performed far from the ICM whenever the blastocyst reaches full expansion. During further culture in the incubator, the natural expansion of the blastocyst elicits TE hatching. Only then is the biopsy fragment finally removed by targeting the junctions between the TE cells with the laser and applying a gentle suction (Video 14.1).

14.6.2.2 Day 3 ZP Opening-Based Trophectoderm Biopsy Protocol

This protocol was described in two papers published in 2004 and 2005 [6, 7]. The embryo is removed from the incubator to open the ZP at the cleavage stage of preimplantation development. The embryo is then cultured to the blastocyst stage and when it starts

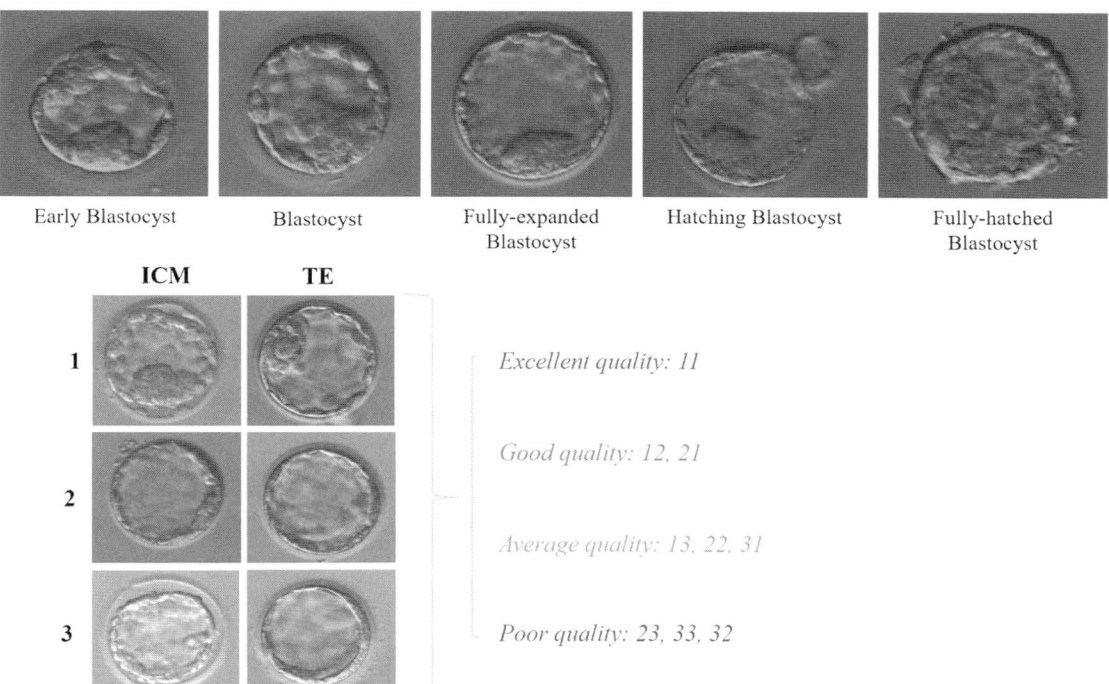

Figure 14.2 The conventional scheme for blastocyst morphological evaluation

expanding some TE cells will hatch from the opening in the ZP. By gentle suction and a few laser pulses targeted to the junctions between TE cells, a few cells are then removed from the blastocyst (Video 14.2). Hopefully the hatched part of the embryo does not involve the ICM, otherwise the biopsy procedure is more difficult. In fact, another hole in the ZP should be produced to retrieve some TE cells opposite to the ICM (as shown in Figure 14.3).

14.6.2.3 Sequential ZP Opening and Trophectoderm Biopsy Protocol

The latest described protocol does not involve any assisted hatching [8]. The operator orients the blastocyst before the procedure so that the ICM is kept as far as possible from the target TE cells. Once the ZP is opened, it is necessary to detach the blastocyst from its inner surface by blowing some media through the hole. Only then does the operator penetrate the ZP and suck the selected cells into the biopsy pipette. Finally, by alternating laser shots directed at the junctions

between the TE fragment and the body of the embryo and gentle suction the fragment is removed (i.e. pulling method; Video 14.3; Figure 14.1).

14.6.2.4 Alternative Method to Remove the Biopsy Fragment: The Flicking Method

Alternatively to the pulling method, the flicking method can be adopted to remove the biopsy fragment. Specifically, after loosening the bonds between the selected TE fragment and the body of the blastocyst with a few laser shots the embryo is released from the holding pipette and positioned on top of it. A quick downward movement of the biopsy pipette containing the selected TE cells is then sufficient to finalize the biopsy (Figure 14.1).

14.6.3 The Focus Issue and the Optimal Blastocyst Orientation

When a TE biopsy is conducted, the most important issue is ensuring that the blastocyst, the ZP opening,

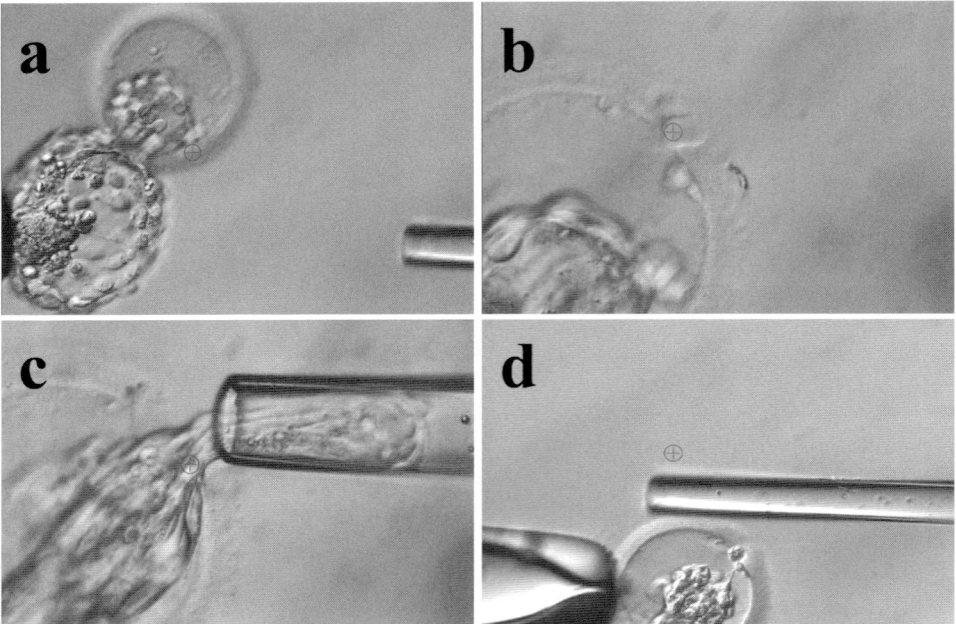

Figure 14.3 Biopsy of an embryo hatching from the inner cell mass after a laser-assisted zona opening at the cleavage stage
a) embryo before the biopsy; b) ZP opening on the opposite side of the former hole; c) the selected trophectoderm cells are sucked into the biopsy pipette and cut with a few laser shots; d) the biopsy is finalized.

and the biopsy pipette are on the same focal plane as the laser objective. Video 14.4 is an example of an operator struggling for this issue. At 20x magnification, secure the embryo to the holding pipette and position it at the bottom of the biopsy dish, orient the blastocyst so that the ICM is visualized at 7 o'clock, focus on the ZP, and move the biopsy pipette on this same focal plane (i.e. the edges of the pipette are dark and the pipette itself is in focus). Only then, switch to the laser objective (pulse time 0.3 ms, 6.5 μm) and position the pointer on the ZP opposite to the ICM.

14.6.4 The Quality of the Retrieved Trophectoderm Fragment

The quality of the biopsy fragments is crucial for the reliability of the molecular analysis downstream. The embryologists should try to retrieve 5–10 cells. However, it is difficult to quantify the exact cellularity at the time of biopsy. Therefore, the evaluation mainly relies on the quality of the fragments (always keep a picture of them). Figure 14.4 shows examples of a desirable, a small, a lysed, and a degenerated fragment at 20x magnification. Neal and colleagues

recently reported that in a range of 1–20 TE cells, only when more than 15 cells are biopsied, might euploid blastocysts suffer a decrease in their reproductive competence [20]. Similarly, inconclusive genetic results are more likely to arise from small biopsy fragments, due to a poor DNA template. Ideally 7–8 TE cells should be retrieved to achieve good amplification with no impact on the embryo [19]. Of note, blastocyst quality does not associate with a conclusive result, while the day of the biopsy (day 6–7 better than day 5) and the experience of the IVF clinic do [19].

14.6.5 Trophectoderm Biopsy: Peculiar Cases and Troubleshooting

Several times the embryologists must face deviations from the ideal TE biopsy. Some peculiar biopsy cases are reported hereafter along with some issues that might be encountered during the procedure.

14.6.5.1 Fully Hatched Blastocyst

When the blastocyst is fully hatched from the ZP, it is important to pay more attention to the aspiration with the holding pipette to avoid harming the

Desirable   Small   Small and lysed   Degenerated

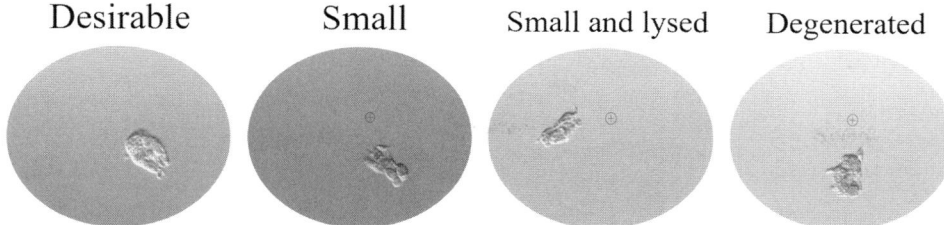

Figure 14.4 Examples of biopsy fragments

embryo, in particular the ICM. Then, by sucking the chosen TE cells into the biopsy pipette, the embryo will collapse and the biopsy procedure might be performed according to the standard protocol (Video 14.5). After the biopsy, blastocyst reexpansion should be prevented, especially since the vitrification procedure might be more stressing for the embryo in the absence of the ZP [18].

14.6.5.2 Poor-Quality Blastocyst

Poor-quality blastocysts (<BB according to Gardner and Schoolcraft's classification) require particular care while removing the biopsied fragment since the TE cells tend to be stickier than normal. The operator should insist on stretching the fragment and using more laser shots until its removal (Video 14.6). In the presence of excluded blastomeres or degenerated cells in the ZP, they should be avoided since their chromosomal content might not represent the ICM.

14.6.5.3 Troubleshooting

Sometimes the biopsied fragment might be lost in the mineral oil or accidentally sucked into a pipette. In the latter case, the biopsy operator should empty the pipette into the washing drop and check whether the biopsy fragment can be recovered. If not, a second biopsy must be taken. Of note, if the blastocyst is completely collapsed and the ICM cannot be distinguished, the operator must return the embryo to the incubator until reexpansion.

For tubing, it is recommended to change the tip of the stripping pipette in between consecutive tubing procedures or at least to thoroughly wash it and completely empty it. Before tubing the biopsy fragment, this must be sucked and released from the stripping pipette in a washing drop a couple of times

to mechanically remove any degenerated or lysed cell debris.

Key Messages

- Three approaches exist to retrieve a sample for PGT purposes: PB, blastomere, and TE biopsy.
- PB biopsy has several limitations, but it is the only feasible approach where embryo biopsy is restricted.
- Blastomere biopsy might impact embryo reproductive potential and suffers from the issues of chromosomal mosaicism and single-cell analysis.
- TE biopsy has not been shown to inhibit reproductive potential and is the gold standard approach at present.
- Three protocols exist to conduct TE biopsy, that seem equivalent in terms of diagnostic and clinical effectiveness.
- Fully expanded good-quality blastocysts (≥BB according to Gardner and Schoolcraft's classification) on day 5–7 postfertilization represent the ideal embryo for TE biopsy. Nevertheless, also fully hatched, in-hatching, and poor-quality blastocysts (<BB) might be biopsied.
- TE biopsy and CCT analysis represent an accurate, cost-effective, and clinically valuable workflow, whose main issue is represented by chromosomal mosaicism.
- Ensuring traceability during the entire biopsy and vitrification/warming procedures is of utmost importance.
- Reexpansion after biopsy and before vitrification should be prevented to improve blastocyst survival after warming.
- Seven-to-eight TE cells are ideal to achieve good DNA amplification outcomes with no impact on embryo reproductive competence.

References

1. Handyside AH, Kontogianni EH, Hardy K, Winston RM. Pregnancies from biopsied human preimplantation embryos sexed by Y-specific DNA amplification. *Nature*. 1990;344:768–70.

2. Scott RT, Jr., Upham KM, Forman EJ, Zhao T, Treff NR. Cleavage-stage biopsy significantly impairs human embryonic implantation potential while blastocyst biopsy does not: a randomized and paired clinical trial. *Fertil Steril*. 2013;100:624–30.

3. Capalbo A, Ubaldi FM, Cimadomo D, Maggiulli R, Patassini C, Dusi L, et al. Consistent and reproducible outcomes of blastocyst biopsy and aneuploidy screening across different biopsy practitioners: a multicentre study involving 2586 embryo biopsies. *Hum Reprod*. 2016;31:199–208.

4. Scott RT, Jr., Ferry K, Su J, Tao X, Scott K, Treff NR. Comprehensive chromosome screening is highly predictive of the reproductive potential of human embryos: a prospective, blinded, nonselection study. *Fertil Steril*. 2012;97:870–5.

5. Veiga A, Sandalinas M, Benkhalifa M, Boada M, Carrera M, Santalo J, et al. Laser blastocyst biopsy for preimplantation diagnosis in the human. *Zygote*. 1997;5:351–4.

6. de Boer KA, Catt JW, Jansen RP, Leigh D, McArthur S. Moving to blastocyst biopsy for preimplantation genetic diagnosis and single embryo transfer at Sydney IVF. *Fertil Steril*. 2004;82:295–8.

7. McArthur SJ, Leigh D, Marshall JT, de Boer KA, Jansen RP. Pregnancies and live births after trophectoderm biopsy and preimplantation genetic testing of human blastocysts. *Fertil Steril*. 2005;84:1628–36.

8. Capalbo A, Rienzi L, Cimadomo D, Maggiulli R, Elliott T, Wright G, et al. Correlation between standard blastocyst morphology, euploidy and implantation: an observational study in two centers involving 956 screened blastocysts. *Hum Reprod*. 2014;29:1173–81.

9. Verlinsky Y, Cieslak J, Ivakhnenko V, Evsikov S, Wolf G, White M, et al. Preimplantation diagnosis of common aneuploidies by the first- and second-polar body FISH analysis. *J Assist Reprod Genet*. 1998;15:285–9.

10. Verlinsky Y, Ginsberg N, Lifchez A, Valle J, Moise J, Strom CM. Analysis of the first polar body: preconception genetic diagnosis. *Hum Reprod*. 1990;5:826–9.

11. Capalbo A, Ubaldi FM, Rienzi L, Scott R, Treff N. Detecting mosaicism in trophectoderm biopsies: current challenges and future possibilities. *Hum Reprod*. 2016;32:492–8.

12. Capalbo A, Rienzi L. Mosaicism between trophectoderm and inner cell mass. *Fertil Steril*. 2017;107:1098–1106.

13. Werner MD, Leondires MP, Schoolcraft WB, Miller BT, Copperman AB, Robins ED, et al. Clinically recognizable error rate after the transfer of comprehensive chromosomal screened euploid embryos is low. *Fertil Steril*. 2014;102:1613–18.

14. Tiegs AW, Hodes-Wertz B, McCulloh DH, Munné S, Grifo JA. Discrepant diagnosis rate of array comparative genomic hybridization in thawed euploid blastocysts. *J Assist Reprod Genet*. 2016;33:893–7.

15. Tiegs AW, Tao X, Whitehead C, Neal SA, Osman EK, Kim J, et al. Does preimplantation genetic testing for aneuploidy (PGT-A) harm embryos? No – a multicenter, prospective, blinded, non-selection study evaluating the predictive value of an aneuploid diagnosis and impact of biopsy. *Fertil Steril*. 2019;115:627–37.

16. ESHRE Special Interest Group of Embryology and Alpha Scientists in Reproductive Medicine. The Vienna consensus: report of an expert meeting on the development of ART laboratory performance indicators. *Reprod Biomed Online*. 2017;35:494–510.

17. Kokkali G, Coticchio G, Bronet F, Celebi C, Cimadomo D, Goossens V, et al. ESHRE PGT Consortium and SIG Embryology good practice recommendations for polar body and embryo biopsy for PGT. *Hum Reprod Open*. 2020;3:hoaa020.

18. Cimadomo D, Capalbo A, Levi-Setti PE, Soscia D, Orlando G, Albani E, et al. Associations of blastocyst features, trophectoderm biopsy and other laboratory practice with post-warming behavior and implantation. *Hum Reprod*. 2018;33:1992–2001.

19. Cimadomo D, Rienzi L, Romanelli V, Alviggi E, Levi-Setti PE, Albani E, et al. Inconclusive chromosomal assessment after blastocyst biopsy: prevalence, causative factors and outcomes after re-biopsy and re-vitrification: A multicenter experience. *Hum Reprod*. 2018;33:1839–46.

20. Neal SA, Franasiak JM, Forman EJ, Werner MD, Morin SJ, Tao X, et al. High relative deoxyribonucleic acid content of trophectoderm biopsy adversely affects pregnancy outcomes. *Fertil Steril*. 2017;107:731–6.

21. Cimadomo D, Ubaldi FM, Capalbo A, Maggiulli R, Scarica C, Romano S, et al. Failure mode and effects analysis of witnessing protocols for ensuring traceability during PGD/PGS cycles. *Reprod Biomed Online*. 2016;33:360–9.

22. Chen SU, Chao KH, Wu MY, Chen CD, Ho HN, Yang YS. The simplified two-pipette technique is more efficient than the

conventional three-pipette method for blastomere biopsy in human embryos. *Fertil Steril.* 1998;69:569–75.

23. Magli MC, Ferraretti AP, Crippa A, Lappi M, Feliciani E, Gianaroli L. First meiosis errors in immature oocytes generated by stimulated cycles. *Fertil Steril.* 2006;86:629–35.

24. Cohen J, Malter H, Fehilly C, Wright G, Elsner C, Kort H, et al. Implantation of embryos after partial opening of oocyte zona pellucida to facilitate sperm penetration. *Lancet.* 1988;2:162.

25. Germond M, Nocera D, Senn A, Rink K, Delacretaz G, Fakan S. Microdissection of mouse and human zona pellucida using a 1.48-microns diode laser beam: efficacy and safety of the procedure. *Fertil Steril.* 1995;64:604–11.

26. Licciardi F, Gonzalez A, Tang YX, Grifo J, Cohen J, Neev Y. Laser ablation of the mouse zona pellucida for blastomere biopsy. *J Assist Reprod Genet.* 1995;12:462–6.

27. Montag M, van der Ven K, Delacretaz G, Rink K, van der Ven H. Laser-assisted microdissection of the zona pellucida facilitates polar body biopsy. *Fertil Steril.* 1998;69:539–42.

28. Verpoest W, Staessen C, Bossuyt PM, Goossens V, Altarescu G, Bonduelle M, et al. Preimplantation genetic testing for aneuploidy by microarray analysis of polar bodies in advanced maternal age: a randomized clinical trial. *Hum Reprod.* 2018;33:1767–76.

29. Magli MC, Montag M, Koster M, Muzi L, Geraedts J, Collins J, et al. Polar body array CGH for prediction of the status of the corresponding oocyte. Part II: technical aspects. *Hum Reprod.* 2011;26:3181–5.

30. Montag M, Koster M, Strowitzki T, Toth B. Polar body biopsy. *Fertil Steril.* 2013;100:603–7.

31. Malter HE, Cohen J. Partial zona dissection of the human oocyte: a nontraumatic method using micromanipulation to assist zona pellucida penetration. *Fertil Steril.* 1989;51:139–48.

32. Dumoulin JC, Bras M, Coonen E, Dreesen J, Geraedts JP, Evers JL. Effect of Ca2+/Mg2+-free medium on the biopsy procedure for preimplantation genetic diagnosis and further development of human embryos. *Hum Reprod.* 1998;13:2880–3.

33. Jones AE, Wright G, Kort HI, Straub RJ, Nagy ZP. Comparison of laser-assisted hatching and acidified Tyrode's hatching by evaluation of blastocyst development rates in sibling embryos: a prospective randomized trial. *Fertil Steril.* 2006;85:487–91.

34. Wang WH, Kaskar K, Ren Y, Gill J, DeSplinter T, Haddad G, et al. Comparison of development and implantation of human embryos biopsied with two different methods: aspiration and displacement. *Fertil Steril.* 2009;92:536–40.

35. Rubio C, Bellver J, Rodrigo L, Castillon G, Guillen A, Vidal C, et al. In vitro fertilization with preimplantation genetic diagnosis for aneuploidies in advanced maternal age: a randomized, controlled study. *Fertil Steril.* 2017;107:1122–9.

Cell-Free DNA Analysis for PGT-A

Luca Gianaroli, Silvia Azzena, and M. Cristina Magli

15.1 Introduction

In humans, the reproductive process is markedly less efficient than that in other mammalian species. Several reasons contribute to this low fecundity including the presence of sexually transmitted diseases, environmental factors, and diseases unique to our species such as, for example, endometriosis. However, the overriding reason for our low fecundity is the high incidence of aneuploidy in oocytes that, even in young women, has an incidence of 20–30% [1].

Since the birth of the first IVF baby in 1978, numerous technological advancements have been introduced, resulting in an increasing number of people now being able to have a child. A particular milestone in the history of assisted reproductive technology was the successful clinical application of pre-implantation genetic testing (PGT) in 1990, when it was proven that blastomere biopsy from a day 3 embryo and testing with fluorescent in situ hybridization (FISH) could determine the sex of the embryo [2]. Following this landmark accomplishment, others began investigating the application of PGT using polar body biopsy in oocytes [3].

Before the introduction of PGT, the only options available for couples, at high reproductive risk, were prenatal diagnosis or childlessness. In case of fetal abnormalities identified with amniocentesis or chorionic villus sampling, prospective parents had to confront the difficult decision between the termination of the pregnancy and the birth of an affected child. Both these options, in addition to the choice of not having their own children, are accompanied by significant emotional distress.

PGT provides an alternative by permitting the selection of embryos before they are transferred to the uterus, thus preventing the potential for more painful and traumatic options when a pregnancy is already ongoing. More specifically, PGT for monogenic diseases (PGT-M) and for structural rearrangements (PGT-SR) allow the selection of healthy embryos to avoid the transmission of hereditary diseases or of unbalanced rearrangements consequent to chromosomal aberrations. PGT for aneuploidy (PGT-A) aims to improve implantation and take-home baby rates by permitting the selection of euploid embryos before transfer.

15.2 Development of PGT-A Technologies

Professor Alan Handyside successfully used PGT on day 3 embryos for the first time in 1990, when it was announced that two patients at risk of transmitting a recessive X-linked disease were pregnant after the transfer of IVF-generated embryos. The report included five patients, who underwent standard IVF. On day 3, embryos were biopsied by aspiration of one or two cells by using a thin microneedle introduced into the perivitelline space after zona pellucida (ZP) opening. Subsequently, Y-chromosome-specific DNA from the biopsies was amplified by PCR. Day 3 embryos identified as females were transferred and two of the patients each had twin pregnancies. The sex of the fetuses was confirmed at 10 weeks gestation by chorionic villus sampling [2].

In the same year, Yury Verlinsky reported a different approach by testing the first polar body to perform preconception diagnosis for autosomal recessive diseases [3]. The same strategy was later applied to test aneuploidy [4]. In the early 1990s, Santiago Munné and his coworkers, while at Cornell University Medical College, focused on assessing whether analysis of individual chromosomes using the FISH technology would enable selection of euploid embryos. The first live birth and correlation between maternal age and chromosome abnormalities was reported in 1995 [5]. The biggest limitation of FISH was the limited number of chromosomes (generally 5–9) that could be analyzed. The first series in which this technique was applied clinically was for a selected group of patients involving a collaboration between the Institute for Reproductive Medicine and Science at St. Barnabas Medical Center (West Orange, NJ, USA) and S.I.S.Me.R., Reproductive Medicine Unit (Bologna, Italy). The first results were published in 1997 [6, 7]. Since these groundbreaking reports using FISH, PGT technology has evolved to cover more than 200 genetic disorders as well as assessment of all 24 chromosomes in hundreds of thousands of embryos around the world.

15.3 Indications for PGT-A

PGT-A is indicated for all cases at high risk of transferring aneuploid embryos, including women of advanced reproductive age, couples with a history of recurrent miscarriages or repeated implantation failures, and couples with severe male factor. The most influential factors predisposing to chromosome missegregation are female age and altered recombination. Recombinant chromosomes are formed during the reciprocal exchanges of DNA between homologous chromosomes (crossover). In addition to sister chromatid cohesion, crossovers link the homologous pairs together during prophase I of meiosis, which takes place during fetal development in females. These linkages persist for decades, as the second round of chromosome segregation only occurs in adult women.

Aneuploidy occurs more frequently during oogenesis than spermatogenesis. Polar body biopsy and subsequent chromosome analysis provided important information about oocyte meiosis. We now know that premature predivision of chromatids rather than nondisjunction of whole chromosomes causes the great majority of errors in the first meiotic division and that more than half of aneuploidies derive from errors in the second meiotic division [8].

In addition to woman's age, aneuploidy has been shown to be associated with other patient characteristics [9]. In a study of 544 infertile couples undergoing 706 IVF cycles presenting with one of the following indications: maternal age $\geq$ 38 years, repeated IVF failures, and recurrent miscarriages, the results showed that the proportion of euploid oocytes was directly correlated with the number of mature oocytes and the establishment of a clinical pregnancy. An inverse correlation was found with female age, some causes of female infertility (endometriosis, miscarriages, ovulatory factor), poor prognosis indications (female age,

number of previous cycles, multiple poor prognosis indications), and number of follicle-stimulating hormone units used in the stimulation per collected oocyte and per mature oocyte [9].

Of note, over time, indications for PGT-A have expanded to include unexplained infertility, polycystic ovary syndrome, and poor responders. As reported in a meta-analysis and in a recent randomized controlled study, the use of PGT-A is indicated for several categories of patients with the aim to reduce the number of IVF cycles and miscarriages, to shorten the time to pregnancy, and to decrease the costs [10, 11]. However, a more recent Cochrane review concludes that the currently available evidence is insufficient to support PGT-A in routine clinical practice, confirming that use of PGT-A in improving IVF outcomes in unselected patients remains controversial [12].

15.4 Biopsy Techniques

Over the years, approaches to PGT have been numerous and varied in terms of biopsy and source of genetic material for analysis. The initial procedures using polar body and cleavage stage biopsy have now evolved to trophectoderm (TE) biopsy. Advances in culture media and the introduction of vitrification have greatly supported this approach. Table 15.1 summarizes the different stages of biopsy for PGT with the corresponding pros and cons.

TE biopsy has several advantages compared to the previously mentioned biopsies: the inner cell mass (ICM) is not touched, more than one cell is available for analysis, and the results obtained represent a more complete and accurate description of the chromosomal structure in preimplantation embryos [13].

At present, although TE biopsy is currently the most used method for PGT-A, it has recently been associated with an increased risk of preeclampsia and hypertensive disorders [14, 15]. It is invasive for the embryo, and efficacy and safety are limited by the embryologist's experience. In fact, as recently reported, the number of biopsied cells not only affects the results of the analysis, but also the implantation rate, especially in cases of poor-quality blastocysts [16].

The above limitations associated with TE biopsy have led to investigations of alternative approaches for identifying euploid embryos. However, neither static morphological evaluations nor time-lapse imaging provide adequate sensitivity for this purpose.

Table 15.1. Pros and cons of the three different procedures of biopsy

Aneuploidy Testing	Pros	Cons – Genetics Lab	Cons – IVF Lab
Polar bodies (PB)	- Less invasive	- Informative only for the maternal counterpart - Moderately predictive of the embryonic status - PB1 involved in both single chromatids and whole chromosomes copy number variations	- High number of biopsy procedures - Sequential biopsies (timing)
Day 3 embryos	- Paternal, maternal, and mitotic contribution to aneuploidy - Usually multiple embryos available	- High level of mosaicism (only one cell analyzed) - High level of chromosome instability - Moderately predictive of the blastocyst chromosome status	- Moderate number of biopsy procedures - More risk of embryo damage
Blastocysts	- Paternal, maternal, and mitotic contribution to aneuploidy - More cells available = more robust diagnosis - Low level of mosaicism - Little (if any) impact on embryo (embryonic mass not reduced)	- Short time for diagnosis (unless cryopreserving) - Unproven Concordance between TE and inner cell mass cells - Evaluation of mosaicism	- Increased workload → cryopreservation and thawing - Concerns over extended embryo culture - Destiny of mosaic embryos

As a result, efforts are currently focused on development of three less invasive techniques for PGT-A. Two of these involve analysis of cell-free DNA (cfDNA) in either blastocyst fluid (BF) [17], or the medium in which embryos have been cultured (spent culture medium, SCM) [18]; and the third involves investigation of miRNAs in the BF and in the SCM [19].

15.5 Blastocyst Fluid: A Source of cfDNA

15.5.1 Principle

After ICM and TE cell differentiation, Na+ ions accumulate on the basolateral side of the TE epithelium. This event creates an osmotic gradient, partially generated by different isoforms of Na+/K+ adenosine triphosphates, that promote the accumulation of water and the subsequent formation of a cavity known as the blastocoele. Tight junctions form between blastomeres as compaction gets underway, which create a seal, preventing leakage of the fluid from the cavity. The progressive accumulation of this fluid inside the blastocyst (BF), causes expansion of the blastocyst and thinning of the ZP. Ultimately,

expansion leads to a breach of the ZP, with natural escape ("hatching") of the blastocyst from the ZP, in preparation for implantation.

In addition to proteins and other factors, the BF also contains embryonic DNA. The cellular origin of the DNA source has yet to be determined. According to some hypotheses, it could be free DNA or enclosed inside microvesicles. Regardless of its form, this DNA can be submitted to amplification and analysis to study the chromosomal status, specific mutations, or genetic diseases [20].

15.5.2 Technique for Blastocentesis

The BF can be aspirated from expanded blastocysts as is routinely performed in many laboratories to collapse blastocysts before vitrification. The procedure is performed at the micromanipulator setup using holding and intracytoplasmic sperm injection (ICSI) pipettes in a dish with drops of buffered medium under paraffin oil (Figure 15.1).

The blastocyst is normally held with the ICM positioned anywhere between 6 and 12 o'clock to avoid a potential contact of the ICSI pipette when entering the cavity. After carefully balancing the

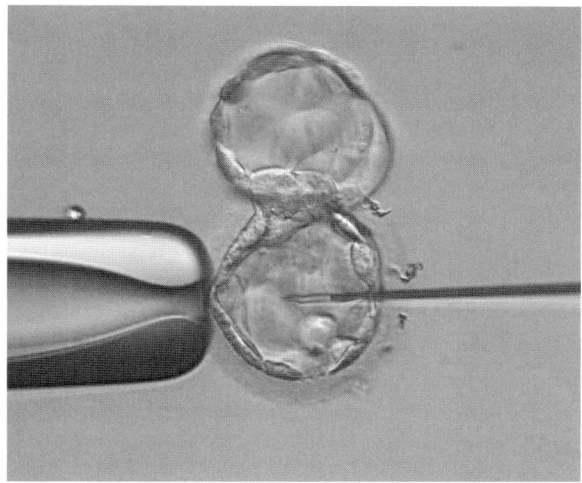

Figure 15.1 Aspiration of the BF from a hatching blastocyst
The ZP was opened on day 3 to facilitate the hatching process. TE cells started to herniate form the breach opened in the ZP that remains thick irrespective of the developmental stage.

ICSI pipette, it is guided into the blastocoelic cavity, entering at the junction between two TE cells. The BF is aspirated until the blastocyst is completely collapsed (Video 15.1). The ICSI pipette is gently withdrawn and the blastocyst is released and immediately cryopreserved. The fluid is transferred into a PCR tube containing 1 μl drop of phosphate buffered saline under microscope view. To do this, the tube is placed horizontally on a dish lid, on the micromanipulator stage. Then, the pipette containing the BF is inserted into the tube and positioned inside the drop and the content is expelled using the microsyringe connected to the ICSI pipette. The tube is closed, briefly spun to lower the drop to the bottom, and frozen for future analysis.

15.5.3 Evidence for cfDNA in BF

The first attempt to characterize the BF content was aimed at studying the metabolic profile of embryos using mass-spectrometry. Research was then focused on genomic DNA that was detected in about 90% of BFs [17]. Other authors showed lower detection rates and, after analyzing 32 samples, 19 displayed no DNA amplification, 4 produced chaotic profiles, and only 9 produced informative results [21]. Of these 9 samples, 3 showed data concordant with the corresponding TE biopsy, 5 were aneuploid while the

corresponding TE biopsy was euploid, and 1 revealed complex aneuploidy while the TE biopsy showed trisomy of chromosome 16 [21]. Nevertheless, more recent studies demonstrate promising utility of BF cfDNA analysis for predicting embryo ploidy (see Section 15.5.4).

15.5.4 Investigations of Concordance between cfDNA in BF and Embryo Chromosome Status by TE Biopsy

We undertook a prospective study to investigate the degree of concordance between the chromosomal status of the BF and that predicted by TE biopsy [13]. The study included 17 couples (maternal age 37.6 ± 3.5 years) undergoing PGT-A for advanced maternal age or repeated IVF failures. The BF was aspirated in 51 blastocysts, whole-genome amplification (WGA) applied, and DNA was detected in 39 BFs (76.5%). The mean amount of DNA after WGA of the BFs was 900.38 ng/μl. In 38 of these 39 BFs, the ploidy condition of TE cells was confirmed resulting in 96.6% of chromosome concordance rate. The results were also evaluated in relation to the ploidy status predicted by polar body and blastomere biopsy, which was confirmed in 93.3% and 100% of cases, respectively.

In 12 of the 51 BF samples analyzed, no informative DNA was detected (23.5%) possibly due to highly fragmented DNA derived from apoptotic cells. As we know, all cells surrounding the blastocoele cavity are metabolically active and secrete various substances. We also know that apoptosis occurs even in good-quality embryos, both in TE and ICM. Therefore, the presence of DNA could be a true reflection of the blastocyst content and could be consequent to its release from apoptotic cells into the blastocoele cavity [13].

More data are available from another study on BF from 116 blastocysts from 51 couples (maternal age 38.1 ± 3.2 years) undergoing 24-chromosome array-comparative genomic hybridization (a-CGH) on polar bodies, blastomeres, or blastocysts. DNA was detected in 95 of the BF samples (82%), of which 85 had strong amplification and 10 had weak amplification. When compared with polar body or blastomere results, BF showed a ploidy concordance of 94.3% in both cases, while the ploidy concordance with TE cells was 97.1% [20] (Figure 15.2).

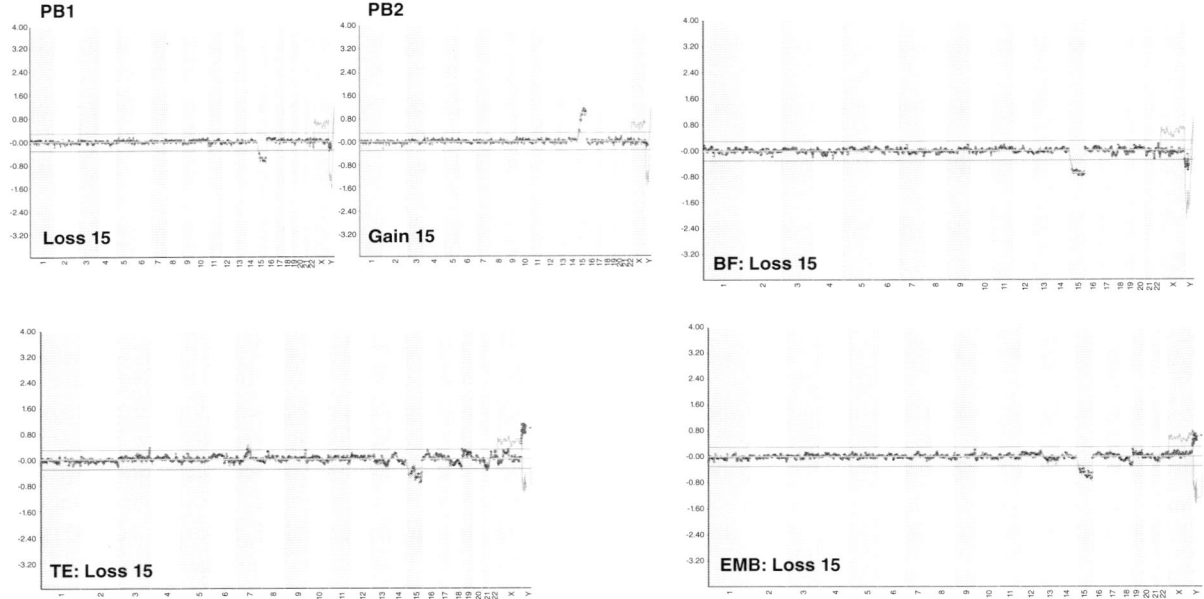

Figure 15.2 Concordance between PB1 and PB2 chromosomal results and those from the corresponding BF, TE, and whole-embryo analyses. Following PB analysis, the embryo is predicted to be monosomic for chromosome 15 as proven by BF, TE biopsy, and by the analysis of the whole embryo.

In a further study, BFs from 256 blastocysts from 91 couples (maternal age 37.7 ± 4 years) were analyzed [22]. According to the TE results, 71 were diagnosed euploid and 185 aneuploid. When the corresponding BFs were submitted to WGA, the incidence of amplification was significantly lower in BFs from TE-euploid blastocysts (45%) when compared with those that were aneuploid (81%, P<0.001). After a-CGH, informative results from BF amplified products were obtained in 172 blastocysts (94.5% of positive amplifications). The total ploidy concordance was 93.6%, while the chromosome concordance was 96%. Comparison between the two TE ploidy groups indicated a difference in incidence of informative results based on ploidy: 97% for aneuploid embryos versus 81% for euploid embryos (P<0.005).

Further analyses were undertaken to investigate whether PGT-A results from BF cfDNA may be utilized for embryo selection. The BF analyses from 53 transferred blastocysts with euploid TE cells were correlated with implantation in a retrospective and in a blinded fashion. In all, 33 clinical pregnancies were obtained, of which 29 were ongoing and 4 miscarried. The ongoing pregnancy rate was significantly higher after the transfer of euploid blastocysts with failed BF

amplification (68%) versus those with positive BF amplification (31.5%, P = 0.01). Interestingly, in the case of one of the miscarriages, the BF from the corresponding blastocyst was found to be aneuploid, which was in discordance with the TE biopsy result, suggesting mosaicism as a possible cause of the miscarriage [22].

An additional observation in this study [22] was that 11 blastocysts showed a partial ploidy discordance. In seven of them, embryos had euploid TE and aneuploid BF as a possible result of the complete elimination of the abnormal cells from the TE into the BF (Figure 15.3). In the remaining four cases, embryos had aneuploid TE and euploid BF, which might reflect a defective transition from the mechanism of DNA repair pathways to the cell cycle control and apoptotic process. While it is unknown why aneuploidy is so frequent in preimplantation embryos, evidence indicates that most errors are not correctable, although several pathways for attempted self-correction exist, including blastomere exclusion, the formation of micronuclei, or cellular fragmentation. At the blastocyst stage, mosaicism is a likely consequence of aneuploidy correction; the possibility of mosaic embryos to develop further depends on the

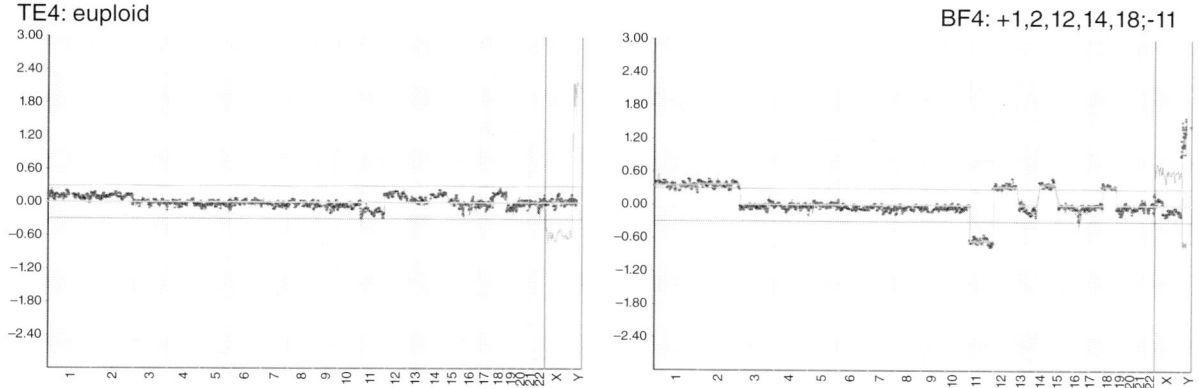

Figure 15.3 **Chromosome analysis by a-CGH in the TE biopsy and corresponding BF**
The blastocyst is called euploid by the software analyzing the TE biopsy, although a modest grade of mosaicism is identified for chromosome 1, 2, 11, 12, 14, and 18. The analysis of the BF reveals a clear aneuploid status by calling an extra copy for chromosomes 1, 2, 12, 14, and 18, and a single copy for chromosome 11. This result supports the role of BF as the collector of aneuploid cells in an attempt by the mosaic embryo to restore an euploid condition.

proportion of euploid/aneuploid cells, on the type of abnormalities, and on the efficiency of the corrective mechanisms.

Taken together, the blastocoelic cavity may represent a "collector" for products from different cells, including those generated by apoptotic processes. As such, we can expect more DNA (possibly apoptotic) in the BF from aneuploid blastocysts [22], which raises the question whether BF-cfDNA analysis can be used for embryo selection. While the balance of evidence indicates that the lack of BF-cfDNA is positively correlated with euploidy and implantation, further research is required to determine whether this PGT-A approach has efficacy in clinic practice.

15.6 SCM: A Source of cfDNA

15.6.1 Principle

Although collection of BF is less invasive than polar body, blastomere, or TE biopsy, the procedure still involves manipulation of the embryo. Standardizing the analysis of cfDNA in SCM would represent a PGT-A approach that is even less invasive.

The presence of cfDNA in blood was documented for the first time in adult serum in 1948 by Mandel and Metais [23]. The source of this DNA was thought to be circulatory lysed cells as well as apoptotic events. Fetal cfDNA was later found in maternal circulation and this prompted researchers to concentrate on study of embryo-derived cfDNA. It was identified in

the amniotic fluid as well as in the yolk sac, suggesting that cfDNA was present in every locale where apoptotic or tissue remodeling activities occur during preimplantation development. These collective observations provided the foundation for the first proof-of-principle report of the successful application of SCM cfDNA for selection of embryos leading to healthy live births [24].

15.6.2 Technique for SCM Collection

The volume of SCM collected for cfDNA analysis will invariably depend on the initial volume of the microdrop used to culture the embryo. However, the ratio of initial microdrop volume to the volume of medium collected has varied among studies. While some investigators have used 25 µL microdrops for culture with collection of only 5 µL of SCM [25], others have used 15 µL microdrops with collection of 10 µl [26] and yet other investigators have utilized 10 µL microdrop volumes for culture with all remaining medium collected after removal of the embryo [27]. Regardless of the microdrop volume for culture, it is recommended that the protocol for SCM collection takes into consideration the fact that there is likely a gradient of cfDNA from the embryo outwards toward the drop perimeter. Therefore, it is inadvisable to pipette the embryo directly from its original position in the drop as the more cfDNA one collects, the more likely one will obtain successful amplification and a result.

A reasonable approach for sample collection is as follows [26]:

- Use 15 µL microdrop volumes for culture.
- Immediately before medium collection, gently nudge the embryo to the edge of the drop with the end of a stripper tip, to create the least possible disturbance of medium in the original location of the embryo.
- Remove the embryo.
- Remove 10 µL of SCM into lysis buffer for cfDNA analysis.

The other metric to be considered for optimized SCM cfDNA analysis is culture duration and over what days the embryo should be cultured. Work by Rubio et al. indicates that culture for more than 48 hours from day 4 to days 6–7 is optimal [27].

15.6.3 Evidence for cfDNA in SCM

Although cfDNA is detectable in the SCM from day 3, day 4, and day 5 culture [25], as mentioned above, results may be more accurate when the SCM is collected following culture of blastocysts from days 6 to 7 [27].

To demonstrate the reliability of cfDNA testing in SCM, the first step was to perform concordance analyses [28]. Table 15.2 shows that the performance of cfDNA testing (i.e. noninvasive PGT-A [niPGT-A]) was higher than that of TE biopsy (i.e. invasive PGT-A [iPGT-A]) in terms of false positive rate, positive predictive value, and concordance for both embryo ploidy and chromosome copy number variation. These data suggest that cfDNA analysis is less prone to errors associated with embryo mosaicism, and is more reliable than TE biopsy.

In another study including 40 morphologically normal day 5 blastocysts donated for research, the concordance data between BF combined with SCM, versus TE biopsy, versus the remaining whole embryos gave five groups of results, as illustrated in Table 15.3 [29]. The results obtained from this study, where the chromosome analysis was performed by next-generation sequencing, showed that DNA from SCM and BF can be amplified and provide information on aneuploidy. However, the differences between the three different types of samples leave the way open to various hypotheses [29]. Similar data were published later, proving again a moderate reliability of this noninvasive technique, compared to traditional protocols [30]. Consistent with these findings, a recent study compared the outcomes following transfer of embryos with euploid TE and euploid SCM results with those having euploid TE with aneuploid SCM. A total of 115 TE biopsies and SCM from 46 patients were analyzed. The ongoing pregnancy rate in the group with euploid TE/euploid SCM showed a threefold increase compared to the group with euploid TE/aneuploid SCM (52.9% vs. 16.7%). Furthermore, in the euploid concordance group no miscarriages were observed, suggesting that this noninvasive technique was highly reliable [27].

Table 15.2. Comparison of the performance of noninvasive PGT-A and TE biopsy for PGT-A from samples collected following blastocyst culture

Performance characteristic	niPGT-A (n = 102)	iPGT-A (n = 100)	p-value
False positive rate	21.7% (5/23)	62.5% (15/24)	0.008
False negative rate	1.3% (1/79)	0.0% (0/76)	1.000
Positive predictive value	94.0% (78/83)	83.5% (76/91)	0.034
Negative predictive value	95.5% (21/22)	100.0% (18/18)	1.000
Sensitivity	98.7% (78/79)	100.0% (76/76)	1.000
Specificity	78.3% (18/23)	50.0% (12/24)	0.069
Concordance for embryo ploidy	94.1% (96/102)	85.0% (85/100)	0.039
Concordance for whole chromosome copy number	81.4% (83/102)	67.0% (67/100)	0.024

Notes: The above comparison includes the three studies assessing performance characteristics of niPGT-A and iPGT-A to the whole embryo, after collection of samples (spent medium with or without BF) at the blastocyst stage (culture day 5 to 6 or day 6 to 7). P-values were derived from Chi square with Fisher's Exact Test with p < 0.05 considered statistically significant.
Published with permission from Elsevier: Table 2 of Racowsky C, in Rubio C et al., *Fertil Steril*. 2021;115(4):841–9.

Table 15.3. Chromosomal information obtained from the analysis of TE cells and SCM combined with BF from 40 expanded blastocysts donated for research. The results were compared against those obtained from the whole embryo

Groups	No. Analyzed	TE	SCM + BF	Whole Embryo	Conclusions
1	11	Euploid	Concordance	Concordance	Full concordance
	4	Aneuploid	Concordance	Concordance	Full concordance
2	2	Aneuploid	Aneuploid	Euploid	Repair activity Mosaicism in TE
3	12	Euploid	Aneuploid	Euploid	Repair activity
4	4	Aneuploid	Euploid	Euploid	Mosaicism in TE
5	7	Discordance	Discordance	Discordance	Full discordance

Notes: Group 1 included 15 cases with total concordance between all three samples: 11 cases were euploid and 4 were aneuploid. Group 2 had 2 cases in which SCM in combination with BF (SCM + BF) and TE biopsy were in agreement for aneuploidy, but differed from the whole embryo sample. Group 3 included 12 cases in which the TE biopsy and whole embryo sample gave the same result, but differed from SCM + BF. Group 4 showed 4 cases with concordance between SCM + BF and whole embryos, but discordance with TE biopsy. Group 5 included 7 cases of absolute discordance between the three samples.
The table summarizes data presented in Li et al., *Sci Rep.* 2018;8:9275.

On the other hand, several authors oppose use of SCM as a PGT-A selection technique due to concerns regarding maternal DNA contamination [31]. Therefore, great care should be taken to remove all cumulus/corona radiata cells before onset of culture.

Collective evidence indicates that further research with more robust datasets is required to clarify the potential use of cfDNA analyses, whether from BF or SCM, for determining embryo ploidy.

15.7 miRNAs and Exosomes as Noninvasive Biomarkers

The presence of miRNAs in culture medium, and their role as embryonic biomarkers, has been postulated [19]. Comparative analysis has been undertaken of miRNAs in the SCM after culture to the cleavage, morula, and expanded morphologically normal blastocyst stages (25 implanted euploid and 28 nonimplanted embryos). Results showed that 96.6% of the miRNAs detected in SCM were expressed from TE cells, and that the SCM taken from cleavage and morula stages did not give the same results [19].

Recently, 89 miRNA and extracellular vesicles (exosomes), were demonstrated in BFs. BF miRNAs reflect the miRNome of preimplantation embryonic cells and these could represent molecular markers of blastocyst quality. DNA fragments were also identified and their derivation could result from the presence of exosomes. Of note, DNA fragments are used to facilitate the diagnosis and prognosis of cancer patients; the possibility exists that their presence in BFs could be used to investigate Mendelian monogenic diseases. Therefore, analysis of miRNAs in BF may provide an additional, minimally invasive approach for predicting embryo quality [32].

15.8 Conclusions

After 30 years of clinical application, PGT is recognized worldwide as a well-established practice to reduce the risk of giving birth to affected children. In the case of aneuploidy testing, most patients, especially if infertile, tend to ethically accept the application of these techniques to decrease miscarriage rates, to shorten time to term pregnancies, and to avoid unnecessary repetitive cycles related to the transfer of undiagnosed embryos. However, the costs and invasiveness of TE biopsy, which in essence is a surgical procedure, are still the major limitations for wider application of PGT.

Research is now required for improving reliability of results from the "less-invasive" BF approach or the "noninvasive" SCM approach for determining the genetic status of human embryos. Several studies in this field are underway, some of them with extremely promising results, especially those using cfDNA in BF combined with SCM. However, these new techniques should first be applied in meticulous and rigorously controlled clinical trials to determine their safety and effectiveness.

Key Messages

- PGT-A plays an important role in select patient populations for embryo selection by identifying euploid embryos.
- TE biopsy is currently the most used method for PGT-A, although mosaicism complicates interpretation of the results.
- Less invasive techniques for PGT-A involve the analysis of cfDNA or of miRNAs in either BF, or the medium in which embryos have been cultured (SCM).
- The analysis of cfDNA in the BF suggests that the blastocoelic cavity may represent a collector for different cell products, including those generated by apoptotic processes. The lack of BF–cfDNA is positively correlated with euploidy and implantation rate.
- The assessment of copy number variation in some cfDNA from SCM may be complicated by contamination due to either the culture medium constituents or cumulus/corona cells.
- miRNAs in BF could represent molecular markers of blastocysts quality.
- Several studies are underway to confirm the possibility of using cfDNA for less or noninvasive techniques for PGT-A. The preliminary results are very promising, especially those combining cfDNA in BF and SCM.

References

1. Franasiak JM, Forman EJ, Hong KH, Werner MD, Upham KM, Treff NR, Scott RT, Jr. The nature of aneuploidy with increasing age of the female partner: a review of 15,169 consecutive trophectoderm biopsies evaluated with comprehensive chromosomal screening. *Fertil Steril*. 2014;101:656–63.

2. Handyside AH, Kontogianni EH, Hardy K, Winston RM. Pregnancies from biopsied human preimplantation embryos sexed by Y-specific DNA amplification. *Nature*. 1990;344:768–70.

3. Verlinsky Y, Ginsberg N, Lifchez A, Valle J, Moise J, Strom CM. Analysis of the first polar body: preconception genetic diagnosis. *Hum Reprod*. 1990;5:826–9.

4. Verlinsky Y, Cieslak J, Ivakhnenko V, Evsikov S, Wolf G, White M, et al. Prevention of age-related aneuploidies by polar body testing of oocytes. *J Assist Reprod Genet*. 1999;16:165–9.

5. Munné S, Alikani M, Tomkin G, Grifo J, Cohen J. Embryo morphology, developmental rates, and maternal age are correlated with chromosome abnormalities. *Fertil Steril*. 1995;64:382–91.

6. Gianaroli L, Magli MC, Munné S, Fiorentino A, Montanaro N, Ferraretti AP. Will preimplantation genetic diagnosis assist patients with a poor prognosis to achieve pregnancy? *Hum Reprod*. 1997;12:1762–7.

7. Gianaroli L, Magli MC, Ferraretti AP, Fiorentino A, Garrisi J, Munné S. Preimplantation genetic diagnosis increases the implantation rate in human in vitro fertilization by avoiding the transfer of chromosomally abnormal embryos. *Fertil Steril*. 1997;68:1128–31.

8. Handyside AH, Montag M, Magli MC, Repping S, Harper J, Schmutzler A, et al. Multiple meiotic errors caused by predivision of chromatids in women of advanced maternal age undergoing in vitro fertilisation. *Eur J Hum Genet*. 2012;20:742–7.

9. Gianaroli L, Magli MC, Cavallini G, Crippa A, Capoti A, Resta S, et al. Predicting aneuploidy in human oocytes: key factors which affect the meiotic process. *Hum Reprod*. 2010;25:2374–86.

10. Dahdouh EM, Balayla J, García-Velasco JA. Comprehensive chromosome screening improves embryo selection: a meta-analysis. *Fertil Steril*. 2015;104:1503–12.

11. Rubio C, Bellver J, Rodrigo L, Castillón G, Guillén A, Vidal C, et al. In vitro fertilization with preimplantation genetic diagnosis for aneuploidies in advanced maternal age: a randomized, controlled study. *Fertil Steril*. 2017;107:1122–9.

12. Cornelisse S, Zagers M, Kostova E, Fleischer K, van Wely M, Mastenbroek S. Preimplantation genetic testing for aneuploidies (abnormal number of chromosomes) in in vitro fertilisation. *Cochrane Database Syst Rev*. 2020;9:CD005291.

13. Gianaroli L, Magli MC, Pomante A, Crivello AM, Cafueri G, Valerio M, Ferraretti AP. Blatocentesis: a source of DNA for preimplantation genetic testing. Results from a pilot study. *Fertil Steril*. 2014;102:1692–9.

14. Zhang WY, von Versen-Höynck F, Kapphahn KI, Fleischmann RR, Zhao Q, Baker VL. Maternal and neonatal outcomes associated with trophectoderm biopsy. *Fertil Steril*. 2019;112:283–90.

15. Makhijani R, Bartels CB, Godiwala P, Bartolucci A, DiLuigi A, Nulsen J, et al. Impact of trophectoderm biopsy on obstetric and perinatal outcomes following frozen-thawed embryo

transfer cycles. *Hum Reprod.* 2021;25:340–8.

16. Zhang S, Luo K, Cheng D, Tan Y, Lu C, He H, et al. Number of biopsied trophectoderm cells is likely to affect the implantation potential of blastocysts with poor trophectoderm quality. *Fertil Steril.* 2016;105:1222–7.

17. Palini S, Galluzzi L, De Stefani S, Bianchi M, Wells D, Magnani M, Bulletti C. Genomic DNA in human blastocoele fluid. *Reprod Biomed Online.* 2013;26:603–10.

18. Shamonki MI, Jin H, Haimowitz Z, Liu L. Proof of concept: preimplantation genetic screening without embryo biopsy through analysis of cell-free DNA in spent embryo culture media. *Fertil Steril.* 2016;106:1312–18.

19. Capalbo A, Ubaldi FM, Cimadomo D, Noli L, Khalaf Y, Farcomeni A, et al. MicroRNAs in spent blastocyst culture medium are derived from trophectoderm cells and can be explored for human embryo reproductive competence assessment. *Fertil Steril.* 2016;105:225–35.

20. Magli MC, Pomante A, Cafueri G, Valerio M, Crippa A, Ferraretti AP, Gianaroli L. Preimplantation genetic testing: polar bodies, blastomeres, trophectoderm cells, or blastocoelic fluid? *Fertil Steril.* 2015;105:676–83.

21. Perloe M, Welch C, Morton P, Venier W, Wells D, Palini S. Validation of blastocoele fluid aspiration for preimplantation genetic screening using array comparative genomic hybridization (aCGH). *Fertil Steril.* 2013;100:S208.

22. Magli MC, Albanese C, Crippa A, Tabanelli C, Ferrarretti AP, Gianaroli L. Deoxyribonucleic acid detection in blastocoelic fluid: a new predictor of embryo ploidy and viable pregnancy. *Fertil Steril.* 2019;111:77–85.

23. Mandel P, Metais P. Les acides nucléiques du plasma sanguin chez l'homme. *C R Seances Soc Biol Fil.* 1948;142:241–3.

24. Xu J, Fang R, Chen L, Chen D, Xiao JP, Yang W, et al. Noninvasive chromosome screening of human embryos by genome sequencing of embryo culture medium for in vitro fertilization. *Proc Natl Acad Sci USA.* 2016;113:11907–12.

25. Ho JR, Arrach N, Rhodes-Long K, Ahmady A, Ingles S, Chung K, et al. Pushing the limits of detection: investigation of cell-free DNA for aneuploidy screening in embryos. *Fertil Steril.* 2018;110:467–75.

26. Huang L, Bogale B, Tang Y, Lu S, Xie XS, Racowsky C. Noninvasive preimplantation genetic testing for aneuploidy in spent medium may be more reliable than trophectoderm biopsy. *Proc Natl Acad Sci USA.* 2019;116:14105–12.

27. Rubio C, Rienzi L, Navarro-Sánchez L, Cimadomo D, García-Pascual CM, Albricci L, et al. Embryonic cell-free DNA versus trophectoderm biopsy for aneuploidy testing: concordance rate and clinical implications. *Fertil Steril.* 2019;112:510–19.

28. Rubio C, Racowsky C, Barad DH, Scott RT, Jr, Simon C. Noninvasive preimplantation genetic testing for aneuploidy in spent culture medium as a substitute for trophectoderm biopsy. *Fertil Steril.* 2021;115:841–9.

29. Li P, Song Z, Yao Y, Huang T, Mao R, Huang J, et al. Preimplantation genetic screening with spent culture medium/blastocoelic fluid for in vitro fertilization. *Sci Rep.* 2018;8:9275.

30. Kuznyetsov V, Madjunkova S, Antes R, Abramov R, Motamedi G, Ibarrientos Z, Librach C. Evaluation of a novel non-invasive preimplantation genetic screening approach. *PLoS One.* 2018;13: e0197262.

31. Vera-Rodriguez M, Diez-Juan A, Jimenez-Almazan J, Martinez S, Navarro R, Peinado V, et al. Origin and composition of cell-free DNA in spent medium from human embryo culture during preimplantation development. *Hum Reprod.* 2018;33:745–56.

32. Battaglia R, Palini S, Vento M, La Ferlita A, Lo Faro MJ, Caroppo E, et al. Identification of extracellular vesicles and characterization of miRNA expression profiles in human blastocoelic fluid. *Sci Rep.* 2019;9:84.

Chapter

16

What Science May Come for Embryo Selection?

Paolo Rinaudo and Eleni Jaswa

16.1 Introduction

Embryo selection methodologies are paramount in the success of IVF cycles. Today, approximately only one-third of patients presenting to a clinic can expect to have a child after one cycle, leaving great room for improvement in our understanding of embryo quality and prediction of pregnancy potential. While current embryo selection technologies are thoroughly described in this book, here we will envision possible new technologies in light of the fact that the current pace of technological advancement is breathtaking.

16.2 Evolution of Assisted Reproductive Technology

Human knowledge is increasing in an exponential fashion. For example, it was estimated that the doubling time of medical knowledge in 1950 was 50 years; in 1980, 7 years; and in 2010, 3.5 years. In 2020 it is projected to be 0.2 years – just 73 days [1]. The assisted reproductive technology (ART) field is witnessing the emergence of a large, novel set of possible interventions. Several novel technologies are making it possible to execute procedures that could not have even been imagined in the past. Overall, we are witnessing an evolution from ART used only for infertility purposes (ART 1.0) to elective indications (ART 2.0) and finally to therapeutic, transformational technologies (ART 3.0, Table 16.1).

ART 3.0 is fueled by breakthrough technological and scientific discoveries. Examples of these technologies include *CRISPR/CAS9* that is a targeted genetic "cut and paste" genome editing tool in which researchers can modify precise regions of DNA. The first birth of CRISPR-edited humans (twin girls) occurred in China in 2018, inciting an intense, ongoing global scientific debate.

In vitro gametogenesis refers to the generation of gametes in culture from embryonic stem cells or inducible pluripotent stem cells. Healthy mouse offspring have been born from sperm and egg cells derived from skin biopsies [2]. If such a technology entered human ART, it would revolutionize not only the clinical ART field but the entire concept of reproduction, by permitting the unlimited creation of gametes.

Flushing of human embryos from the uterus, a technique performed in the early days of IVF, could allow genetic testing of embryos conceived naturally [3].

While *molecular cloning* refers to the process of making multiple copies of molecules or DNA, *Reproductive cloning* involves the creation of an entire cloned human, instead of just specific cells or tissues. While multiple animal species have been cloned and it is theoretically possible to clone a human, this has not been done and is considered illegal because of the significant ethical implications [4]. Of note, monozygotic twins are genetically identical and therefore each one represents a "clone" of the other; this occurs in 0.04% of live births following natural conception and in up to 2–3% following ART, likely because the increased gamete and embryo manipulation processes facilitate embryo splitting.

Mitochondrial transfer involves the transfer of healthy donor mitochondria to replace those of the intended mother, via a variety of techniques including maternal spindle transfer and pronuclear transfer. This intervention is primarily indicated for families with hereditary mitochondrial disease; however, it is also being controversially explored as an adjunctive measure for age-related infertility.

Finally, it is worth mentioning the rapidly advancing work on *blastocyst complementation* between different species (for example, combining a pig blastocyst deficient of some key genes with a human blastocyst). This technology could generate a mammalian chimera (e.g. a pig with a human heart) that could provide unlimited organs for transplantation [5].

Table 16.1. Evolution of ART

		Timeline
ART 1.0	Infertility-based. Provided only to infertile couples	Based on the pioneering work of Robert Edwards and Patrick Steptoe (1960, now)
ART 2.0	Elective: gamete and embryo banking in individuals without a history of infertility	Since ~2010 an increasing number of patients use elective procedures
ART 3.0	Therapeutic. Examples include: • Mitochondrial transfer • Use of CRISPR/CAS9 • In vitro gametogenesis • Flushing of in vivo embryos from the uterus for testing • Cloning	These techniques are feasible in animals now. The theoretical capability exists to execute these procedures in humans as well

Importantly, these novel technologies might require new and more sophisticated gamete and embryo selection tools, to assess the changes induced by the technologies themselves.

16.3 Novel Technologies for Embryo Selection

Technologies for embryo selections are rapidly evolving. Significant progress can be expected from the adoption of new technologies or the refinement of currently existing ones. For example, novel biomarkers describing the metabolic fitness of a gamete or embryos might become critically important for selecting a healthy embryo to transfer.

While current technologies select embryos based on their implantation potential, we can imagine a future in which embryos could be selected not only for the implantation potential but also based on the expected future health of the individual (Table 16.2). This could be important, since the ultimate goal of improving IVF efficiency should be rapid identification of an embryo that will generate not only a healthy singleton newborn, but also a healthy adult.

16.3.1 Use of Artificial Intelligence for Embryo Selection

Artificial intelligence (AI) represents technologies designed to recapitulate human-like intelligence, that is, the ability to learn, reason, and self-correct, in machines such as computers.

Basic terminology of relevant data science concepts is found in Table 16.3 and Figure 16.1. Machine learning is one feature of AI that describes the learning capacity of technological systems, such that they might iteratively make predictions from datasets without explicit external programming. In a simplified conceptual view, a machine learning model is trained using a sample of a dataset (the training dataset) on which it creates a "fit" (i.e. learns to make predictions); the model is subsequently validated against the remaining data from the dataset (the validation dataset) for accuracy.

Potential use cases of AI in ART include:

- Assessment of gametes and embryo quality from images. AI is especially efficient in image processing, using algorithms such as convolutional neural networks
- Massive data processing to enhance fertility diagnostics and to inform clinical predictions
- Personalization of treatment regimens

There are several potential advantages of using AI in ART. First, it is believed that AI might remove the subjectivity in interpreting data (for example, in assessing the morphology of an embryo), allowing for unbiased selection procedures. Second, the automated nature of AI is expected to reduce costs and increase efficiency and quality control. Finally, thanks to increasing computational power, AI might be able to incorporate very large datasets from an IVF cycle (e.g. patient demographics, medical history, stimulation regimens, follicular response, endocrine parameters, retrieval characteristics, embryo morphology,

Table 16.2. Technologies for embryo selection

Aimed at identifying embryos with higher implantation potential		
Type of technology	**Usage**	**Evidence of utility**
Morphology	Routinely used	70% PPV
Time lapse	Frequently used	Insufficient evidence whether more or less effective than conventional morphology
Analysis of chromosomal ploidy (preimplantation genetic testing)	Frequently used but controversial	Controversial; older randomized controlled trials (RCTs) suggested benefit while a more recent RCT failed to repeat this
Metabolomic of embryos	Performed but still experimental	Unknown
Mitochondria number	Experimental	Unknown
Gene expression profiling of embryos or granulosa cells	Experimental	Unknown
Use of novel imaging techniques	Experimental	Unknown
Use of artificial intelligence to select embryos	Experimental	Unknown
Selection of male germ cells by cell sorting	Experimental	Unknown
Aimed at assessing implantation and future health of the embryos		
Selection of embryos based on predisposition to develop adult-onset diseases	Experimental	Unknown
Selection of embryos based on epigenetic/imprinting fingerprint	Experimental	Unknown

time-lapse imaging) to yield a greater understanding and prediction of cycle outcomes than ever before, by connecting dots invisible to humans.

While societal concerns have been voiced about AI replacing humans and jobs, proponents of the technology suggest that by removing the automatable, "mindless" tasks, AI might instead free humans to perform work that is more creative, interesting, and human.

However, limitations of machine learning remain. The "black box" concept represents the idea that the calculations performed between input and output by some machine learning systems often cannot be discerned or understood by humans, even the system programmers. This introduces the potential for unintended biases in the systems, particularly in the setting of skewed training datasets. As our understanding of machine learning grows, we will need to impose reporting standards and statistically sound criteria for publication. Finally, conventional peer review is limited both by the highly technical nature of AI, and the fact that companies developing these technologies are not subject to the same peer review processes and traditional academic institutions.

Currently, published evidence of leveraging AI to benefit ART is limited but increasing. For example, while only two total abstracts incorporating AI and machine learning were presented at the annual ASRM and ESHRE conferences in 2017, 16 projects were presented in 2019 [6]; most remain unpublished at the time of writing.

One of the largest published endeavors using AI to select high-quality embryos implemented a neural network-based framework (STORK) founded on Google's Inception model [7]. Approximately 50 000 images from 10 148 embryos captured via

Table 16.3. Basic concepts in data science

AI	The science and engineering of creating human-like intelligence in computer systems, to achieve goals like reasoning, learning, and self-correction
Machine learning	A subset of AI representing computers' ability to learn from data without being explicitly programmed
Deep learning	A subset of machine learning based on artificial neural networks, in which data passes through multiple transformations allowing software to train itself to perform a variety of tasks
Supervised learning	Trial-and-error machine learning based on labeled data, allowing the algorithm to compare its output with the correct output during training
Unsupervised learning	Machine learning involving unlabeled datasets; the algorithm looks for patterns to create its own categories of data
Artificial neural network	Computer systems inspired by biological neural networks, comprising a system of interconnected units or nodes
Convolutional neural network	A neural network especially adept at image recognition; involves breaking images into overlapping tiles using filters in hierarchical layers of complexity and then pooling data into smaller parts
Data science	Understanding and interpreting data
Big data	Extremely large datasets (terabytes and larger) requiring new technologies and techniques for interpretation
Training dataset	The sample of data from which the model learns, and is fit to generate predictive algorithms
Validation dataset	The sample of data from which the trained model is validated and tuned

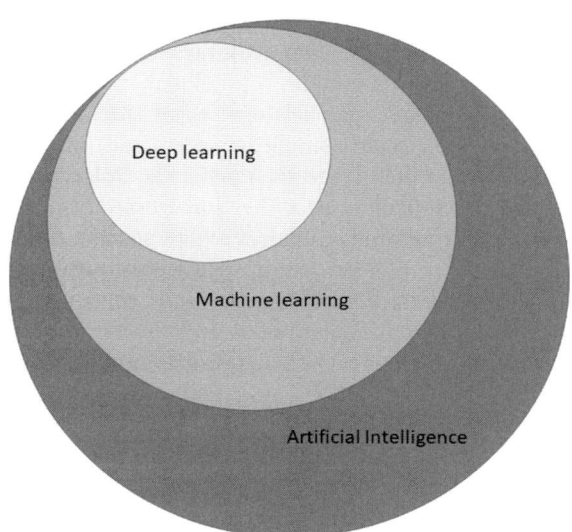

Figure 16.1 Relationship between artificial intelligence, machine learning, and deep learning
AI encompasses the science and engineering of creating human-like intelligence in computer systems. Machine learning is a type of AI, while deep learning is a further subdivision of machine learning based on artificial neural networks.

time-lapse imaging were studied. STORK discerned patterns and iteratively learned from the training set of images without preprogrammed features informed by the researchers. Ultimately, the model was able to predict embryo quality better than human embryologists with an area under the curve of >0.98 [8]. When combined with patient age, the model generated various likelihoods of pregnancy based on an interaction between patient age and quality. Of note, STORK was unable to directly predict pregnancy or positive versus negative live birth from morphology alone [7]. Yet, this research remains a proof-of-concept that machine learning using large datasets might yield fully automated blastocyst quality assessments that rival or exceed conventional microscopy-based human-performed methods.

The future will illuminate how AI is further leveraged in reproductive medicine.

16.3.2 Selecting Male Gametes by Cell Sorting

The importance of selection in ART is not limited to embryos. Upstream gamete selection tools are also currently in development. For example, cell sorting techniques are being explored for sperm selection, as these gametes typically exist in surplus in comparison to oocytes.

Magnetic-activated cell sorting (MACS) is one technology under investigation. MACS involves incubating spermatozoa in a buffer containing annexin V-conjugated microbeads. Annexin V has a high affinity for the externalized phosphatidylserine phospholipids on the cell membranes of apoptotic sperm cells. Exposure of the spermatozoa in this buffer to a magnetic field in an affinity column allows for separation of the nonapoptotic from apoptotic cells. However, this technique did not improve clinical outcomes of intracytoplasmic sperm injection (ICSI)–oocyte donation cycles [9]. When combined with traditional modalities of swim-up and density-gradient, MACS did not improve semen parameters and further was deleterious to total and rapidly progressive sperm counts [10]. Thus, MACS has yet to demonstrate any benefit over conventional sperm separation methods.

Microfluidic sperm sorting is another emerging gamete selection technique. A microfluidic sorting chip allows for rapid sorting of raw semen samples, avoiding centrifugation and the related oxidative stress, to produce clinically usable sperm. One blinded, controlled laboratory study using the microfluidic "sperm chip" determined that this cell sorting technique yielded highly motile sperm with virtually undetectable DNA fragmentation [11]. If and how a reduction in sperm DNA fragmentation index might translate into improved live birth rate is yet to be established.

16.3.3 Label-Free Microscopy: A Noninvasive Tool to Assess Gametes and Embryo Quality

The cornerstone of gamete and embryo grading today relies upon the use of conventional light microscopy. This technique has been used in the IVF laboratory for decades and is limited by its ability to provide only two-dimensional information about three-dimensional structures, offering rudimentary images of complex structures. Furthermore, staining techniques used to distinguish cellular structures are incompatible with clinical use in the IVF lab, since labeling could damage gametes and embryos.

A variety of novel microscopy techniques are being explored to improve gamete and embryo

selection. These recent advances harness emerging technologies in optics as well as data processing computer algorithms. Overall, these techniques are aimed at providing additional information about gametes, embryos, and the cellular processes within, without disrupting the viability of these structures. The additional information yielded by advanced imaging techniques may advance our understanding of reproductive biology. Whether novel microscopy methods will enable advances in gamete and embryo selection and be routinely deployed in the IVF lab remains to be determined. However, these are exciting developments to closely monitor.

Novel microscopy techniques for gamete and embryo selection include the following:

- polarization microscopy
- interferometric phase microscopy
- confocal Raman spectroscopy
- hyperspectral fluorescence lifetime imaging
- gradient light interference microscopy

Polarization microscopy includes optical microscopy techniques utilizing polarized light (i.e. light waves in which the vibrations occur in a single plane). It allows for enhanced visualization of structures with birefringence. Birefringence, also called "double refraction," indicates the property of a material to reflect incident light into two rays taking slightly different paths. Examples of cellular birefringent structures include parallel bundles of microtubules (such as the oocyte spindle or sperm tail) and the inner layer of the oocyte zona pellucida. Polarization microscopy initially used a filter and crossed compensator, revealing only structures with a specific orientation (i.e. perpendicular) in relation to the filter. A new polarized microscope was invented in 1995 using a circumpolar polarizer, allowing for visualization of birefringent structures having any orientation [12].

Polarization microscopy has been used to visualize the location of the oocyte spindle. Several studies have investigated the relevance of the spindle orientation for IVF/ICSI, in order to avoid potential injury on injection of sperm. A meta-analysis has correlated visualization of the spindle with improved fertilization and embryo development compared with nonvisualization [13]. Spindle dynamics have also been explored to understand oocyte meiotic maturation. In addition, another use case of polarization microscopy has been to determine whether imaging of the oocyte zona pelucida might influence ART success rates; early data suggest there may be a correlation between high birefringent intensity of structures in gametes and IVF/ICSI outcomes [14]. Finally, polarization microscopy is an emerging technique for sperm selection, as birefringence has been correlated with morphology, DNA integrity, and potentially embryo implantation.

Interferometric phase microscopy (IPM), also referred to as digital holographic microscopy, is being investigated as a method to enhance sperm imaging. Sperm imaging by traditional bright field microscopy is limited by the low contrast existent between the optical properties of the spermatozoa and the ones of the surrounding field. The human eye is unable to perceive the very minor delay in light passing through the sperm compared to the surrounding. In contrast, IPM uses different techniques to translate phase delays into visualized contrast. In particular, computer algorithms are used to generate a phase map in which each pixel indicates the thickness of the sperm at a specific point (shown by differing colors), yielding a 3D model of the structure. This technique enables detection and quantitative measurements of the sperm nucleus, acrosome, vacuoles, and dry mass, without requiring labeling that is used in conventional bright field microscopy. 3D sperm imaging may further improve assessments of motility. Whether these additional data augment the current World Health Organization semen analysis approach in assessing clinical outcomes remains to be seen [15, 16].

Confocal Raman spectroscopy is a laser-based microscopy technique that allows for label-free, non-invasive, 3D imaging. The submicrometer spatial resolution affords visualization of macromolecular structures within cells. This technique has been used to observe the meiotic maturation of living murine oocytes from the germinal vesicle through the metaphase II stage. In vivo imaging revealed differences between fixed oocytes and in vivo oocytes in terms of organelle distribution, nuclear organization, and mitochondrial architecture, emphasizing the importance of imaging of living cells for our understanding of reproductive processes [17]. Future research may perhaps extend such findings to human oocytes, with the goal of identifying oocytes with higher ability to fertilize and develop, an especially important fact given the current trend to cryopreserve oocytes.

Hyperspectral fluorescence lifetime imaging (FLIM) is a tool for visualizing fluorescent structures based on the decay rate of the fluorescence in the sample. In biology this tool has been used to assess the metabolic state of cells and tissues, because nicotinamide adenine dinucleotide and flavin adenine dinucleotide, two key metabolic cofactors, are naturally fluorescent; thus no special labels are needed. FLIM can be coupled with time-correlated single photon counting, in which very rapid detectors record the arrival of each photon from a laser. This technique has been used in a mouse model to assess mitochondrial function of oocytes, revealing differences between young and old oocytes, as well as those derived from wild type versus knockout mice as a model of oocyte dysfunction [17]. In addition, FLIM-based metabolic imaging of an experimental mouse model was able to detect metabolic changes through embryo development to the blastocyst stage, suggesting this tool may add value in embryo selection in future ART [18].

Gradient light interference microscopy (GLIM) is a technique that allows for 3D rendering of live embryos. By controlling the path length over which light travels, thick multicellular structures such as embryos can be probed in a noninvasive way and multiple unlabeled image slices composited into a 3D model. This technique was first demonstrated in bovine embryos, revealing their 3D structure and internal composition [19]. Because the GLIM technique is offered as an add-on module to conventional microscopes, ready deployment may be available to ART laboratories [19]. The future will establish whether GLIM imaging offers an advantage to human embryo selection in IVF.

16.3.4 Selection of Embryos Based on Predisposition to Develop Adult-Onset Diseases

The 1997 movie *Gattaca* depicted a society in which ART will be the only method of reproduction. Further, blastomere testing would allow choosing an embryo based on the risk of developing adult diseases and fitness.

The likelihood of using such technology is still in the distant future. As an example, genome-wide association study technology, which analyzes the DNA sequence for evidence of genes predisposing to diseases, has not proven to be significantly helpful. For example, at least 18 loci have been linked to predispose to type 2 diabetes, yet these loci explain only about 6% of diabetes occurrence. On the other hand, it is conceivable that we will be able to select embryos based on their transcriptomic and epigenetic signature of stress. Evidence for this has its origin in the work of Henry Leese who proposed the so-called quiet embryo hypothesis, later modified into the so-called Goldilocks hypothesis [20]. Basically, embryos with higher implantation potential will be the ones that will show an intermediate level of metabolic activity, without evidence of too much or too little stress. Novel embryo selection technology might therefore aim to define parameters of stress in the embryo and then will select embryos that will score in the optimal physiologic range. The strategy to select embryos with optimal stress might be particularly important, since animal studies show that embryos with evidence

of high stress might result in adults with increased predisposition to adult diseases, like diabetes and hypertension.

The Barker hypothesis postulates a mechanism to explain the correlation between in utero (and in this case, preimplantation) stress and adult health [21]. When an embryo or fetus encounters a stressful environment, it will activate survival pathways to adapt to the environmental conditions encountered. While this will confer a survival advantage in the short term, it will subsequently predispose to adult disease. This concept is very important, because it would suggest that embryo with lower stress should be selected for transfer.

This is well explained in a series of experiments (Figure 16.2) where mouse embryos were generated

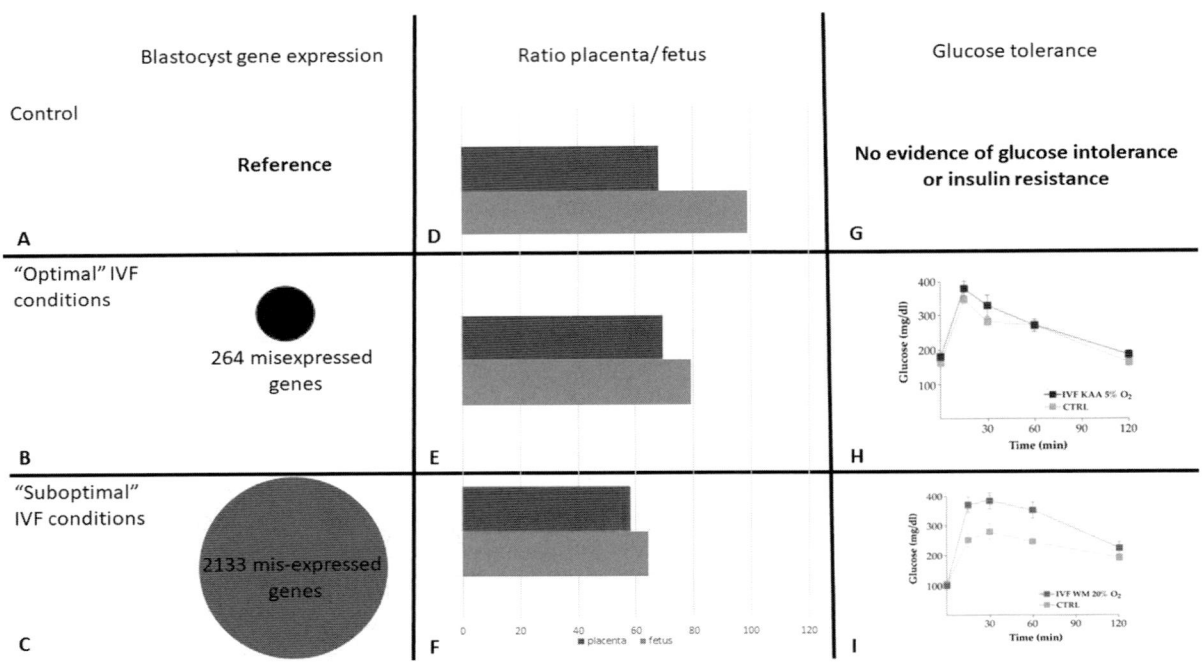

Figure 16.2 Selecting embryos with less stress might result in healthier offspring
To measure embryonic stress, blastocyst gene expression was measured by microarray technology. Compared to control mouse embryos flushed out of the uterus at the blastocyst stage (**A**), blastocysts generated by IVF and cultured in optimal conditions have 264 misexpressed genes (**B**). Blastocysts that were cultured in suboptimal conditions have nearly 10-fold misexpressed genes (n = 2 133, **C**). The size of the circle is proportional to the number of abnormal genes. (Data are from Feuer SK et al., *Reprod.* 2016;153:107–22.)
Importantly, the embryonic stress is memorized: at mid-gestation (day 12.5 in mice), fetuses generated in vitro in optimal conditions have lower weight and larger and heavier placentae (**E**) when compared to in vivo embryos (**D**); this effect is even more evident in embryos that were cultured in suboptimal conditions (**F**). (Data are from Delle Piane L et al., *Hum Reprod.* 2010;25:2039.)
Finally, adult mice generated by IVF in optimal conditions have normal glucose levels when tested with a glucose tolerance test (GTT) (**H**), although they have higher fasting insulin levels (indicating insulin resistance – data not shown). On the contrary, mice generated by IVF in stressful conditions are glucose intolerant when tested by GTT (**I**). Data are from Feuer SK et al., *Endocrin.* 2014;155:1956.
These data suggest that limiting stress to embryos (for example by minimizing the number of procedures done to gametes and embryos) might benefit the future health of the individual.

by IVF in either optimal conditions (i.e. cultured in potassium simplex optimized medium with amino acids and 5% oxygen atmosphere) or in suboptimal conditions (i.e. embryos cultured in Whitten's medium and 20% oxygen) and then transferred to unstimulated pseudopregnant recipient mice. In different experiments, the embryos' in utero growth and adult health were assessed. Control blastocysts were flushed out of the uterus after superovulation and natural mating and then transferred to unstimulated pseudopregnant recipients.

Overall, compared to control, mouse embryos cultured in optimal conditions showed: (a) altered blastocyst gene expression (264 misexpressed genes), (b) fetuses had lower weight and larger placenta at mid-gestation, and (c) the resulting offspring showed increased fasting insulin level (a marker of insulin resistance) but normal glucose tolerance when tested with a glucose tolerance test. On the contrary, blastocysts cultured in suboptimal conditions showed nearly 10 times as many misrepresented genes compared to control. Fetal weight was progressively smaller and the placenta larger, indicating abnormal growth. Finally adult IVF offspring show clear evidence of glucose intolerance.

Other researchers, by analyzing imprinted genes' expression and methylation, have similarly shown that increased manipulation of gametes and embryos results in increased misexpression and abnormal methylation of imprinted genes with subsequent abnormal placentation.

These findings suggest that embryo selection based on the response of gametes and embryos to the culture environment might become increasingly relevant in the future.

16.4 The Need for Debate and Safety

As novel technologies for embryo selection emerge and evolve, there is a critical need for ethical guidance. At present, in the United States, new approaches to embryo selection are regulated primarily at the institutional level under the discretion of institutional review boards. Although human reproduction is an intensely politicized issue, there is no federal governing body with explicit oversight of deployment of ART technologies for embryo sorting in IVF clinics across the country. The Ethics Committee of the American Society for Reproductive Medicine has taken position on some interventional technologies (e.g. by defining human cloning unethical), however no document guides the choice of nascent embryo selection techniques. At present clinicians have a significant and appropriate amount of autonomy regarding the choice of ART technologies to offer to patients. However, the ramifications of such individual decisions are significant for patients and societies; unanticipated side effects of embryo manipulation procedures might be compounded as children age and reproduce. Guidance is clearly needed to ensure that novel technologies are adopted thoughtfully and with explicit consideration of efficacy and, importantly, safety to patients and offspring conceived.

16.5 Conclusion

Embryo selection technologies will certainly continue to evolve at a rapid pace. It is possible and likely that yet-unknown technologies will appear and provide great benefit to patients. One critical message for all practitioners involved in ART is that avoiding excessive gamete and embryo manipulation remains a key goal.

Key Messages

- The pace of technological advancement is breathtaking. Novel technologies, like in vitro gametogenesis, might require novel tools for embryo selection.
- AI is poised to be extensively used in the field of ART.
- Improvement of existing technologies (like assessment of metabolism of gametes or embryos) might provide a new tool for embryo selection.
- Novel noninvasive imaging technologies are rapidly emerging.
- Use of noninvasive technologies for embryo selection will become preferred.
- Independent of the technology chosen to select gametes and embryos, there is a critical need to limit stress to the embryos, as reprogramming of the genome can occur with unknown long-term consequences.
- An ongoing ethical dialogue to guide development of new technologies is crucial.

References

1. Densen P. Challenges and opportunities facing medical education. *Trans Am Clin Climatol Assoc*. 2011;122:48–58.

2. Larose H, Shami AN, Abbott H, Manske G, Lei L, Hammoud SS. Gametogenesis: a journey from inception to conception. *Curr Top Dev Biol*. 2019;132:257–310.

3. Nadal A, Najmabadi S, Addis B, Buster JE. Novel uterine lavage system for recovery of human embryos fertilized and matured in vivo. *Med Devices (Auckl)*. 2019;12:133–41.

4. ASRM. Human somatic cell nuclear transfer and reproductive cloning: an Ethics Committee opinion. *Fertil Steril*. 2016;105(4): e1–4.

5. Suchy F, Nakauchi H. Lessons from interspecies mammalian chimeras. *Annu Rev Cell Dev Biol*. 2017;33:203–17.

6. Curchoe CL, Bormann CL. Artificial intelligence and machine learning for human reproduction and embryology presented at ASRM and ESHRE 2018. *J Assist Reprod Genet*. 2019;36(4): 591–600.

7. Khosravi P, Kazemi E, Zhan Q, Malmsten JE, Toschi M, Zisimopoulos P, et al. Deep learning enables robust assessment and selection of human blastocysts after in vitro fertilization. *NPJ Digit Med*. 2019;2:21.

8. Matsunari H, Nagashima H, Watanabe M, Umeyama K, Nakano K, Nagaya M, et al. Blastocyst complementation generates exogenic pancreas in vivo in apancreatic cloned pigs.

Proc Natl Acad Sci U S A. 2013;110(12):4557–62.

9. Romany L, Garrido N, Motato Y, Aparicio B, Remohí J, Meseguer M. Removal of annexin V-positive sperm cells for intracytoplasmic sperm injection in ovum donation cycles does not improve reproductive outcome: a controlled and randomized trial in unselected males. *Fertil Steril*. 2014;102(6):1567–75.e1.

10. Cakar Z, Cetinkaya B, Aras D, Koca B, Ozkavukcu S, Kaplanoglu I, et al. Does combining magnetic-activated cell sorting with density gradient or swim-up improve sperm selection? *J Assist Reprod Genet*. 2016;33(8):1059–65.

11. Quinn MM, Jalalian L, Ribeiro S, Ona K, Demirci U, Cedars MI. Microfluidic sorting selects sperm for clinical use with reduced DNA damage compared to density gradient centrifugation with swim-up in split semen samples. *Hum Reprod*. 2018;33(8):1388–93.

12. Oldenbourg R, Mei G. New polarized light microscope with precision universal compensator. *J Microsc*. 1995;180(Pt 2):140–7.

13. Petersen CG, Oliveira JBA, Mauri AL, Massaro FC, Baruffi RLR, Pontes A, et al. Relationship between visualization of meiotic spindle in human oocytes and ICSI outcomes: a meta-analysis. *Reprod Biomed Online*. 2009;18 (2):235–43.

14. Montag M, Köster M, van der Ven K, van der Ven H. Gamete competence assessment by polarizing optics in assisted reproduction. *Hum Reprod Update*. 2011;17(5):654–66.

15. Haifler M, Girshovitz P, Band G, Dardikman G, Madjar I, Shaked

NT. Interferometric phase microscopy for label-free morphological evaluation of sperm cells. *Fertil Steril*. 2015; 104(1):43–7.e2.

16. Mirsky S, Barnea I, Shaked N. Label-free quantitative imaging of sperm for in vitro fertilization using interferometric phase microscopy. *J. Fertil. Vitr.-IVF-Worldw. Reprod Med. Genet. Stem Cell Biol*. 2016;4(3): 1000190.

17. Heraud P, Marzec KM, Zhang QH, Yuen WS, Carroll J, Wood BR. Label-free in vivo Raman microspectroscopic imaging of the macromolecular architecture of oocytes. *Sci Rep*. 2017;7(1):8945.

18. Sanchez T, Venturas M, Aghvami SA, Yang X, Fraden S, Sakkas D, Needleman DJ. Combined noninvasive metabolic and spindle imaging as potential tools for embryo and oocyte assessment. *Hum Reprod*. 2019;34(12): 2349–61.

19. Nguyen TH, Kandel MK, Rubessa M, Wheeler MB, Popescu G. Gradient light interference microscopy for 3D imaging of unlabeled specimens. *Nat Commun*. 2017;8(1):210.

20. Leese HJ, Guerif F, Allgar V, Brison DR, Lundin K, Sturmey RG. Biological optimization, the Goldilocks principle, and how much is lagom in the preimplantation embryo. *Mol Reprod Dev*. 2016;83(9): 748–54.

21. Barker DJP, Winter PD, Osmond C, Margetts B, Simmonds SJ. Weight in infancy and death from ischaemic heart disease. *Lancet*. 1989;2:577–80.

Epilogue

The ability to determine the viability of an embryo created by IVF remains key to achieving successful clinical outcomes. While this has been the case since the early days of assisted reproductive technology (ART), the improved efficiency of ovarian stimulation regimens and in vitro fertilization and culture techniques means that the responsibility for selection lies less on nature and more with the embryologist.

As a commercial enterprise, bringing newer and better selection techniques to the market remains an attractive proposition, and much has been written about the responsibility of embryologists and clinicians to ensure that innovations in the field are properly validated before being widely introduced, even with the pressures to use them before this has been achieved. This has perhaps been one of the key challenges in embryology during the last 10 years.

What of the next 10 years? From an embryologist's point of view, it might be understandable to see the next decade as presenting an existential challenge to the profession. Artificial intelligence and automation are words that could be reasonably expected to induce anxiety in the IVF lab. However, we would argue that while they may change the tasks of the embryologist, their successful development and implementation will only increase the importance of the embryologist's role in the effective and safe treatment of infertility. Perhaps an analogy can be found in the cockpit of a commercial airliner. Advances in technology mean that an aeroplane can be made airborne, flown to a precise distant destination, and safely landed without the involvement of the pilot. But they remain necessary because in the end humans have faith and trust in human intervention more than in technology when life is at stake. People entrusting their hopes and plans for having their family to fertility clinics will still need the pilots to be in the cockpit.

Moreover, while algorithms increasingly find their way into clinical and laboratory practice, the complexity of biology and the profound importance of reproduction for achieving contentment and purpose in life means that embryos will always represent more than products and recipients of care: they, like their "parents," are our patients. Individual patients require individual care: assisted by algorithms yes, but not managed by them.

We believe that this book presents a comprehensive state of the ART in this field. We are grateful to the expert contributors who have recounted what has been achieved and what still requires development. They have reminded us too of the profound responsibilities that the embryologist has toward those seeking help to build their families.

Index